BMA

Practical Pathology of Serous Membranes

Practical Pathology of Serous Membranes

Edited by

Alberto M. Marchevsky
Cedars–Sinai Medical Center, Los Angeles, USA

Aliya N. Husain
University of Chicago, USA

Françoise Galateau-Sallé
MESOPATH National Reference Center & Cancer Center Leon Berard, Lyon, France

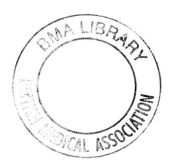

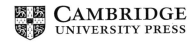
CAMBRIDGE
UNIVERSITY PRESS

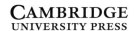

University Printing House, Cambridge CB2 8BS, United Kingdom

One Liberty Plaza, 20th Floor, New York, NY 10006, USA

477 Williamstown Road, Port Melbourne, VIC 3207, Australia

314–321, 3rd Floor, Plot 3, Splendor Forum, Jasola District Centre,
New Delhi 110025, India

79 Anson Road, #06-04/06, Singapore 079906

Cambridge University Press is part of the University of Cambridge.

It furthers the University's mission by disseminating knowledge in the pursuit of
education, learning and research at the highest international levels of excellence.

www.cambridge.org
Information on this title: www.cambridge.org/9781107119642
DOI: 10.1017/9781316402009

First published 2018

Printed in the United Kingdom by Clays, St Ives plc

A catalogue record for this publication is available from the British Library

Library of Congress Cataloging-in-Publication Data
Names: Marchevsky, Alberto M., editor. | Husain, Aliya N., editor.
Title: Practical pathology of serous membranes / edited by Alberto M. Marchevsky,
    Aliya N. Husain.
Description: Cambridge, United Kingdom ; New York, NY : Cambridge University
    Press, 2018. | Includes bibliographical references and index.
Identifiers: LCCN 2017061264 | ISBN 9781107119642 (hardback : alk. paper)
Subjects: | MESH: Serous Membrane – pathology | Mesothelioma – pathology |
    Mesothelioma – diagnosis
Classification: LCC QP90.5 | NLM QS 532.5.E7 | DDC 612/.01522–dc23
LC record available at https://lccn.loc.gov/2017061264

ISBN 978-1-107-11964-2 Mixed Media
ISBN 978-1-108-47298-2 Hardback
ISBN 978-1-316-40200-9 Cambridge Core

. . . .

Contents

Contributors

Fadi W. Abdul-Karim, MD
Cleveland Clinic, Cleveland, OH, USA

A. Valeria Arrossi, MD
Cleveland Clinic, Cleveland, OH, USA

Richard Attanoos, MD
Department of Cellular Pathology, University Hospital of Wales, Cardiff, UK

Bonnie Balzer, MD, PhD
Cedars-Sinai Medical Center, Los Angeles, CA, USA

Shikha Bose, MD
Cedars-Sinai Medical Center, Los Angeles, CA, USA

Lucian R. Chirieac, MD
Dana-Farber/Harvard Cancer Center, Brigham and Women's Hospital, Harvard Medical School, Boston, MA, USA

Eugene A. Choi, MD
Dan L Duncan Comprehensive Cancer Center, Baylor Clinic, Houston, TX, USA

Nicole A. Cipriani, MD
Department of Pathology, University of Chicago, Chicago, IL, USA

Jane Cunningham, MBBC
Department of Radiology, Brigham and Women's Hospital, Harvard Medical School, Boston, MA, USA

Sanja Dacic, MD, PhD
Department of Pathology, University of Pittsburgh Medical Center, Pittsburgh, PA, USA

Manuel Fernández-Bruno
Oncology Department, Hospital de Mataró, Barcelona, Spain

Silvia Fernández, MD
Oncology Department, Hospital de Mataró, Barcelona, Spain

Françoise Galateau-Sallé, MD
MESOPATH National Reference Center & Cancer Center Leon Berard, Lyon, France

Allen Gibbs, MD
University Hospital Llandough, Penarth, UK

Ritu R. Gill, MD, MPH
Department of Radiology, Brigham and Women's Hospital, Harvard Medical School, Boston, MA, USA

Macarena González
Oncology Department, Hospital de Mataró, Barcelona, Spain

Aliya N. Husain, MD
Department of Pathology, University of Chicago, Chicago, IL, USA

Marina Ivanovic, MD
Department of Pathology, University of Iowa Carver College of Medicine, Iowa City, IA, USA

Thomas Krausz, MD, FRCPath
Department of Pathology, University of Chicago, Chicago, IL, USA

Pilar Lianes, MD, PhD
Oncology Department, Hospital de Mataró, Barcelona, Spain

Alberto M. Marchevsky, MD
Cedars-Sinai Medical Center, Los Angeles, CA, USA

Stephanie M. McGregor, MD, PhD
Department of Pathology and Laboratory Medicine, University of Wisconsin, Madison, WI, USA

Peter Pytel, MD
Department of Pathology, University of Chicago, Chicago, IL, USA

Jordi Remon, MD
Oncology Department, Hospital de Mataró, Barcelona, Spain

Wickii T. Vigneswaran, MD
University of Chicago Medicine, Chicago, IL, USA

Sean C. Wightman, MD
MacLean Center for Clinical Medical Ethics, University of Chicago, Chicago, IL, USA

Preface

The pleura, peritoneum, and less often other serous membranes can present practicing pathologists with a variety of diagnostic challenges, but there are relatively few books that provide an up-to-date review of the pathology of lesions affecting these areas. This volume attempts to provide a comprehensive yet concise review of the large number of non-neoplastic and neoplastic conditions that can involve the serous membranes. The book includes an initial chapter describing the embryology, anatomy, and selected aspects of the biology of serous membranes. This is followed by a detailed classification of neoplastic and non-neoplastic lesions that can affect the pleura, peritoneum, pericardium, and other serous membranes. This chapter adopts the classification proposed by the World Health Organization (WHO) in 2015. Drs. Cunningham and Gill, experienced radiologists at the Brigham and Women's Hospital in Boston, MA, summarize for pathologists and illustrate the most important aspects of various imaging studies that are very important for the diagnosis and classification of various lesions, particularly of malignant mesothelioma. This is followed by two chapters that describe the various methods currently used to diagnose malignant mesothelioma and other lesions on biopsy specimens and cytological specimens. These chapters include a detailed description of the various immunostains that are used for diagnosis and a critical review of various diagnostic pitfalls in the interpretation of histopathologic findings and the results of ancillary tests. The following two chapters describe the practical problems that can arise during the diagnosis of the multitude of non-neoplastic conditions that can involve the serous membranes. Although many of these lesions are described in more detail in general surgical pathology textbooks, the chapters attempt to summarize the problems that are more likely to be encountered in practice for pathologists dealing with biopsies or other diagnostic samples taken from serous membranes.

The reminder of the volume provides a detailed description with multiple illustrations of the pathology of the various benign and malignant neoplasms that can arise in the pleura and peritoneum, and less often in other serous membranes. In particular, the book includes a comprehensive review of the pathology of malignant mesothelioma, with a brief review of the epidemiology and etiology of these lesions, detailed description of immunohistochemistry, molecular methods and other novel diagnostic tools and discussion about the prognostic implications of various pathologic findings. This is followed by two chapters written by experienced thoracic surgeons at the University of Chicago and oncologists in Spain that describe the practical detail needed by pathologists in the surgical treatment of pleural and peritoneal mesothelioma and the current modalities being used for the treatment of these neoplasms with chemotherapy and radiation therapy. The reminder of the volume describes the pathology of other neoplasms that can involve the serous membranes, including primary carcinomas, malignant lymphomas, and a wide variety of benign and malignant mesenchymal tumors.

We hope that this book will provide an up-to-date, clearly written, and practical review of the surgical pathology of serous membranes, and that it will help surgical pathologists diagnose the multitude of neoplastic conditions and tumors that they can encounter during the evaluations of surgical and cytologic specimens from these areas. The book is also intended to help radiologists, surgeons, oncologists, and pulmonologists who may need a quick reference to the pathology of the pleura, peritoneum, and other serous membranes.

Alberto M. Marchevsky, MD
Aliya N. Husain, MD
Françoise Galateau-Sallé, MD

The Mesothelium
Embryology, Anatomy, and Biology

Thomas Krausz and **Stephanie M. McGregor**

Introduction

Using only dissection and gross inspection, Xavier Bichat first described the serous membranes of the coelomic body cavities in 1799 (1):

> Every serous membrane represents a sack without any opening, spread over the respective organs which it embraces, and which are sometimes very numerous, as in the peritoneum, sometimes single, as in the pericardium, covering these organs in such a manner that they are not contained in its cavity, and so that if it were possible to dissect out their surface, we should obtain this cavity entire. This sack exhibits, in this respect, the same disposition as those caps doubled in on themselves, which are worn at night; a trivial comparison, but which gives an exact idea of the conformation of these membranes.

Despite not using a microscope – because he felt they were of limited utility – Bichat described over 20 different tissue types and noted the resemblance of the serous membranes to the lining of the lymphatics; subsequent authors likened the serous membranes to epithelial surfaces (2). Then, in the late nineteenth century, Minot demonstrated that despite these characteristics, the cells lining the body cavities are mesodermal in derivation (3). For this reason, Minot proposed the term "mesothelium" to convey this apparent paradox of epithelial function stemming from mesodermal roots. It is fairly intuitive that the epithelium-like mesothelium can provide a barrier function, and when paired with a smooth, fluid-bathed surface, one can readily extrapolate that these sheets of cells are also capable of minimizing friction so as to protect their encased vital organs even further. However, while serving as a slippery surface may be the most conspicuous purpose of the mesothelium, ongoing studies continue to reveal myriad unexpected functions of these seemingly humble cells, many with notable pathophysiologic significance.

Gross Anatomy of the Body Cavities and Serous Membranes

Humans possess four serous membranes: the pleura, the pericardium, the peritoneum, and the tunica vaginalis, with the latter existing only in males. Each membrane is essentially continuous, covering both the outer aspect of the cavity and the components within it, as the parietal and visceral mesothelium, respectively (Figure 1.1). As such, each membrane can be

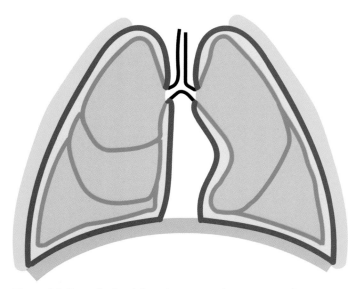

Figure 1.1 The parietal and visceral serous membranes consist of a continuous sheet of mesothelium. In the setting of the lung, the visceral pleura (green) is apposed directly to the lung parenchyma (gray) and reflects onto the chest wall (pink) and the diaphragm (brown) as the parietal pleura (purple); housed by these mesothelial cells is a true space, namely the pleural cavity (lavender).

viewed as a reflection of the other, but with a different underlayment, and can be likened to a fisted hand compressing the central aspect of an inflated balloon. In the case of the pleura, the distinction between parietal and visceral mesothelium occurs at the lung hilum, with the visceral pleura adherent to the lung and the parietal pleura coating the inner aspect of the chest wall (endothoracic fascia) and superior aspect of the diaphragm; the parietal pleura is frequently subdivided into the costal, mediastinal, diaphragmatic, and cervical (superior to first rib) regions, which demonstrate some distinguishing features. The parietal peritoneum coats the abdominal cavity as a whole, including the superior aspect of the retroperitoneal organs, such as the uterus and urinary bladder. The transition from parietal to visceral peritoneum occurs at many locations; for example, at the junction of the diaphragm with the superior aspect of the liver, or the reflection from the posterior abdominal wall onto the root of the small intestine mesentery (Figure 1.2). The human peritoneum is so expansive, with an estimated total surface area of approximately 1.8 m², that it is comparable to the skin in extent (4). The terminology relating to the pericardium can be inconsistent between sources and therefore somewhat

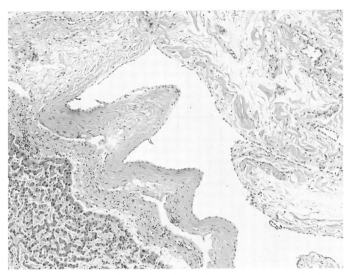

Figure 1.2 Peritoneal reflection from liver to diaphragmatic connective tissue. Visceral peritoneum lines the liver capsule (bottom left) and reflects onto the connective tissue lining the diaphragm (top right), where it is regarded as parietal peritoneum.

confusing; the visceral pericardium is more commonly known specifically as the "epicardium," and the seemingly general term "pericardium" is used by some in a more limited sense referring to the parietal pericardium. All of these cavities have in common that in the physiologic state there exists between the parietal and visceral membranes only enough fluid to prevent stress on the protected organs, making them true – as opposed to potential – spaces.

Basic Embryology of the Serous Membranes

The serous membranes develop in association with their underlying organs in an intimate manner that is highly conserved throughout vertebrates. Early in the third week of human ges-

tation there is a division in the dorsal–ventral axis of the lateral plate mesoderm that carves out a space, i.e., the coelom, which will shortly thereafter be lined by mesothelium (Figure 1.3). The superficial layer produced by this separation forms the parietal (somatic) mesoderm, which combined with the immediately overlying ectoderm is known as the somatopleure and will form the body wall and parietal mesothelium; the deep layer constitutes the visceral (splanchnic) mesoderm, which can be viewed in combination with the underlying endoderm as the splanchnopleure and ultimately forms the organs of the coelomic cavities and the visceral mesothelium. It is exactly this emergence from a central division within a solid group of cells that results in the maintenance of physical continuity between the parietal and visceral mesothelium. The resulting coelom then exists as a single cavity until the fifth week of gestation, when septae begin laying the foundation that defines the future pleural, pericardial, and peritoneal cavities. The tunica vaginalis later forms from the processus vaginalis, which is a transiently patent extension of the peritoneum which is eventually obliterated in its central aspect to form a discrete cavity surrounding the testes.

The coelomic space is always bound by mesoderm throughout development, but mesothelium proper is not clearly established at the time the coelom is formed (5). Details of these processes stem from work done in model organisms, but it can be estimated that the mesothelium is established in the fifth to sixth weeks of human gestation. In vertebrates mesothelial development has been studied most thoroughly in the context of the epicardium, which is derived from the proepicardium (also known as the proepicardial serosa). The proepicardium is a transient, extracardiac primordium that contributes not only to the epicardium but also develops the coronary vasculature, cardiac fibroblasts, and smooth muscle of the cardiac vasculature (6). It begins as an epithelioid outgrowth from the sinus venosus and then courses through the pericardial coelom. In its earliest state the proepicardium demonstrates gene expression

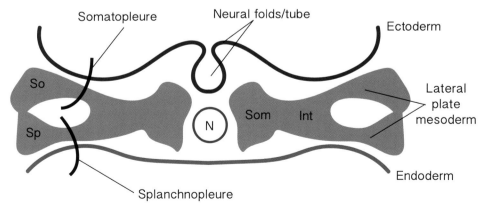

Figure 1.3 Mesothelial embryology. The lateral plate mesoderm divides into the somatic (So) and splanchnic (Sp) mesoderm, which partially comprise the somatopleure and splanchnopleure in combination with the ectoderm and endoderm, respectively (N, notochord; Som, somite; Int, intermediate mesoderm).

profiles characteristic of mesothelium, including genes such as *WT1*, even before it has finished coating the outer surface of the heart, and it harbors distinct progenitor populations distinguished by marker gene expression such as the transcription factor Tbx18. The proepicardium forms a coat around the heart from a combination of direct migration and transpericardial seeding, i.e., shedding, from villous or bleb-like protrusions, with subsequent contributions to the tissues of the heart proper; these protrusions exist not only at the sinus venosus but also develop at the roof of the pericardial cavity near the cardiac outflow tract, where they likely also establish the epicardium surrounding the great vessels (6).

There has been speculation that a process similar to that forming the epicardium occurs in the context of the visceral peritoneum (serosa) covering the intestinal mesentery, because mesothelial features are first identified at the root of the dorsal mesentery of the intestine and can subsequently be observed more broadly; however, recent work suggests that the processes governing serosal development are very different from those of the epicardium (5,7,8). Elegant experiments using chick–quail chimeras have demonstrated that rather than originating from an exogenous migratory population, the intestinal serosa is established from mesothelial progenitors scattered throughout the splanchnic mesoderm that differentiate *in situ*. Moreover, although the pleura and pancreatic mesothelium develop in close proximity to the proepicardium, they both demonstrate "organ-intrinsic" mesothelial development like that seen in the intestinal serosa (9). Therefore, to date, the epicardium is the only known mesothelial membrane that develops from recruitment of exogenous migratory precursors, and organ-intrinsic mesothelial progenitors may be the common mechanism of mesothelium formation.

Functional Anatomy and Fluid Dynamics

Despite being in continuity, there are subtleties between the parietal and visceral mesothelium in the functional anatomy to justify that they be considered as separate structures; and while the serous membranes are essentially sacs that are impermeable to the outside world – with the exception of the fallopian tubes – they are not completely impervious but rather connected to the lymphatics. Von Recklinghausen first demonstrated openings between mesothelial cells in 1863 using silver stains, and multiple subsequent investigators questioned his findings (10,11). Over time, studies using electron microscopy confirmed the disruptions and it is agreed that "stomata" do exist between the mesothelium and the lymphatics, ranging from 2 to 11 μm in diameter (12). Stomata first appear late in ontogeny and increase postnatally. While it was initially thought that stomata only exist in the diaphragmatic peritoneum, there are reports of stomata in the majority of mesothelial sites, with some controversy as to whether they exist in the pelvis. It has also been demonstrated that there are stomata between the serous membranes themselves, thus joining the pleural cavity to the

peritoneal and pericardial cavities. These connections may explain the phenomenon of asbestos fibers reaching beyond the pleural cavity to places they would not be expected to deposit due to inhalation (13).

More prominent openings of the mesothelium can also be found at "milky spots," which are much larger than stomata on average, ranging from 0.5 to 3.5 μm^2 (12). Milky spots are so named because of their white appearance stemming from their abundant lymphoid content. Not surprisingly, they have a direct connection to the underlying large lymphatic vessels – lymphatic lacunae as well as a rich capillary network. In place of a surface mesothelium, milky spots are lined by macrophages, which presumably facilitate immune function and uptake of any foreign particles. While milky spots are most prominent in the omentum, they are also present in numerous other locations, including the pleura and various peritoneal sites, such as the broad ligament.

In a normal resting state, each of the coelomic cavities contains just enough fluid to maintain an essentially frictionless environment. In the pleural cavity, this fluid is estimated to be approximately 0.3 ml/kg and is hypo-oncotic in nature, consisting essentially of a plasma ultrafiltrate that is derived primarily from the systemic circulation supplying the parietal pleura (14). Using Starling forces, Neergard proposed in 1927 that pleural fluid dynamics are a function of the difference between hydraulic and colloidosmotic pressure. However, an increased understanding of the pleural anatomy in mammalian model systems over time has revealed the presence of interstitial spaces and lymphatics in the pleura, which undoubtedly contribute to the maintenance of fluid homeostasis (Figure 1.4). Consistent with this original hypothesis, it does appear that pleural liquid is derived from the vasculature of the parietal pleura as previously believed, but it travels through the extrapleural interstitium prior to entering the pleural space. Nearly all fluid drainage in turn proceeds through the lymphatics of the parietal pleura, which contain valves that ensure unidirectional flow and presumably contribute to volume control. These stomata to the pleural lymphatics are most prominent in the mediastinal and diaphragmatic regions, resulting in drainage of the pleura to the hilar, retroperitoneal, and lower mediastinal lymph nodes; given that pleural fluid is derived primarily from the apical aspects, it therefore seems that there is some degree of circulation within the pleural cavity (14,15).

Histology and Structural Biology

While mesothelial cells exhibit both epithelial and mesenchymal features – and it is this very ability to transition from one state to the other, i.e., to undergo epithelial–mesenchymal transition, that makes them such an interesting subject of study – mesothelial cells primarily demonstrate epithelioid morphology in their mature state forming the serous membranes. Normal resting mesothelial cells exist as a monolayer with apical–basolateral polarization overlying a basal lamina,

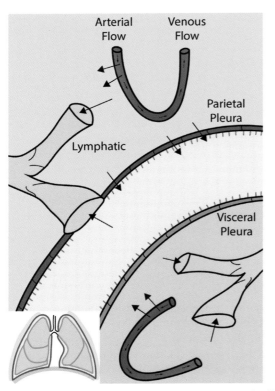

Figure 1.4 Pleural fluid dynamics. Pleural fluid is produced as an ultrafiltrate of the systemic circulation that first passes through the extrapleural interstitium. Drainage of the pleural cavity then occurs through lymphatics in the extrapleural tissues via stomata within the parietal pleura. The visceral pleura is not thought to contribute to the pleural fluid.

with the vast majority exhibiting the flat character of squamous cells (Figure 1.5a,b). These squamoid mesothelial cells are approximately 20–25 μm in diameter and characteristically have a centrally placed nucleus with a relative paucity of organelles that are primarily perinuclear in distribution or just overlie the nucleus (12). Interspersed among them to varying degrees, depending on location, are cuboidal mesothelial cells; there is a higher proportion of cuboidal cells in the mediastinal pleura, peritoneal diaphragm, liver, spleen, and "milky spots" of the omentum. These cuboidal cells have a diameter of only 8 μm on average and have markedly different features than squamoid mesothelial cells beyond their smaller footprint. They feature a larger nucleus with a prominent nucleolus, more numerous and complex microvilli, more developed organelles, increased mitochondrial content, and a different enzymatic profile that is more active than that of their squamoid counterparts. In addition to these two extremes of squamoid and distinctly cuboidal, cells with intermediate features exist and can even be the dominant cell type in some sites (12,16).

Like epithelium, mesothelial cells have a variety of specialized features, perhaps most notably microvilli (Figure 1.6). The microvilli of mesothelial cells were studied in great detail in the 1950s by Odor using the rat oviduct as a model system, and then in 1970, Stoebner declared that microvilli are perhaps the most useful defining feature of the mesothelium

(17,18). Mesothelial microvilli are covered by a film of negatively charged, hyaluronic acid-rich glycoprotein – the glycocalyx – that is thought to aid in fluid adsorption, to provide a defense function against infection, and to protect against formation of adhesions; the hyaluronic acid can be demonstrated by Alcian blue staining (pH 2.5) and is sensitive to digestion with hyaluronidase (13). While the microvilli *per se* cannot be visualized by light microscopy alone under most circumstances, their abundance results in an apparent gap between cells, forming a sort of "window" that is readily visualized in cytologic preparations; in some preparations, e.g., Giemsa staining performed on an air-dried slide, metachromatic staining can highlight the microvilli as a unit (Figure 1.7). By electron microscopy, it is evident that the microvilli of mesothelial cells are diverse, but overall long and slender (up to 3 μm in length, compared to approximately 1 μm in the intestine), with the potential to increase the peritoneal surface area approximately 20-fold (12,19,20). Moreover, the mesothelial microvilli have known plasticity and can increase in concentration or alter their surface charge in response to changes in the environment. It is currently hypothesized that the main function of microvilli is to trap proteins from the serosal fluid to maintain mesothelial integrity (13).

Microvilli are only one feature of mesothelial cells that is reminiscent of epithelium (12,13). Multiple mechanisms contribute to the epithelium-like barrier function of mesothelium, including tight junctions (zonula occludens), adhering junctions (zonula adherens), and desmosomes (macula adherens). The adhering junctions of mesothelial cells contain E, N, and P cadherins, but in contrast to the E-cadherin-predominant epithelium, N-cadherin is dominant in mesothelial junctions. Mesothelial cells also produce their own underlying basement membrane materials, communicate with one another via gap junctions, and actively engage in transport of both fluids and particulate matter using pinocytic transport. In some cases, namely the visceral peritoneum overlying the spleen and liver, there is a prominent layer of elastin beneath the basal lamina (12). Like microvilli, pinocytic vesicles can be demonstrated by electron microscopy in mesothelial cells, where they are seen primarily in association with the plasmalemma on the luminal surface; their functionality has been demonstrated by tracer studies. Multiple additional findings reflecting diverse function of normal mesothelial cells have been demonstrated, including lamellar bodies, lipid droplets, cytofilaments, glycogen accumulation, and occasionally primary cilia.

Postnatally, the inherent mesenchymal features of mesothelial cells are most apparent in reactive states; in the resting state their mesenchymal character is revealed primarily through special studies demonstrating expression of intermediate filaments that are characteristic of mesenchymal lineages (vimentin and desmin) in addition to those characteristic of epithelium (keratins), with the extent of coexpression varying according to context (Figure 1.5c,d). The mesenchymal features of mesothelial cells also become evident in culture, where they lose their polygonal character and take on a spindle appearance; *in vivo* these

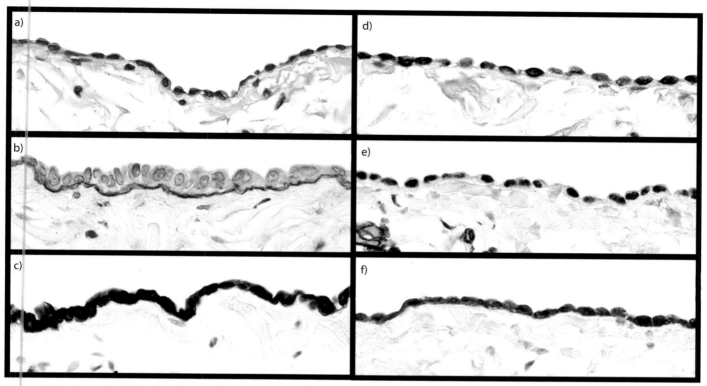

Figure 1.5 Basic mesothelial histology. Hematoxylin and eosin-stained section (a) demonstrates single-layer of mesothelial cells that rest on a basal lamina (b, laminin). Mesothelial cells express both keratins (c, CAM5.2) and intermediate filaments of mesenchymal cells (d, desmin) and can be identified by a variety of immunohistochemical markers with various localization (e, WT-1 in nucleus; f, calretinin in nucleus and cytoplasm).

features are most pronounced prenatally and in states of repair, which are discussed below. There are a variety of immuno-histochemical markers that are characteristically expressed in mesothelial cells, both with epithelioid and spindle morphology; these include WT-1, calretinin, D2–40 (podoplanin), and keratins, with CK5/6 being the most frequently utilized clinically (Figure 1.5e,f).

Mesothelial Regeneration

Disrupted epithelial surfaces are known to heal from the edges of a wound, and it was thereby assumed for some time that mesothelium must undergo a similar process. Indeed, while normal mesothelium is not mitotically active ($<$ 0.5 percent of cells dividing at rest), up to 80 percent of mesothelial cells can be demonstrated to be cycling at a wound edge (15). However, while cells at the wound edge develop spindle morphology and migrate into the wounded area and undoubtedly contribute to wound healing, as a whole, mesothelium regeneration appears to occur largely via an alternate mechanism. In the 1950s to 1970s, multiple investigators reported findings indicating that healing time for mesothelial wounds is not related to their size and rather that mesothelial wounds heal across the entire surface in such a manner that healing occurs within 7–10 days,

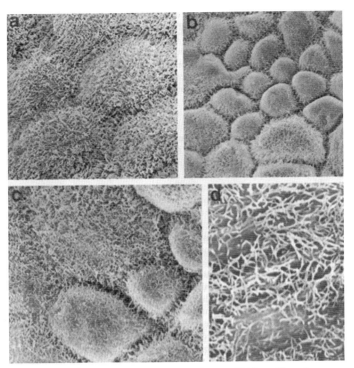

Figure 1.6 Scanning electron microscopy of microvilli. Microvilli can be so dense as to obscure cell boundaries (a, ×200), but can be variable in distribution (b, ×150; c, ×200). Panel (d) demonstrates a high-power view of microvilli (×3000). [With permission from Michailova & Usunoff, 2006, Springer.]

irrespective of size, thus arguing at a minimum that mechanisms other than healing from the wound edge must also be at play (21). Multiple theories have been proposed to explain this finding, including origination from residents beneath the mesothelium, settling of mesothelial cells having previously

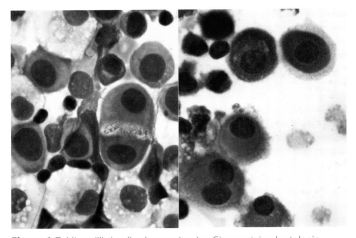

Figure 1.7 Microvilli visualized as a unit using Giemsa-stained cytologic preparations. Abundant microvilli form a "window" between adjacent mesothelial cells (left) that can in some preparations be recognized as a unit by metachromatic staining that rings the cell (right).

detached from another site, pre-existing free-floating serosal progenitors, and transformation from bone marrow-derived populations, including macrophages and pluripotent precursors (13,15,21).

Overall studies favor that a free-floating serosal progenitor is responsible for much of the mesothelial healing process (13). Findings in favor of this theory include recovery of healing with the addition of peritoneal lavage cells, and conversely, impaired healing following peritoneal lavage that presumably removes said progenitors. Direct analysis of peritoneal fluid has also demonstrated an increase in the amount of free-floating mesothelial cells following injury, and tracing studies have directly demonstrated incorporation of mesothelial cells introduced by lavage. It is postulated that free-floating mesothelial cells are able to take hold of the components of the exposed extracellular matrix. It should also be noted that mesothelial cells secrete a variety of growth factors that facilitate healing, including transforming growth factor-beta, fibroblast growth factors, and platelet-derived growth factors among others, as well as extracellular matrix components, such as collagen types I, III, and IV, elastin, fibronectin, and laminin (13). Bone marrow-derived and submesothelial precursors are essentially excluded by rescue with lavage in the setting of irradiation to the bone marrow or wound, respectively.

Manifestations of Mesothelial Cells in the Development of Other Mesenchymal Tissues

As mentioned previously, the mesenchymal features of mesothelial cells are evident in culture, as demonstrated by loss of their usual polygonal shape and acquisition of spindled morphology reminiscent of fibroblasts. Beyond this spindled appearance, for some time it has been known that true myofibroblastic differentiation, e.g., expression of smooth muscle actin, can be induced in mesothelial cells in culture (22). However, it has become increasingly clear that this function has biological relevance both embryologically and in the context of various states of injury, as mesothelial cells generate other cell lineages (23). One of the first observations of this phenomenon was identified using quail–chick chimeras, in which epicardial mesothelium was identified as differentiating into endothelium and smooth muscle through a process akin to the epithelial–mesenchymal transition (EMT) (24). Mesothelial cells are of course not truly epithelial despite their many shared features, and for this reason, the more specific term "mesothelial–mesenchymal transition (MMT)" also appears in the literature. Using lineage-tracing studies, such results of an EMT/MMT have since been observed in numerous contexts, including the myocardium, smooth muscle of the airways and vasculature, endothelium, hepatic stellate cells, fibroblasts, perivascular mesenchyme, gut tube anlage, and visceral adipocytes (23,25). Similarly, in the context of myocardial infarction, mesothelial cells are able to proliferate and migrate into the heart where they differentiate into fibroblasts, vascular smooth muscle, endothelial cells, and potentially even cardiomyocytes (23).

Mesothelium in Immunity

Given that mesothelial cells are capable of uptake of particulate matter, it is not a huge leap to accept that they are also capable of phagocytosis. However, there are reports indicating that mesothelial cells can also perform antigen presentation and produce cytokines. For example, following phagocytosis of bacteria, mesothelial cells can release interleukin-8 (26). In fact, they can produce a variety of chemokines and cytokines, including IL-1, IL-6, IL-15, G-CSF, M-CSF, GM-CSF, IL-8, MCP-1, and RANTES, among others (13). In some cases these mediators are released as the result of phagocytosis of either foreign material or an organism by the mesothelial cell itself, and in others it is a response to other mediators in the cellular milieu that have been released by other cells with a more classic role in immunity, such as macrophages or T cells. Mesothelial cells also express a range of adhesion molecules that can be used to facilitate leukocyte migration. By serving as a dock for leukocytes and releasing various effectors of immune function in a polarized manner – i.e., into the body cavity – mesothelial cells are able to facilitate recruitment of leukocytes to the site of need.

Mesothelium in Coagulation and Fibrinolysis

Mesothelial cells actively influence the steady state between coagulation and fibrinolysis. Procoagulant activity is facilitated by (1) release of tissue factor, which is the essential activator of the extrinsic pathway of the coagulation cascade, (2) physical assembly of the prothrombinase complex on the cell surface, and (3) secretion of plasminogen activator inhibitor (PAI-1 and PAI-2) (13). To counter this activity, fibrinolysis is facilitated primarily by release of tissue plasminogen activator (tPA) but also by urokinase plasminogen activator (uPA), both of which are capable of digesting fibrin. In the absence of tissue insult, these two processes exist in a delicate balance; following injury, it appears that the fibrinolytic activity of the mesothelium is increased (21). However, in many cases this may not be sufficient, and adhesions can result. There is work ongoing to address the possibility of harnessing these processes to reduce adhesions in the peritoneum.

Therapeutic Applications of Mesothelial Cells

Omental grafting has been used for many years in a variety of surgical settings as a means of facilitating wound healing, and additional applications are continually being developed (27–29). The cellular processes underlying the success of omental grafting are largely unclear, at least in part due to the variety of cell types that make up the omentum. Grafts obtained from cultures of isolated mesothelium have provided evidence that mesothelial cells are likely responsible for at least some of

this success, with possible mechanisms including the generation of vasculogenic cells and/or paracrine secretion of growth factors that promote the process of neovascularization (16,30). Such potential for differentiating into a variety of lineages, both in the embryo and in the adult, makes the mesothelium an appealing target for tissue engineering. Potential applications include prevention and treatment of peritoneal adhesions, peritoneal restoration following dialysis, vascular grafting, and nerve regeneration (16,31). The vast majority of studies are preclinical at this stage, but there is abundant potential in this line of study that will be of interest in upcoming years.

Comparative Anatomy and Embryology

While the basic arrangement of somatopleure, the coelom, and splanchnopleure is conserved throughout true coelomates, as one may expect, there are some striking differences in the serous membranes between species (5). There is one notable and striking exception to the considerable similarity of the body cavities even within mammals, which is seen in the elephant. Embryologically, the pleural cavity of the fetal elephant is quite similar to that of the human, but it is obliterated late in gestation (32–35). This "congenital pleuridesis" completely obliterates the pleural space, thus raising the question as to the true necessity of having a pleural space in humans; this question also arises in the context of therapeutic pleuridesis, in which the pleural space is intentionally obliterated in order to prevent recurrent pleural effusion. It is thought that the elephant obliterates the pleural space as a means of handling the pressures associated with snorkeling at depth. Indeed, the obliteration cannot simply be a result of the size of the organism or the pressure of the water, as whales have normally developed pleural spaces.

In addition to structural differences between species, developmental processes can vary even when the resulting structure is essentially the same. The epicardium is structurally conserved among all vertebrates, but the manner in which it develops is fairly variable, despite the fact that the proepicardium can be demonstrated even in the fairly primitive dogfish (6,36). In dogfish, it appears that all of the epicardium is seeded in a transpericardial fashion, with patches eventually coalescing to form a complete membrane. In contrast, experiments in amphibian and avian embryos have demonstrated that most epicardium is formed by progenitors spreading across a tissue bridge between the villous protrusions of the proepicardium and the dorsal aspect of the ventricles, although transpericardial seeding also occurs. Perhaps surprisingly, transpericardial seeding is the predominant mechanism in mammals. It is hypothesized that this difference stems from the closed nature of the pericardial cavity in dogfish and mammals, whereas the pericardial cavity communicates with the extraembryonic coelom in avian embryos, which could result in loss of the seeded progenitors from their intended location.

The fallopian tubes are the only connection between the serous cavities and the outside world in humans. In contrast, the peritoneum of fish has a well-established and large connection to the outside world that is used for the excretion of fluid and cells. Interestingly, while microvilli have been designated as a hallmark feature of mesothelial cells, they are not present in the peritoneum of fish. Various functions have been attributed to the microvilli that abundantly coat the human mesothelium, among them protection from frictional contact. Such a function is congruent with the absence of microvilli in the peritoneum of fish, where the membranes are not subject to abrasion, but float rather freely in a pool of water.

References

1. Bichat X. *A treatise on the membranes in general, and on different membranes in particular*. Paris: Richard, Caille & Ravier; 1799: 266 pp.

2. Hajdu SI. A note from history: landmarks in history of cancer, part 3. *Cancer*. 2011;118(4):1155–68.

3. Minot CS. The mesoderm and the coelom of vertebrates. *Amer Natur*. 1890;24(286):877–98.

4. Wittmann DH, Iskander GA. The compartment syndrome of the abdominal cavity: a state of the art review. *J Intens Care Med*. 2000;15(4):201–20.

5. Winters N, Bader D. Development of the serosal mesothelium. *J Dev Biol*. 2013;1(2):64–81.

6. Männer J, Pérez-Pomares JM, Macías D, Muñoz-Chápuli R. The origin, formation and developmental significance of the epicardium: a review. *Cells Tissues Organs*. 2001;169(2):89–103.

7. Winters NI, Thomason RT, Bader DM. Identification of a novel developmental mechanism in the generation of mesothelia. *Development*. 2012;139(16):2926–34.

8. Wilm B, Ipenberg A, Hastie ND, Burch JBE, Bader DM. The serosal mesothelium is a major source of smooth muscle cells of the gut vasculature. *Development*. 2005;132(23):5317–28.

9. Winters NI, Williams AM, Bader DM. Resident progenitors, not exogenous migratory cells, generate the majority of visceral mesothelium in organogenesis. *Dev Biol*. 2014;391(2):125–32.

10. Recklinghausen Von FT. Zur Fettresorption. *Arch Path Anat Physiol*. 1863;26:172–208.

11. Allen L. The peritoneal stomata. *Anat Rec* 1936;67(1):89–103.

12. Michailova KN, Usunoff KG. *Serosal membranes (pleura, pericardium, peritoneum). Normal structure, development and experimental pathology*. Advances in Anatomy, Embryology and Cell Biology Vol. 183. Berlin: Springer; 2006: 144 pp.

13. Mutsaers SE. Mesothelial cells: their structure, function and role in serosal repair. *Respirology*. 2002;7(3):171–91.

14. Miserocchi G. Physiology and pathophysiology of pleural fluid turnover. *Eur Respir J*. 1997;10(1):219–25.

15. Husain AN, Krausz T. Morphologic alterations of serous membranes of the mediastinum in reactive and neoplastic. In: Marchevsky AM, Wick M, editors. *Pathology of the Mediastinum*. Cambridge: Cambridge University Press; 2014: 356 pp.

16. Herrick SE, Mutsaers SE. Mesothelial progenitor cells and their potential in tissue engineering. *Int J Biochem Cell Biol*. 2004;36(4):621–42.

17. Odor LD. Observations of the rat mesothelium with the electron and phase microscopes. *Am J Anat*. 1954;95(3):433–65.

18. Stoebner P, Miech G, Sengel A, Witz JP. [Notions of pleural ultrastructure. I. Mesothelial hyperplasia]. *Presse Med*. 1970;78(26):1179–84.

19. Sumigray KD, Lechler T. Desmoplakin controls microvilli length but not cell adhesion or keratin organization in the intestinal epithelium. *Mol Biol Cell*. 2012;23(5):792–99.

20. Andrews PM, Porter KR. The ultrastructural morphology and possible functional significance of mesothelial microvilli. *Anat Rec*. 1973;177(3):409–26.

21. Ryan GB, Grobéty J, Majno G. Mesothelial injury and recovery. *Am J Pathol*. 1973;71(1):93–112.

22. Yang AH, Chen JY, Lin JK. Myofibroblastic conversion of mesothelial cells. *Kidney Int*. 2003;63(4):1530–39.

23. Dixit R, Ai X, Fine A. Mesothelial progenitors in development, lung homeostasis, and tissue repair. In: Firth A, Yuan JX-J, editors. *Lung Stem Cells in the Epithelium and Vasculature*. Totowa, NJ: Humana Press; 2015: 193–201.

24. Pérez-Pomares J-M, Carmona R, González-Iriarte M, Atencia G, Wessels A, Muñoz-Chápuli R. Origin of coronary endothelial cells from epicardial mesothelium in avian embryos. *Int J Dev Biol*. 2002;46(8):1005–13.

25. Rinkevich Y, Mori T, Sahoo D, Xu P-X, Bermingham JR, Weissman IL. Identification and prospective isolation of a mesothelial precursor lineage giving rise to smooth muscle cells and fibroblasts for mammalian internal organs, and their vasculature. *Nature Cell Biol*. 2012;14(12):1251–60.

26. Visser CE, Steenbergen JJ, Betjes MG, Meijer S, Arisz L, Hoefsmit EC, et al. Interleukin-8 production by human mesothelial cells after direct stimulation with staphylococci. *Infect Immun*. 1995;63(10):4206–09.

27. Pederson WC. Revascularization options for terminal distal ischemia. *Hand Clinics*. 2015;31(1):75–83.

28. Shah OJ, Bangri SA, Singh M, Lattoo RA, Bhat MY. Omental flaps reduces complications after pancreaticoduodenectomy. *HBPD INT*. 2015;14(3):313–19.

29. Rafael H. Omental transplantation for neuroendocrinological disorders. *Am J Neurodegener Dis*. 2015;4(1):1–12.

30. Shelton EL, Poole SD, Reese J, Bader DM. Omental grafting: a cell-based therapy for blood vessel repair. *J Tissue Eng Regen Med*. 2013;7(6):421–33.

31. Kawanishi K, Nitta K, Yamato M, Okano T. Therapeutic applications of mesothelial cell sheets. *Ther Apher Dial*. 2015;19(1):1–7.

32. West JB. Why doesn't the elephant have a pleural space? *News Physiol Sci*. 2002;17:47–50.

33. West JB. Snorkel breathing in the elephant explains the unique anatomy of its pleura. *Respir Physiol*. 2001;126(1):1–8.

34. West JB, Fu Z, Gaeth AP, Short RV. Fetal lung development in the elephant reflects the adaptations required for snorkeling in adult life. *Respir Physiol Neurobiol*. 2003;138(2–3):325–33.

35. Eales NB. The anatomy of a foetal african elephant, *Elephas africanus* (*Loxodonta africana*). Part III. The contents of the thorax and abdomen, and the skeleton. *Trans R Soc Edinb*. 1929;56(1):203–46.

36. Cano E, Carmona R, Muñoz-Chápuli R. Evolutionary origin of the proepicardium. *J Dev Biol*. 2013;1(1):3–19.

Chapter 2

Classification of Neoplastic and Non-neoplastic Lesions of the Serosal Surfaces

Alberto M. Marchevsky

The pleura, pericardium, peritoneum, and other serous membranes described in Chapter 1 can be the site of origin of a wide variety of inflammatory, neoplastic, and other conditions. In addition, the serous membranes are often involved by metastatic carcinomas, lymphomas, sarcomas and other malignancies. Chapter 6 of this volume describes the clinicopathologic aspects of acute and chronic pleuritis, pericarditis, and peritonitis, as well as a variety of other non-neoplastic conditions listed in Table 2.1. Some of these conditions such as pleuritis, pericarditis, pneumothorax and others are relatively frequent, while the benign and low-grade malignant tumors of mesothelial origin listed in Table 2.2 are unusual. Adenomatoid tumors are occasionally found in the tunica vaginalis of the testis and much less frequently in other locations. Multicystic mesothelioma and well-differentiated papillary mesothelioma are rare neoplasms.

The most common primary malignant tumor of mesothelial origin is malignant mesothelioma. Most of these lesions are diffuse, but infrequent examples of localized malignant mesothelioma have been described in the pleura and peritoneum.

Table 2.1 Non-neoplastic conditions of the pleura, pericardium, and peritoneum

Inflammatory conditions
Pleuritis
Pericarditis
Peritonitis
Pneumothorax
Reactive and atypical reactive mesothelial hyperplasia
Other non-neoplastic lesions of the pleura
Parietal pleural plaques
Rounded atelectasis
Amyloidosis
Atypical mesothelial hyperplasia
Other non-neoplastic lesions of the peritoneum
Peritoneal cysts
Endometriosis and endosalpingiosis
Deciduosis
Trophoblastic implants
Walthard rests
Splenosis
Melanosis
Gliomatosis peritonei
Omental–mesenteric myxoid hamartoma
Tumor-like conditions of the serosal membranes
Calcifying pseudotumor
Others

Table 2.2 Benign and low-grade malignant tumors of mesothelial origin

Adenomatoid tumor
Multicystic mesothelioma of the peritoneum
Well-differentiated papillary mesothelioma

Table 2.3 shows a classification of malignant mesothelioma which adds a list of growth patterns to the widely accepted World Health Organization (WHO) classification of the disease (1,2).

Serosal membranes are often the site of metastasis from carcinomas, melanomas, and other neoplasms. However, rare primary carcinomas of the pleura have been described. The peritoneum can be the site of origin of more frequent serous papillary carcinomas that show identical pathologic features to those developing in the ovaries. Table 2.4 lists various epithelial and germ cell tumors that can occur in the pleura, pericardium, and/or peritoneum.

Serosal membranes are periodically involved by Hodgkin and non-Hodgkin systemic lymphomas, but are less often the site of origin of lymphoid malignancies, such as primary effusion lymphomas, diffuse large B-cell lymphoma and other lesions listed in Table 2.5.

Table 2.3 Malignant tumors of mesothelial origin and their growth patterns

Diffuse malignant mesothelioma of the pleura
Epithelioid mesothelioma
Growth patterns
Solid
Tubulo-papillary
Trabecular
Micropapillary
Adenomatoid
Clear cell
Transitional
Deciduoid
Small cell
Lymphohistiocytoid
Pleomorphic
Sarcomatoid mesothelioma
Desmoplastic mesothelioma
Sarcomatoid mesothelioma with heterologous elements
Biphasic mesothelioma
Localized malignant mesothelioma
Epithelioid
Sarcomatoid
Desmoplastic
Biphasic

Table 2.4 Carcinomas and germ cell tumors involving the pleura, pericardium, and/or peritoneum

Carcinomas
   Primary
      Primary carcinoma of the pleura
      Serous papillary carcinoma of the peritoneum
   Metastatic
      Ovarian
      Gastric
      Pancreatic
      Colonic
      Pseudomyxoma peritonei
      Others
Germ cell tumors
   Teratomas
   Yolk-sac tumor

Table 2.5 Lymphoid malignancies of the pleura and peritoneum

Primary effusion lymphoma

Diffuse large B-cell lymphoma

Hodgkin lymphoma

Myeloma

Other
   Secondary
      Chronic lymphocytic leukemia
      Others

Table 2.6 Mesenchymal tumors and tumor-like conditions of the pleura and peritoneum

Solitary fibrous tumor
   Malignant solitary fibrous tumor

Schwannoma

Inflammatory myofibroblastic tumor

Desmoid-type fibromatosis

Lipoma and liposarcoma

Synovial sarcoma

Leiomyosarcoma
   Leiomyomatosis peritonealis disseminata

Angiosarcoma and epithelioid hemangioendothelioma

Desmoplastic small round cell tumor
Pleuropulmonary blastoma

PNET/Ewing sarcoma (Askin tumor)

Others

Finally, the serosal membranes can be the site of origin or metastasis of a variety of mesenchymal tumors and tumor-like conditions such as solitary fibrous tumor, synovial sarcoma, desmoid-type fibromatosis, and other lesions listed in Table 2.6.

References

1. Galateau-Sallé F, Churg A, Roggli V, Travis WD, World Health Organization Committee for Tumors of the Pleura. The 2015 World Health Organization Classification of Tumors of the Pleura: advances since the 2004 classification. *J Thorac Oncol.* 2016;11:142–54.

2. Travis WD, Brambilla E, Burke AP, Marx A, Nicholson AG. Introduction to the 2015 World Health Organization Classification of Tumors of the Lung, Pleura, Thymus, and Heart. *J Thorac Oncol.* 2015;10:1240–42.

Chapter 3

Multi-modality Imaging of Pleural and Peritoneal Disease

Jane Cunningham and Ritu R. Gill

Introduction

The normal pleurae are exceptionally thin, measuring 0.2–0.4 mm and imperceptible on standard radiologic imaging (1). On chest radiographs the healthy parietal pleurae are never seen; however, the visceral pleura may be visualized as it invaginates the lung along the oblique or transverse fissures or where the right and left pleural cavities meet the junctional lines. On CT, the normal fissures can be identified as avascular, curvilinear bands with a paucity of adjacent lung markings extending medially from the hilum to the chest wall laterally. The exact appearance can vary depending on the orientation plane of the fissures relative to the plane and thickness of the CT slice (2). The minor fissure is typically seen as a lucent area with triangular morphology with its apex at the hilum. Multiplanar reformats, including coronal and sagittal sequences, are especially helpful in improving identification of the fissures in health and disease. Thin-section CT images allow identification of the intercostal stripe which describes a 1–2-mm line composed of the visceral pleurae, physiologic pleural fluid, parietal pleura, endothoracic fascia, and the innermost costal muscles and extend along the paravertebral margin to the lateral aspect of the adjacent ribs (3). The relationship of the pleura to adjacent anatomic structures has important implications for the spread of disease.

The peritoneum is composed only of a solitary layer of mesothelial cells and subjacent connective tissue containing collagen, elastic tissue, blood vessels, and lymphatics (4). Therefore, in healthy individuals the peritoneum is not identifiable on radiologic imaging; abnormal accumulation of fluid, air, or soft tissue within the peritoneal spaces allows visualization of the normal peritoneal recesses (5). These include the interconnecting bilateral paracolic gutters, the lesser sac, Morison's pouch, the subphrenic space, and the retrovesical space in men or Pouch of Douglas in women. The supra- and infra-mesocolic compartments are divided by the transverse mesocolon (4). Intercommunication of the peritoneal spaces allows ascites to accumulate in the most dependent recesses of the peritoneal cavity – recto-uterine or retrovesical pouches in the erect position; however, in supine patients small volumes of intraperitoneal fluid are usually seen in the hepatorenal space, or Morison's pouch. Conversely, air rises to accumulate in the superior, non-dependent portion of the peritoneal cavity and changes in patient position.

Table 3.1 Imaging characteristics and associations of pleural pathologies

Pathology	Imaging characteristics	Associations
Exudative effusion	MRI: high T2, low T1	Infection, PE, and malignancy
Transudative effusion	MRI: high T2, low T1	Cardiac or hepatic failure
Hemothorax	CT: high density > 35 HU	Trauma, postoperative
Chylothorax	CT: low density < 0 HU	Thoracic duct injury, LAM
Empyema	CT/MRI: split pleura sign	Bacterial, tuberculosis
Pneumothorax	CXR: visceral pleural line	Bronchopleural fistula, COPD
Tension pneumothorax	CXR: contralateral shift of mediastinum, flat diaphragm	Trauma, PEA cardiac arrest
Pleural thickening	CT: diffuse, enhancing, 3–10 mm	Fibrosis post pleuritis or empyema radiation therapy, pleurodesis
Diffuse calcification	CT: unilateral high-density	Prior TB empyema, old hemothorax
Focal calcification	CT: bilateral calcified pleural plaques, basal predominant	Asbestos exposure, round atelectasis
Solitary fibrous tumor	MRI: low T1 and low T2 signal enhance, vascular pedicle in 40 percent	Hypoglycemia via IGF II
Lipoma	MRI: high T1, fat-sat signal drop	
Mesothelioma	CT: circumferential pleural rind, effusion, fissural nodules	Asbestos exposure

Radiologic Manifestations of Pleural and Peritoneal Diseases

A *pleural effusion* refers to the abnormal accumulation of fluid in the pleural space, and can be a manifestation of a wide variety of pathologies (Tables 3.1 and 3.2). Broadly, pleural effusions are classified as either transudate or exudate. Exudative effusions are secondary to increased capillary permeability due to infection, thromboembolic disease, or malignancy. Transudative pleural effusions occur when the osmotic pressure in the

Table 3.2 Imaging characteristics and associations of pleural pathologies

Pathology	Imaging characteristics	Associations
Ascites	CT: fluid density < 15 HU	Cirrhosis, malignancy, CHF, bladder dome rupture
Hemoperitoneum	CT: high density > 30 HU	Hepatic or splenic lacerations, sentinel clot sign
Pneumoperitoneum	Erect CXR: subdiaphragmatic Lucent air. PFA: Rigler's sign	Postoperative, bowel perforation
Carcinomatosis	CT: thickened, nodular, enhancing peritoneum. Omental infiltration	Advanced malignancy, ovarian, GI
Sarcomatosis	CT: thickened, nodular, enhancing peritoneum Omental infiltration	Metastatic sarcomas
Lymphomatosis	CT: thickened, nodular, enhancing peritoneum. Omental infiltration	Advanced lymphoma
Tuberculous peritonitis	CT: enhancing, thickened peritonum. Loculated ascites	May have fibrotic nodular form
Encapsulating peritoneal sclerosis	CT: thickened bowel wall and peritoneal lining due to fibrosis	Peritoneal dialysis in CKD, radiation causes bowel obstruction
Desmoplastic small round cell tumor	PET-CT: markedly FDG-avid soft-tissue peritoneal masses	Malignant ascites
Pseudomyxoma peritonei	CT: gelatinous ascites, scalloped hepatic and splenic contour	Ruptured mucinous tumors, appendiceal mucocele

pleural space exceeds the serum oncotic pressure, thereby causing fluid to shift passively from the circulation into the pleural cavity, in hepatic failure or nephrotic syndrome. Alternatively, transudates can occur in cardiac failure due to increased circulatory hydrostasis causing fluid shift (6). The majority (42–77 percent) of exudative effusions are caused by malignancy (1,2). Distinction between transudative and exudative pleural effusions is therefore an important first step towards establishing a diagnosis and can be achieved by thoracentesis and measuring biochemical indices in accordance with Light's Criteria. Imaging can be useful in identifying the presence of associated findings such as consolidation, mass, and/or pleural thickening, characterizing the nature of pleural fluid; however, imaging findings can be non-specific and inconclusive.

Blunting of the posterior or lateral costophrenic sulci on lateral or frontal radiographs suggests the presence of pleural effusion (7,8). Other features of pleural effusions on radiographs include apical capping, decreased visibility of the lower lobe vasculature, and accentuation of the minor fissure. Fluid can encapsulate in interlobar fissures, most commonly the transverse fissure, giving it a biconvex lenticular shape with well-defined margins when seen in profile on lateral radiographs and which can be mistaken for a mass – the so-called vanishing or pseudotumor (Figure 3.1) (9).

Subpulmonic effusions have distinct radiographic appearance; the pleural fluid initially accumulates between the inferior aspect of the lung and the diaphragm without spilling over into the costophrenic sulci. This leads to the apparent elevation of the ipsilateral hemidiaphragm, with a more laterally positioned apex of the diaphragm and sharper than usual lateral slope downward to the costophrenic angle (8,10). When present on the left side, increased distance (> 2 cm) between the lung base and the gastric bubble can also be seen. Infrequently, very

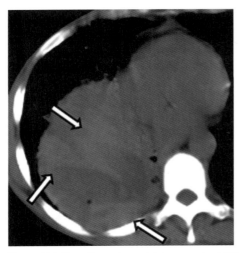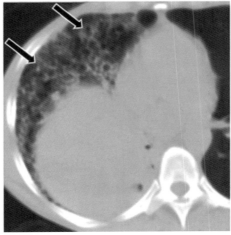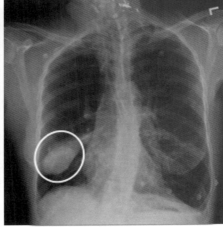

Figure 3.1 Pleural hematoma. Axial non-contrast CT images with lung and soft-tissue window settings demonstrate heterogeneous right posterior pleural collection with areas of high attenuation consistent with blood in this patient with right pleural hematoma (white arrows). There is also pulmonary parenchymal hemorrhage in the adjacent right lung evidenced by ground glass opacification (black arrows). Chest radiograph performed months later shows pseudotumor projected over the right lower zone correlating with evolution and loculation of the hematoma (encircled).

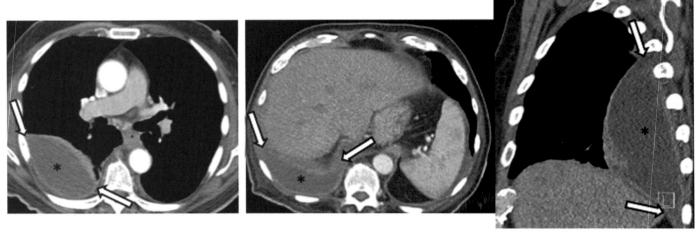

Figure 3.2 Empyema. Axial and sagittal images from contrast-enhanced chest CT in a patient with leukemia who presented with fever and chest pain demonstrate a loculated right basal pleural effusion (*) with thickening and ehancement of the pleura (white arrows). The appearance is consistent with the "split pleura sign" of empyema.

large effusions can invert the diaphragm such that it is convex inferiorly and moves paradoxically with respiration on fluoroscopy (10).

Image guidance is particularly advantageous in cases of small or loculated pleural effusions (11). It allows identification of the largest pocket of fluid and provides guidance for aspiration. Similarly, imaging can guide the most appropriate site for chest tube or indwelling pleural catheter placement and increase the sensitivity and specificity of pleural biopsies (8,11–13). Barnes et al. found lower pneumothorax rates and associated requirement for chest tube insertion of 5 percent and 0.7 percent, respectively, when ultrasound was employed compared to 10 percent and 4 percent without ultrasound (13).

Ultrasound can satisfactorily distinguish between pleural fluid and thickening (14). Simple pleural effusions are seen as homogeneous black or anechoic fluid collections (15). Pleural fluid gives a color signal on Doppler imaging, which is especially useful in increasing sensitivity in minimal effusions (16).

Exudative effusions are sequelae of intense pleural inflammation, associated with a history of hemothorax, empyema, or tuberculous pleuritis and presence of septations and adhesive fibrin bands.

CT is more sensitive than ultrasound for the detection of pleural fluid, and can help characterize the fluid based on density (12). Simple pleural effusions generally measure < 15 Hounsfield Units (HU), hemorrhagic fluid is > 35 HU, and serosanguinous or proteinaceous fluid ranges between 15 and 35 HU. Chylothorax, secondary to thoracic duct injury or in cases with lymphoma, can have effusions with lower or even negative HU suggestive of high lipid concentration. However, biochemical analysis remains the gold standard, as CT attenuation values cannot reliably distinguish transudative from exudative effusions.

CT provides information on other ancillary findings such as diffuse thickening and enhancement. These features can be associated with empyema (Figure 3.2), which also tends to cause loculated fluid collections that are seen as lenticular rim-enhancing, non-dependent fluid collections of fixed position in the pleural space (Figure 3.3). Pleural nodularity or masses can also be accurately identified with CT and may be indicative of primary or secondary malignant involvement. The sensitivity and specificity of the features suggestive of malignancy in 146 patients with pleural effusions were as follows: nodularity (37 percent and 97 percent), rind (22 percent and 97 percent), mediastinal pleural involvement (31 percent and 85 percent), thickening > 1 cm (35 percent and 87 percent) (17).

On MRI, pleural effusions are characterized by their water content and are therefore of low signal intensity on T1-weighted sequences and high signal intensity on T2-weighted sequences. MRI has been considered superior to CT to classify the type of effusion, both by assessing the signal intensity on T1- and T2-weighted sequences, enhancement characteristics, and by measuring apparent diffusion coefficient on diffusion-weighted MRI (18). Exudates have increased diffusion restriction when compared with transudates (4). Blood in the pleural space can be recognized by the *concentric ring sign* characterized by a high T1 signal intensity centrally due to methemoglobin and a dark outer hemosiderin ring (1,12,19).

Gupta et al. evaluated the utility of FDG-PET imaging in distinguishing benign from malignant pleural effusions in lung cancer patients. Pleural cytology, biopsy, and clinical follow-up for ≥ 1 year was the reference standard. The sensitivity, specificity, and accuracy was 89 percent, 94 percent, and 91 percent, respectively, with PET accurately identifying malignant pleural disease in 16 of 18 patients and correctly excluding pleural malignancy in 16 of 17 patients (20).

Occasionally pleural fluid can be difficult to distinguish from ascites, especially when present in the posterior costophrenic recess adjacent to the diaphragm. Features more suggestive of pleural origin include: *the displaced crus sign* – if

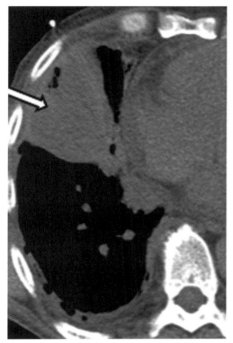 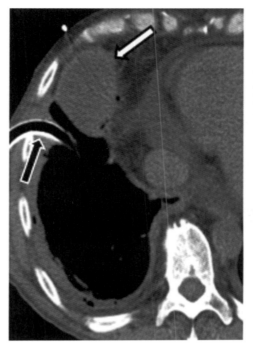 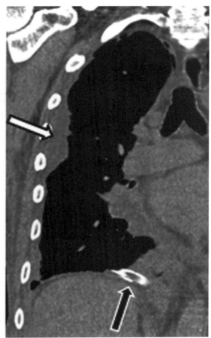

Figure 3.3 Empyema. Axial and coronal non-contrast CT images of the right hemithorax reveal loculated fluid in the anterolateral pleural space with associated thickening of the pleura (white arrows). Morphology, relatively high attenuation (20 HU) as well as locules of air are concerning for empyema. There is a right basal chest tube *in situ* (black arrows), which may account for some of the air foci seen in the pleural space.

the crus is pushed away from the spine by the fluid it is in the pleural space whereas ascites lies anterior and lateral to the crus; *the diaphragm sign* – fluid outside the diaphragm is pleural fluid and inside the diaphragm is ascites; and the *bare area sign* – restriction of ascites by the coronary ligaments indicates ascites is present (12).

A similar mechanism explains fluid accumulation in the peritoneal space due to bowel perforation. The gastrointestinal serosa is formed by the visceral peritoneum so a breach of this layer allows bowel contents including fluid and air to enter the peritoneal cavity. The distribution of fluid can indicate its source; for example, hemorrhagic ascites which has accumulated in the right subphrenic space, Morison's pouch, the lesser

Ascites

Pathologic accumulation of excess fluid in the peritoneal cavity is termed ascites (Figure 3.4). The composition of ascites varies with the underlying etiology. Plain radiography is not sufficiently sensitive for the detection of ascites and has been superseded by other modalities. Ultrasound can detect even trace volumes of free fluid typically in the recto-uterine pouch or peri-hepatic ascites. Generally, simple ascites is seen as a black area devoid of echoes outlining the contour of the adjacent peritoneal recess or organ. Complex ascites is associated with internal echogenic debris and/or internal septations. Following trauma, hemoperitoneum can occur if there is laceration of the capsule of the liver or spleen. As the breached capsule is due to a tear of the visceral peritoneum lining the organ, this allows direct spread of blood from the injured viscus into the peritoneal cavity (21). Hemorrhagic ascites can be recognized on CT as fluid of increased attenuation, typically > 30 HU. With narrow window display settings fluid–fluid levels due to dense hemorrhage layering dependently can be more easily appreciated.

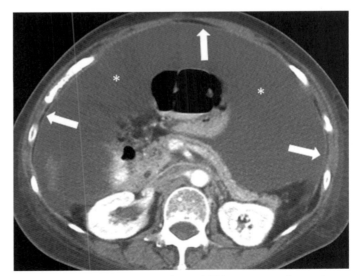

Figure 3.4 Ascites. Axial contrast-enhanced CT demonstrates a large volume of ascites (*) with peritoneal thickening and enhancement (arrows). The differential diagnosis is broad and includes malignant ascites, infectious ascites such as spontaneous bacterial peritonitis, or tuberculous ascites.

sac and the right paracolic gutter is likely to have come from the liver. Conversely, splenic hemorrhage would probably be seen in the left subphrenic space, left paracolic gutter, and gastrohepatic space (21). The *sentinel clot sign* whereby the dense clot is seen adjacent to the organ responsible for the bleeding has helped identify the site of bleeding. Anatomically, the peritoneum reflects along the dome of the bladder; therefore, injury at that site results in intraperitoneal accumulation of urine in the paravesical and paracolic recesses; rupture at other sites leads to subperitoneal urine leaks.

Peritoneal fluid has a recognized flow pattern that contributes to typical patterns of spread of disease within this compartment (21). This has implications for metastatic peritoneal tumor dissemination and also influences the spread of infection within the peritoneal cavity and location of abscess formation. Organized infections are common in the dependent pelvic recesses and from there extend along the right paracolic gutter to the right subphrenic space or Morison's pouch. The falciform ligament limits flow from the right to the left subphrenic space. Left-sided abscesses can communicate via the left subphrenic space with the gastrohepatic and perisplenic spaces. Inflammatory fluid and enzymes in pancreatitis can spread via the lesser sac, the gastrosplenic, and the gastrocolic ligaments to involve the stomach and colon. The left kidney and liver can be affected by inflammatory dissemination along the splenorenal and hepatoduodenal ligaments, respectively (22). Ascites is seen as high T2 signal fluid on MRI. Motion artifacts in the fluid occur due to prolonged scan times, which can limit assessment.

Pneumothorax

Pneumothorax refers to the presence of air in the pleural space, which may occur due to a bronchopleural fistula, spontaneous rupture of a bulla, trauma, iatrogenic injury following biopsy or surgery, infection by gas-forming organisms in the pleural space, or rupture of the esophagus. Identification of a pneumothorax on chest radiographs relies on recognition of the visceral pleural line, which can be seen as a very thin, sharply defined line that divides the lucent intrapulmonary air from the lucent air in the pleural space. The absence of lung parenchymal markings beyond this line affirms the diagnosis. Diagnostic uncertainty can be resolved with a lateral decubitus film performed with the side of the suspected pneumothorax superiorly, as the air in the pleural space rises and increases the distance between the lung and the chest wall (23).

One must have a high degree of suspicion of the possibility of this diagnosis in ventilated patients in the ICU and review the most frequent locations of pneumothorax in supine patients which differ from upright studies due to the positional nature of air accumulation in the least-dependent anteromedial pleural recess, followed by subpulmonic, apicolateral, and posteromedial sites. Therefore, radiographic signs associated with supine pneumothorax include: very deep lucent costophrenic sulcus, a lucency over the right or left upper quadrant, and much sharper appearance of hemidiaphragm possibly with the presence of a

visceral pleural line above the diaphragm (24). Tension pneumothorax occurs when the pressure in the pleural space remains positive throughout the respiratory cycle, which compromises cardiac output due to decreased venous return, and it is essential that it be expeditiously treated by prompt needle aspiration of the affected side.

Ultrasound has a limited role for evaluating pneumothorax; however, the *pleural gliding/lung sliding sign* has been described as a way to identify pneumothorax occurring at the time of ultrasound-guided thoracentesis (11,25).

Pneumoperitoneum

The most frequent cause of air entering the peritoneal cavity, apart from deliberate iatrogenic/surgical pneumoperitoneum, is rupture of gastrointestinal organs. The distribution of intraperitoneal air is affected by patient position. Chest radiographs performed in the upright position are frequently utilized to evaluate for pneumoperitoneum. When present, air can be seen as curvilinear lucencies underneath and outlining the contour of the diaphragm, the thickness of which can vary with the volume of free air. On abdominal radiographs free air outlines the bowel wall, which is seen as a thin line surrounded by lucency due to adjacent intra- and extra-luminal gas. This is referred to as *Rigler's sign*. Alternatively, free air can outline structures like the falciform ligament. The cause of pneumoperitoneum may be identifiable on radiographs; for example, small bowel obstruction seen as dilated bowel loops, incarcerated hernias or necrotic bowel as evidenced by pneumatosis or air in the bowel wall.

Cross-sectional imaging with CT is more sensitive both to detect the presence of intraperitoneal air and to elucidate the cause. CT is performed with patients in the supine position and therefore air is typically seen in the anterior upper abdomen, especially when large volumes are present. Localized foci of gas may indicate the site of perforation, for example adjacent to sigmoid diverticulitis or inflamed appendix.

Pleural and Peritoneal Thickening and Enhancement

Focal or diffuse patterns of pleural thickening can occur due to benign or malignant etiology. Pleural thickening is usually a fibrotic response to inflammation or pleuritis. Fibrosis of the visceral pleura can follow pleural effusion with adhesions to the parietal pleura. This can be sequelae of *Mycobacterium tuberculosis* infection, empyema, connective tissue diseases, trauma, radiation therapy, or chemical or talc pleurodesis (Figure 3.5). Some typical imaging features are recognized; for example, unilateral dense sheets of calcification with prominent volume loss and parenchymal fibrosis in those with a history of TB. Post-traumatic or post-surgical hemothoraces also tend to be associated with unilateral calcification; however, associated findings of rib fractures or median sternotomy are usually present to suggest these etiologies.

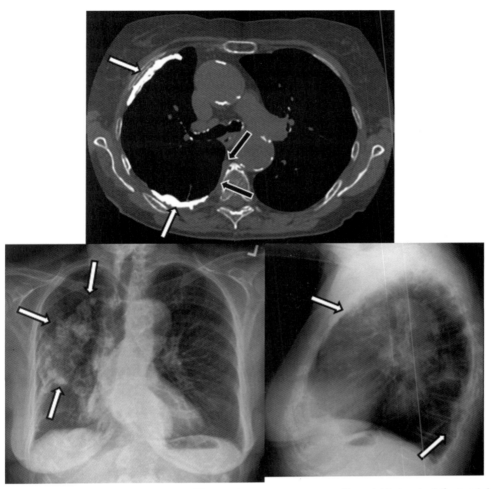

Figure 3.5 Fibrothorax. Axial non-contrast CT image demonstrates coarse curvilinear right pleural calcification (white arrows) and thickening (black arrows) consistent with calcified fibrothorax. This may result from prior empyema, especially tuberculous empyema, or hemorrhagic effusion. PA chest radiograph shows well-defined, holly leaf-like calcification projected over the right hemithorax (white arrows). Lateral chest radiograph assists in localizing the calcification (white arrows) to the anterior and posterior pleura consistent with fibrothorax.

Peritoneal thickening and enhancement may also be localized or generalized and is frequently encountered in oncologic imaging studies due to peritoneal carcinomatosis (Figure 3.6). Infectious or inflammatory etiologies may be responsible and can mimic tumor infiltration.

On normal chest radiographs no line is visible between the inside of the chest wall and the outer border of the lung, but if the pleura is thickened it can be seen as a 1–10 mm linear opacity along the lateral margin of the lung and possibly extending into the interlobar fissure. It is more common along the basal visceral pleural surface where inflammatory mediators accumulate, which can explain the loss of visualization of the costophrenic sulci in cases of pleural thickening (10). Tuberculosis is suspected in the setting of apical pleural thickening, and may be more prominent with increasing age (26,27). Asymmetry should raise concern for superior sulcus tumors.

In cases of severe inflammation in conditions such as hemothorax, pyothorax, or tuberculous pleuritis, there is increased degree and extent of pleural thickening that may calcify, and can measure in excess of 2 cm and surround the entire lung. Decortication can be considered in these circumstances to alleviate associated symptoms if the lung remains functional (10). Even though pleural thickening can be seen on chest radiographs, it is more readily identified on cross-sectional imaging studies. Ultrasound can help in distinguishing pleural effusion from pleural thickening. Diffuse pleural thickening is defined on CT as a thickness of $\geq$ 3 mm extending over a distance of $\geq$ 5 cm (1). CT can be useful to characterize smooth peripheral density seen on chest radiographs, which could be mistakenly interpreted as pleural thickening, as subcostal fat deposition in obese patients, which is very low-density between the ribs and parietal pleura (12).

Peritoneal tuberculosis can have a variety of imaging appearances including loculated ascites with thickened, enhancing peritoneum, and septated, non-contiguous peritoneal fluid collections. Another form is due to a fibrotic response to infection and is manifest by peritoneal or omental

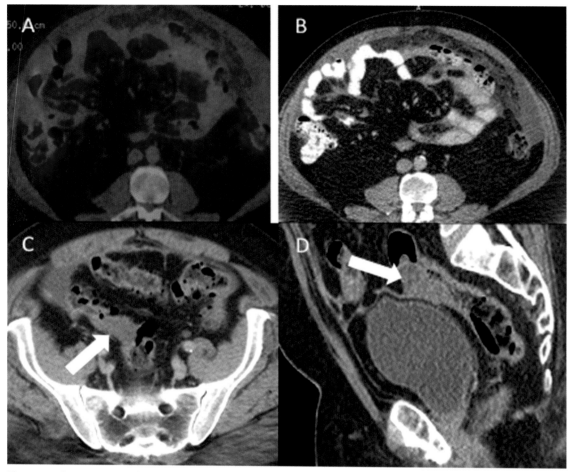

Figure 3.6 Primary peritoneal carcinomatosis. FDG PET-CT (A) and axial (B,C) and sagittal (D) CT post-oral and IV contrast of a male with primary peritoneal carcinomatosis. (A,B) Tracer uptake is seen along the tumor infiltration of the peritoneum, greater omentum and bowel serosa. (C,D) Serosal tumor implant along sigmoid colon (arrows).

soft tissue masses and matting of bowel loops with or without associated obstruction (28).

Encapsulating peritoneal sclerosis is a rare condition characterized by progressive inflammatory fibrosis of the peritoneum, which may be associated with peritoneal dialysis in chronic kidney disease (CKD), radiation enteritis, previous abdominal surgery, endometriosis, or cirrhosis (29). This causes constriction of the bowel serosa and consequent obstruction, which may have insidious onset. Imaging demonstrates thickening of the bowel wall and peritoneal lining.

Asbestos-related Pleural Plaques and Diffuse Pleural Thickening

Generalized or localized thickening of the parietal rather than visceral pleura occurs as a result of asbestos. Localized foci of thickened pleura are referred to as plaques, which are the most common imaging feature seen in those with a history of asbestos exposure (Figure 3.7). There is generally a long latency period, in the region of 30 years, between initial asbestos exposure and the appearance of pleural plaques, which are usually bilateral with basal predominance and follow the contours of the ribs (30,31). Pleural plaques tend to be asymptomatic, but patients with diffuse pleural thickening may experience symptoms related to restrictive pattern of pulmonary function tests.

The plaques often become calcified, which allows them to be seen as linear or geographic opacities on chest radiographs predominantly located along the domes of the diaphragm and mediastinum. However, CT is more sensitive for identifying asbestos-related pleural thickening, which rarely calcifies. Round atelectasis can be seen in cases of asbestos-related pleural thickening and refers to focal subpleural atelectasis due to cicatrized pleural disease (10). However, it is not specific to asbestos and can also occur in the setting of pleural thickening due to chronic infection, trauma, or connective tissue diseases. A classic comet-tail sign represents the parenchymal vessels and bronchi curving into the rounded focal area of lung collapse. Histopathologically the plaques are composed of dense hyaline

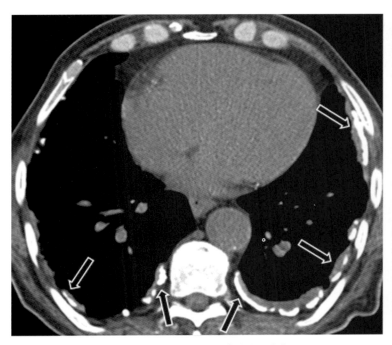
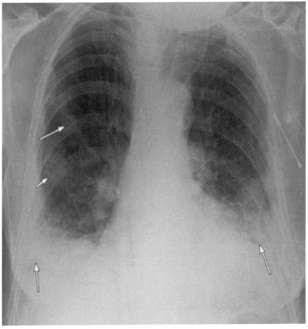

Figure 3.7 Calcified pleural plaques. Bilateral calcified pleural plaques are seen on non-contrast chest CT (black arrows). On PA and lateral chest radiograph the plaques have classic geographic, holly leaf-like appearance (white arrows).

collagen and therefore are of low signal intensity on T1- and T2-weighted MRI sequences.

Pleural and Peritoneal Nodularity

Similar to pleural thickening, pleural nodules may be solitary or multiple and are either of benign or malignant potential. However, malignant pleural nodularity is most frequently due to metastatic disease (Figure 3.8). Peritoneal nodularity occurring due to malignant infiltration is termed peritoneal carcinomatosis (Figure 3.9). The pattern of peritoneal fluid flow influences the distribution of peritoneal tumor deposits. Low infra-diaphragmatic pressure draws pelvic fluid into the upper abdomen, via the right paracolic gutter, to the right subphrenic space and Morison's pouch and onward into the lesser sac via the epiploic foramen. Fluid then transits back

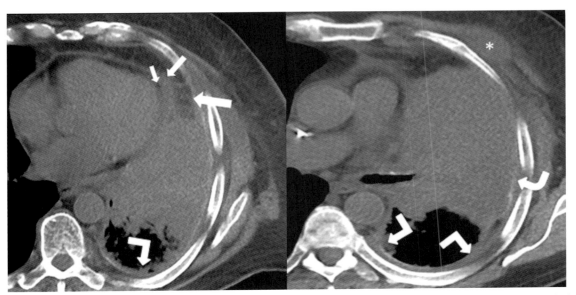

Figure 3.8 Pulmonary adenocarcinoma with pleural mestastases. Axial non-contrast CT thorax images show soft-tissue mass in the left hemithorax due to advanced pulmonary adenocarcinoma. There is malignant infiltration of the pleura with thickening and trace effusion (curved arrows) and invasion of the musculature of the left chest wall (*). Invasion of the pericardial fat, pericardium, and epicardial fat is also evident (large, medium, and small arrows, respectively).

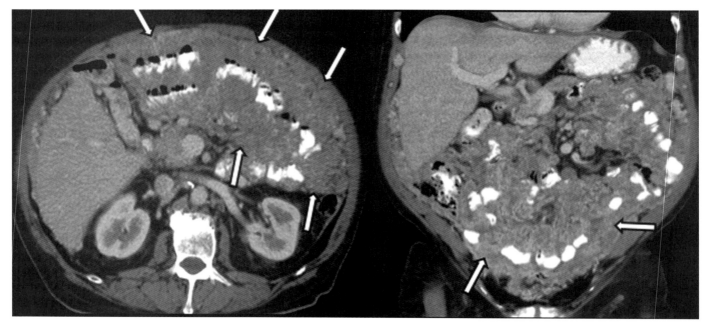

Figure 3.9 Metastatic gastrointestinal stromal tumor. Axial and coronal CT images with oral and intravenous contrast show diffuse peritoneal and omental tumor infiltration (white arrows) in this patient with metastatic gastrointestinal stromal tumor.

from the infracolic abdomen into the pelvis due to gravitational influences (21).

Morphologic features on cross-sectional imaging can help to distinguish benign from malignant entities. Fortier et al. reviewed the MR imaging appearances of chest wall lesions in 45 patients and found that well-defined, smooth margins, although not entirely specific, were associated with benignity; present in 12 of 14 benign lesions and only identifiable in 10 of 31 malignant lesions ($p < 0.05$). Also, a capsule or pedicle was only seen in benign lesions (32). Features associated with malignancy included irregular, poorly defined margins and invasion of local structures. For most lesions signal intensity on MRI was not specific, with the exception of characteristic signal intensity in lipoma and arteriovenous malformation. Indicators of chest wall invasion by tumor on MRI include disruption of the high-signal extrapleural fat on T1-weighted images or abnormal foci of high signal extending into the chest wall musculature on T2-weighted sequences. Evaluation of sagittal and coronal reformats is particularly useful to identify chest wall invasion. MR helps to visualize osseous invasion by tumor, seen as low and high signal in the marrow on T1- and T2-weighted sequences, respectively (18). Vascular encasement by soft tissue is a sign of tumor involvement.

Transperitoneal spread of disease can be seen in various malignancies and refers to the extension of tumor from the subperitoneal space across the peritoneal lining to involve the peritoneal cavity. Such spread has an anatomical basis; for example, the pancreas lies immediately posterior to the lesser sac so pancreatic adenocarcinoma can breach the posterior peri-

toneal lining of the lesser sac and can give rise to peritoneal carcinomatosis (21). The omentum is frequently involved by peritoneal carcinomatosis. Omental studding by tumor occurs when neoplastic cells in the peritoneal cavity cross the thin visceral peritoneum lining the omentum, usually via lymphatic channels, and deposit in the omental fat (Figure 3.10). Progressively increased volumes of soft tissue tumor infiltration lead to omental caking.

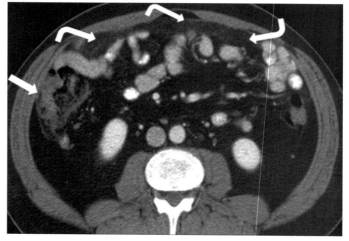

Figure 3.10 Colon adenocarcinoma with omental metastases. Axial contrast-enhanced CT demonstrates primary cecal adenocarcinoma (arrow) with metastatic infiltration of the greater omentum (curved arrows).

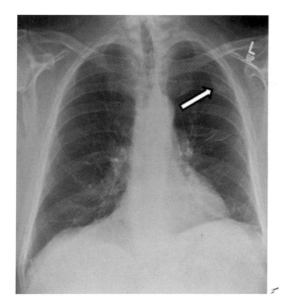

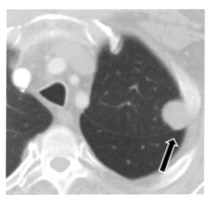
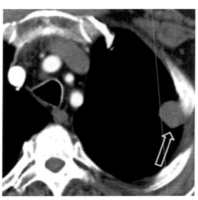
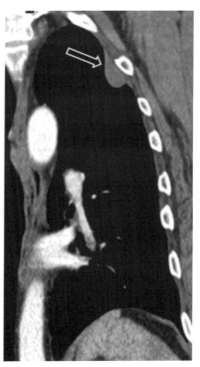

Figure 3.11 Solitary fibrous tumor of pleura. PA chest radiograph demonstrates a well-defined peripheral opacity in the lateral left upper hemithorax (white arrow). The lesion has obtuse angles with the chest wall suggestive of pleural origin. The axial and coronal CT images confirm the soft-tissue mass arises from the left superolateral pleura and contacts the left oblique fissure (black arrows). This was proven to be a solitary fibrous tumor of the pleura.

Primary Pleural and Peritoneal Neoplasms

Fibrous Tumor of the Pleura

Fibrous tumor of the pleura is an uncommon pleural neoplasm that typically arises from mesenchymal cells in the visceral pleural layer (Figure 3.11). They occur slightly more frequently in female patients, with a mean age of 50 years at presentation (1,33,34). They are mostly solitary, but occasionally there can be multiple, and are very slow-growing. A peculiar clinical association with hypoglycemia occurs in approximately 4 percent of cases due to a mechanism involving insulin-like growth factor II.

The typical appearance is of a smooth or lobulated mass close to the diaphragm and frequently (up to 40 percent) with a vascular pedicle connecting the mass to the pleural surface, which can contribute to its mobility on some imaging studies. As expected, given its fibrous composition, these tumors are of low signal on T1- and T2-weighted sequences. Central necrosis or myxoid degeneration can account for areas of T2 high signal in these lesions. These neoplasms are highly vascular and therefore show avid homogeneous contrast enhancement following gadolinium administration (1). The malignant fibrous tumors are avid on F18-FDG PET unlike the benign counterpart. The malignant fibrous tumors are hyperintense on T2-weighted images and iso or low signal on T1-weighted images and show intense enhancement. The malignant potential in these tumors is determined by the amount of mitosis and even the benign counterparts can recur and metastasize to distant sites throughout the body.

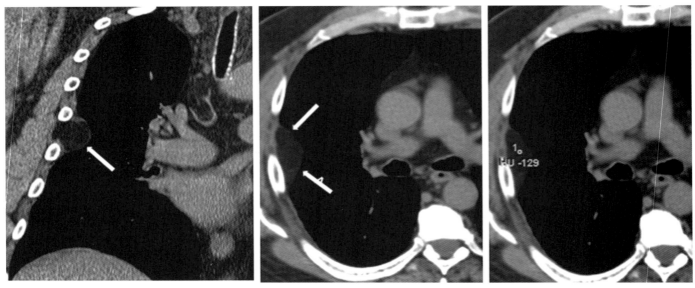

Figure 3.12 Pleural lipoma. Non-contrast CT images of the right hemithorax in axial and coronal plane show a well circumscribed pleural mass along the right costal surface (white arrows), which is of very low attenuation with Hounsfield Units consistent with fat density. Note the oblique angles this lipoma makes with the chest wall confirming its pleural origin.

Benign and Malignant Lipomatous Tumors

Lipomas are another rare benign pleural neoplasm with imaging appearances typical of adipose tissue; they exhibit high signal intensity on T1-weighted images and lose signal on fat-suppressed sequences (1,34,35). On CT lipomatous lesions measure negative Hounsfield Unit attenuation (Figure 3.12). In contrast to the smooth, well-defined, homogeneous appearance of lipomas, liposarcomas tend to be large, ill-defined, and

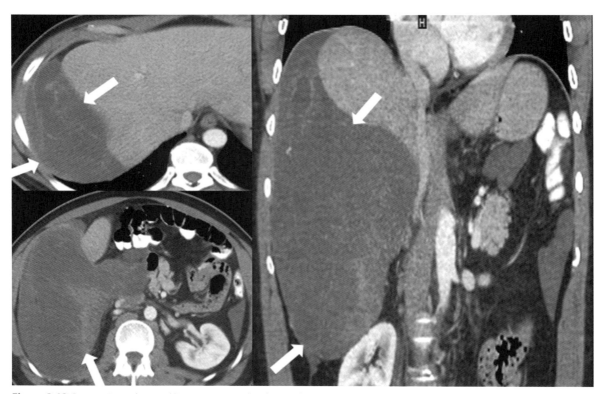

Figure 3.13 Retroperitoneal myxoid liposarcoma. Axial and coronal CT images demonstrate extensive, large right retroperitoneal mass with fat and soft-tissue composition consistent with retroperitoneal myxoid liposarcoma (arrows).

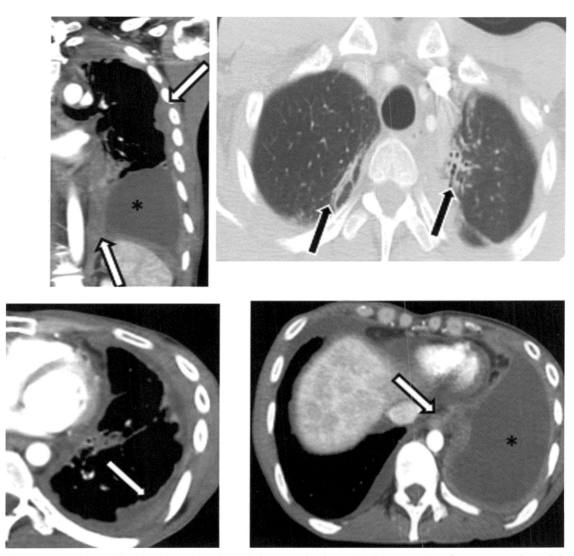

Figure 3.14 Radiation-induced malignant pleural mesothelioma. Axial and coronal soft-tissue windows from contrast-enhanced chest CT show circumferential, rind-like, and nodular thickening of the left pleura (white arrows) and a moderate left pleural effusion (*). Axial image on lung windows at the level of the upper lobes show bilateral, medial volume loss and traction bronchiectasis consistent with prior radiation therapy. The pleural abnormality was a radiation-induced mesothelioma.

infiltrative. They are composed of both fat and soft-tissue elements and therefore have a heterogeneous appearance on imaging studies. Even after contrast enhancement they tend to have low attenuation (< 50 HU) on CT (Figure 3.13) (1,36). On MRI they can show high T2 signal due to myxoid degeneration.

Malignant Pleural Mesothelioma

Malignant pleural mesothelioma (MPM) is an aggressive primary neoplasm arising from mesothelial cells of the pleura associated with previous asbestos exposure. Although rare, with an incidence in the US of 2500 to 3000 cases annually, it has been increasing worldwide due to widespread environmental exposure to asbestos (37–39). In North America alone, it was estimated that there would be $> 80,000$ new cases by 2024 (38,40).

Therefore, in developing nations where there has been continued, unregulated exposure it seems likely that more cases will be seen in these countries in the future (41,42). Typically exposure is associated with occupation – for example, men working in shipyards or women in the textile industry – but generalized daily environmental exposure can also increase prevalence, such as in Egypt where accordingly there are a greater proportion of young patients affected (43).

Histopathologically, malignant mesothelioma is classified into three subgroups: epithelioid which is the most common, followed by the biphasic pattern, and lastly the rare sarcomatoid variant. Desmoplastic mesothelioma is an even rarer subtype of sarcomatoid mesothelioma (44). Patients with epithelioid type have better survival with tri-modality therapy than those with biphasic or sarcomatoid histology (45). It would therefore

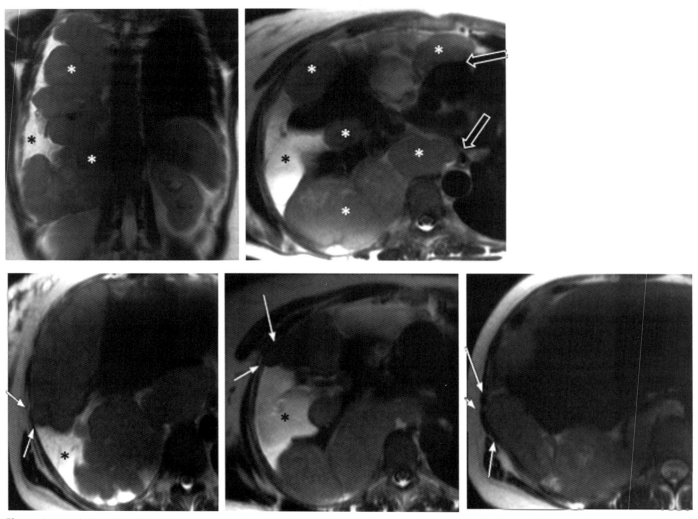

Figure 3.15 Malignant pleural mesothelioma. Axial and coronal T2 Haste MRI images reveal circumferential, bulky, lobulated right pleural masses and nodules encasing the right hemithorax and extending along the fissures, mediastinal, costal and diaphragmatic pleural surfaces consistent with malignant mesothelioma (white *). There is also a moderate-volume loculated right pleural effusion (black *). The tumor invades the mediastinal fat and abuts the ascending and descending aorta and esophagus without invasion (black arrows). There are foci of endothoracic fascial involvement (white arrows) but no chest wall invasion. The diaphragm is also involved, but there is no transdiaphragmatic spread of tumor.

be advantageous to accurately determine the exact histology of MPM preoperatively to help therapeutic strategic decisions. Open pleural biopsy is often needed to optimally classify these tumors prior to surgery (45).

CT is the prime imaging modality that is employed for evaluation of MPM (46,47). Imaging manifestations of MPM include ipsilateral pleural effusion, interlobar fissural and mediastinal pleural thickening and nodularity, circumferential rind-like nodular pleural thickening, and encasement with volume reduction of the involved hemithorax and associated ipsilateral mediastinal shift and rib destruction(48–50) (Figure 3.14). Aggressive local spread characterizes the behavior of MPM (51,52). It can invade the visceral and parietal pleura as well as the adjacent chest wall, mediastinum, and diaphragm. Pleural mesothelioma can invade and involve the peritoneum through direct diaphragmatic extension. On MRI, the imaging char-

acteristics of MPM include signal intensity, which is intermediate or mildly increased compared to intercostal muscles on T1-weighted sequence and moderately high signal intensity on T2-weighted sequence (1,12,36,47). Following administration of gadolinium intravenous contrast, malignant mesothelioma enhances and T1-weighted fat-suppressed sequences are associated with the highest sensitivity for detection of local invasion or malignant pleural nodularity, especially in the fissures (1). Metastatic spread of disease by lymphatics is frequent in MPM; studies have shown incidences between 25 percent and 57 percent (53–55) (Figure 3.15). Often the disease can involve mediastinal nodes that are not typically affected by other intrathoracic malignancies (51). Distant metastases are unusual at presentation of the epithelioid subtype, but osseous metastases are not infrequent in patients with the more aggressive sarcomatoid and biphasic variants. Hematogenous spread is generally a late

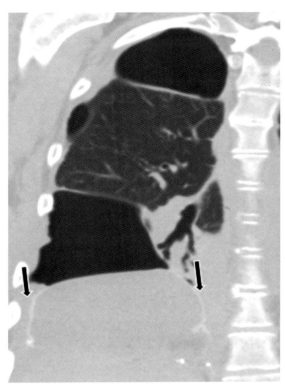
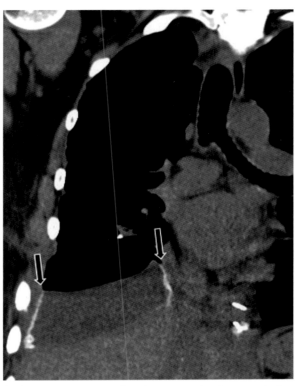

Figure 3.16 Malignant pleural mesothelioma post pleurectomy, diaphragmatic resection and mesh reconstruction. Postoperative images demonstrate pleurectomy, diaphragmatic reconstruction (black arrows), and moderate-volume hydropneumothorax.

feature of the disease (52). As the disease progresses, metastases can occur in the lungs, liver, and adrenal glands (44).

The extent of primary tumor is an important factor in overall survival (56). Overall, MPM has a poor prognosis, with 50 percent of affected patients succumbing to the disease within 2 years irrespective of treatment, usually as a result of progressive pulmonary encasement and respiratory failure (50,57,58). Without treatment, survival time ranges from 4 to 12 months (59). Factors associated with poor prognosis in mesothelioma include non-epithelioid or sarcomatoid histology, age > 70 years, male gender, poor performance status, high white cell count and CRP at baseline (58,60). Scherpereel et al. state that patient performance status and histologic subtype are the most clinically important prognostic factors (61). Measurement of standardized uptake value (SUV) can have relevance to patient prognosis. Flores et al. found that a high SUV in the primary tumor correlated with N2 disease in MPM (62).

Clinical staging in MPM does not predict prognosis and correlation with pathological stage is dismal. The most commonly used clinical staging system in use was proposed by the International Mesothelioma Interest Group. Nakas et al. found deficiencies in the IMIG staging system and substantial discrepancies when they compared clinical staging by imaging to pathologic staging in 164 MPM patients. cT stage differed from pT stage in 56 percent of patients, with 46 percent understaged. cN stage differed from pN stage in 44 percent, understaged in 31 percent (63). Overall survival was not found to be associated with pT stage. Rusch et al. analyzed the IASLC database to inform the upcoming revisions to the MPM staging system (58). Currently there are no size-based criteria, the T stage is determined by assessing invasion of adjacent structures by the tumor, and the N criteria are similar to those of lung cancer staging and are based on the IASLC map (64).

By combining information obtained from CT and PET imaging with mediastinoscopy or even EBUS-TNA, more accurate and comprehensive preoperative staging should be achievable. Erasmus and colleagues found that by combining PET with CT, the T stage was accurately classified in 63 percent of patients, of whom 25 percent had non-resectable T4 disease. Heelan and colleagues compared CT and MRI in staging MPM and found that MRI was more accurate at demonstrating invasion of the diaphragm and endothoracic fascia or solitary resectable foci of chest wall invasion.

The presence of lymph node metastases is a poor prognostic indicator of survival in MPM (65,66), but currently accurate prediction of nodal involvement by any and even a multi-modality approach is limited. Even though cervical mediastinoscopy is part of the diagnostic work up, evaluation of nodal stations such as internal mammary, hilar and diaphragmatic stations is not possible using this approach (67,68). Rice et al. highlighted the potential utility of invasive staging, in this case with extended surgical approach including laparoscopy, peritoneal lavage as well as mediastinoscopy to identify the group of patients with unresectable disease not classified as such

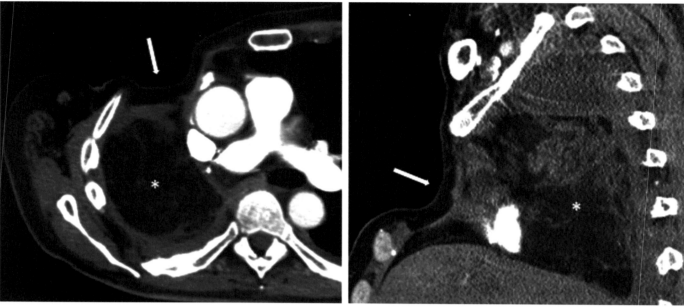

Figure 3.17 Closure of Clagett window with omental flap. Axial and sagittal images from chest CT with intravenous contrast demonstrate omental flap (*) closure of right anterior chest wall Clagett window (white arrows), which was created as part of treatment of a bronchopleural fistula with superimposed infection of the right hemithorax following right extra-pleural pneumonectomy for malignant mesothelioma.

by imaging and thereby avoid potential high risks associated with radical resection (69).

Imaging is also of paramount importance for evaluating the disease after implementation of a given treatment strategy (Figures 3.16 and 3.17). Local recurrence is the most frequently implicated in cases with progressive disease that fail tri-modality therapy consisting of a combination of extrapleural pneumonectomy, chemotherapy and radiation therapy (70,71). In their study of 46 patients, 35 percent first recurred in the ipsilateral hemi-thorax, making it the most common site of failure followed by abdominal in 26 percent, contralateral thorax in 17 percent, and other distant locations in 8 percent, with the remainder recurring in multiple synchronous sites.

Restaging following systemic therapy, which aims to improve both symptoms and survival, has unique challenges given the diffusely infiltrative growth pattern of MPM. Acknowledging resultant limitations of standard radiologic approaches to response assessment in MPM, Byrne et al. proposed a modified RECIST (response evaluation criteria in solid tumors) criteria for restaging of MPM (72). This involves six measurements of tumor thickness parallel to the mediastinum or chest wall, two on each of three selected axial slices on the CT chest. These are summated to give one pleural unidimensional measurement. They proposed that a decrease of 30 percent on two occasions on scans with an interval of 4 weeks apart represented a partial response, and progressive disease, an increase of 20 percent over the nadir. They validated their proposal by demonstrating statistically significant correlation with survival and lung function measured by forced vital capacity (FVC). Armato and coworkers looked at interobserver variability in the measurement of changes in mesothelioma thickness over time; in particular, they compared the measurements made by four individual readers when measurements made on the baseline imaging were displayed and when follow-up measurements were made using the prior report (73,74). They concluded that the method by which baseline results are made available to readers influences the measurements they acquire at restaging and therefore could affect classification of tumor response and potentially limit consistency of results.

Other studies have evaluated the role of serial PET imaging for restaging of MPM following chemotherapy. Gerbaudo et al. showed that MPM had high metabolic tumor rate as evidenced by areas of increased FDG uptake seen on PET scans (Figure 3.18). Kaira et al. explain the biologic basis for utility of FDG-PET in MPM (75). Francis and colleagues quantified the total glycolytic volume (TGV) of tumor on ^{18}F-FDG-PET scans performed before and after one cycle of chemotherapy. They found that the median TGV fell to 30 percent of baseline after treatment in all patients classified as partial responders by RECIST CT evaluation (76). In addition to this potential role of early prediction of response to chemotherapy, they demonstrated a statistically significant association between a fall in TGV and improved survival ($p = 0.015$), which was not the case for reduction in SUVmax or CT.

Malignant Peritoneal Mesothelioma

The serous membrane of the peritoneum may be primarily or secondarily affected by mesothelioma (Figure 3.19). Up to 30 percent of malignant mesothelioma originates in the peritoneum (5). Similar to its pleural counterpart, it is an aggressive malignancy with a poor prognosis, but unlike pleural

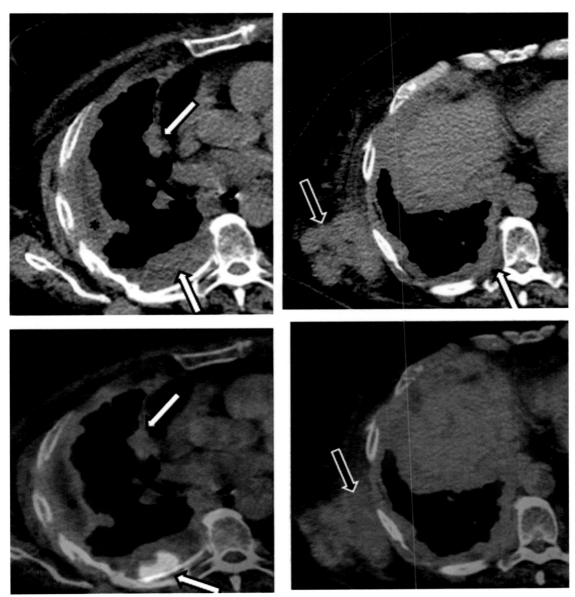

Figure 3.18 Sarcomatoid malignant pleural mesothelioma subtype. Axial non-contrast and fused images from FDG PET-CT demonstrate circumferential rind-like right pleural thickening with prominent nodularity (white arrows) and loculated pleural effusion (*). The solid components are FDG-avid and consistent with pathologically proven sarcomatoid mesothelioma. The fluid is not FDG-avid but still represents part of the malignant disease process. There is a nodular soft-tissue mass which is also FDG-avid in the right posterolateral chest wall possibly due to direct invasion or seeding of tumor at site of previous biopsy or chest drain.

disease, peritoneal mesothelioma is not typically associated with asbestos exposure or calcified plaques (77). Appearances on cross-sectional imaging are characterized by either ascites with diffuse or nodular peritoneal thickening or peritoneal tumor masses with scalloping or mass effect on adjacent organs. Differentiation between peritoneal carcinomatosis and peritoneal mesothelioma can be difficult on imaging and the diagnosis will often need diagnostic paracentesis.

Desmoplastic Small Round Cell Tumor

This is a relatively recently recognized, highly aggressive malignancy that most commonly involves the peritoneal cavity, espe-cially the paravesical space in young patients (Figure 3.20). Disseminated, often large, peritoneal heterogeneous masses with central areas of low attenuation or necrosis are seen on imaging. There may be associated ascites (77).

Papillary Serous Carcinoma

Typical imaging features of this rare primary peritoneal malignancy include occurrence in post-menopausal women, multifocal distribution of disease including omental infiltration and extensive calcification in the absence of an ovarian mass to suggest metastatic papillary serous carcinoma, which has identical histology (Figure 3.21) (78).

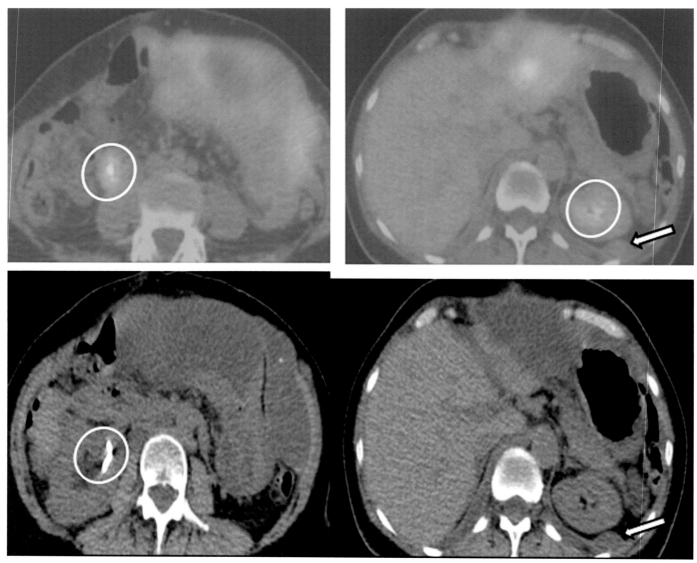

Figure 3.19 Peritoneal mesothelioma. Non-contrast CT and fused axial images from FDG PET-CT show increased tracer uptake in abdominal and pelvic soft-tissue masses consistent with increased metabolic activity in peritoneal mesothelioma. There is a mildly FDG-avid focal soft-tissue nodule in the left posterior retroperitoneum consistent with mesothelioma deposit (white arrows). FDG avidity within white circles is related to tracer excretion in the urinary tract. There is a partially visualized ureteric stent on the right.

Metastatic Pleural and Peritoneal Infiltration

Pleural involvement by metastatic disease accounts for the majority or 90 percent of cases of malignant pleural thickening; only 10 percent of cases are due to primary pleural malignancy (Figures 3.22 and 3.23) (79). The most common neoplasms to involve the pleura include lung, breast, ovarian, gastric, and lymphoma (Figure 3.24) (1,80). Although relatively rare, invasive thymoma or thymic carcinoma has a high propensity for contiguous or drop pleural metastases (Figure 3.25). In addition to hematogenous or lymphatic spread to the pleura, direct local invasion can occur, for example, superior sulcus tumor invasion (19,81). Similarly, metastatic tumor infiltration is the most common cause of malignant peritoneal disease (Figure 3.26). Intra-abdominal primary neoplasms most frequently implicated are gastric, ovarian, colon, and pancreatic adenocarcinomas (Figure 3.21). Lymphoma and sarcoma can also infiltrate and spread via the peritoneum (Figures 3.27 and 3.28).

While pleural infiltration can be suspected on the basis of the chest radiography appearance, CT or MRI is necessary to assess whether it is benign or malignant. Features that are worrisome for malignant involvement on contrast-enhanced CT include ≥ 1 cm nodular or circumferential thickening of the parietal pleura and involvement of the diaphragmatic and mediastinal surfaces (50). An advantage of CT is that it may also elucidate the primary neoplastic source or other sites of

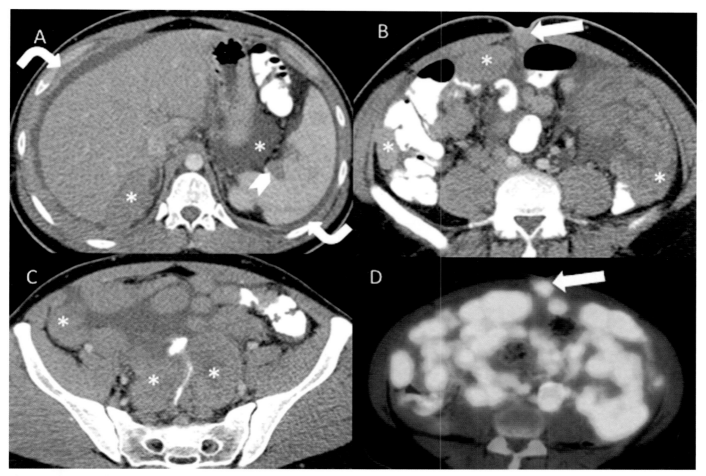

Figure 3.20 Desmoplastic small round cell tumor. (A–C) Axial abdominopelvic CT images with oral and IV contrast show diffuse peritoneal and retroperitoneal soft-tissue masses (*) with intense metabolic activity on FDG PET-CT (D). Umbilical tumor implant consistent with Sr. Mary Joseph metastasis (arrows). Peritoneal thickening, enhancement, and ascites due to peritoneal carcinomatosis (curved arrows). Invasion of the splenic hilum by peritoneal implant (arrowhead).

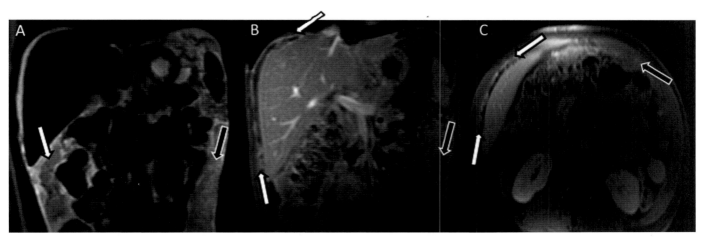

Figure 3.21 Metastatic serous ovarian carcinoma with peritoneal carcinomatosis. (A–C) T2 and T1 post-gadolinium coronal and axial images, respectively, show peritoneal thickening, nodularity (white arrows), and tumor infiltration of the omentum (black arrows).

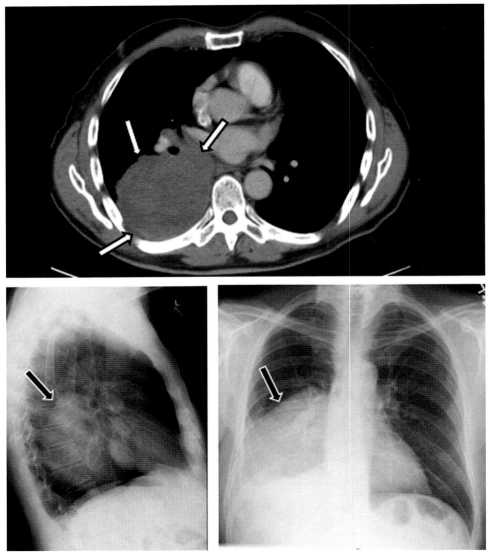

Figure 3.22 Synovial sarcoma of pleura. PA and lateral chest radiograph demonstrate a large mass-like opacity in the right posteroinferior hemithorax (black arrows). Axial non-contrast chest CT demonstrates a heterogeneous soft-tissue mass in the posterior right hemithorax with pleural involvement (white arrows). The mass has irregular margins anteriorly and was consistent with a synovial sarcoma of the pleura.

metastatic disease. MRI may be better in distinguishing benign from malignant pleural disease (1,82) by combining information on morphology as well as signal intensity characteristics. It has been published (1,36) that pleural thickening of lower signal intensity than adjacent intercostal muscles on T2-weighted sequences is indicative of benign etiology.

The increased sensitivity of CT for the detection of malignant peritoneal thickening, enhancement, nodularity and fluid is critical to allow more accurate radiologic preoperative tumor staging and resectability assessment as well as restaging following therapy and surveillance for recurrent disease (83). Multi-detector CT allows accurate detection of peritoneal implants even under 1 cm in size, although locations with decreased sensitivity for identification include the lesser omentum, the left hemidiaphragm, the bowel serosa,

and the root of the mesentery (84). For peritoneal tumor deposits of > 1 cm, performance of MRI is generally comparable with MDCT (84). Following gadolinium administration, the enhancement of the peritoneum should be less than or equivalent to normal hepatic enhancement. Contrast enhancement greater than the liver parenchyma is suggestive of peritoneal pathology (84). Continued improvement in MR techniques facilitates identification of smaller tumor deposits (< 5 mm) and those in locations that prove challenging for detection on CT, including serosal, mesenteric, and subphrenic sites (84). Metastatic peritoneal nodules are typically low signal on T1- and intermediate to high signal on T2-weighted imaging and are best appreciated with fat-suppressed T2 and delayed fat-suppressed T1 sequences with contrast (84).

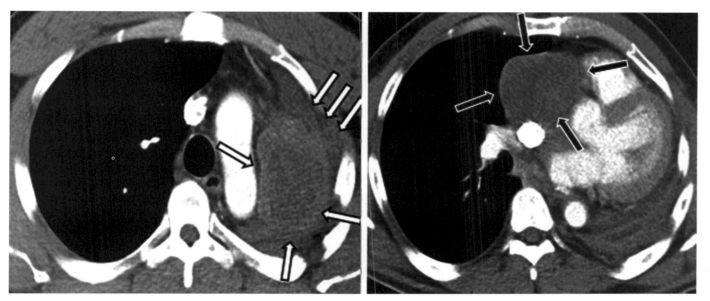

Figure 3.23 Malignant peripheral nerve sheath tumor. Axial images from contrast-enhanced CT thorax show a heterogeneous left apical pleural metastasis (white arrows) and mediastinal tumor invasion (black arrows) in this patient with prior left pneumonectomy for pulmonary metastases from a malignant peripheral nerve sheath tumor.

There are distinct differences in imaging appearance of metastatic peritoneal involvement by each of three cancer cell lines, namely, carcinoma, lymphoma, and sarcoma (85,86). Peritoneal carcinomatosis is characterized by ascites, peritoneal thickening, and omental caking more frequently than measurable nodules, which are more frequently associated with sarcomatosis and typically have a well-defined, smooth outline (85). Lymphomatous peritoneal involvement is more likely to infiltrate the omentum and mesentery

and is associated with lymphadenopathy and splenomegaly (Figure 3.29) (86).

Pseudomyxoma Peritonei

Pseudomyxoma peritonei describes the accumulation of gelatinous ascites in the peritoneal space following rupture of a mucinous tumor, typically mucocele of the appendix. Less commonly, mucinous colorectal, ovarian, gastric, or urachal

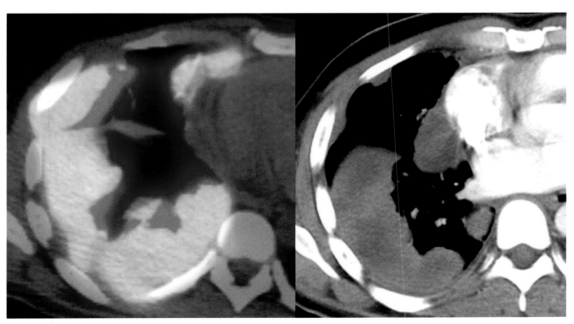

Figure 3.24 Pleural lymphoma. Axial fused and non-contrast images from FDG PET-CT in a patient with non-Hodgkin lymphoma demonstrate marked FDG-avidity in large right pleural masses consistent with lymphomatous infiltration.

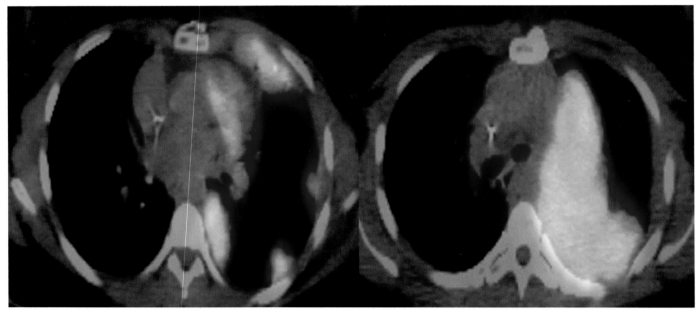

Figure 3.25 Pleural metastases from invasive thymoma. Fused axial images from FDG PET-CT in a patient with previous resection of thymoma shows multiple FDG-avid pleural masses and nodules consistent with recurrent thymoma with pleural metastases.

tumors are responsible. Radiologic studies demonstrate loculated ascites with scalloping of adjacent organs (87).

Future Directions of Imaging Pleural and Peritoneal Diseases

Multi-parametric MRI is likely to have an ever-increasing contribution in evaluation of both pleural and peritoneal diseases.

Diffusion-weighted imaging (DWI) is well established in the assessment of several malignancies (88,89). DWI assesses the motion of water molecules that increases the conspicuity of tissue with restricted diffusion, such as tumor or abscess which are seen as bright foci on DWI images and which can be quantified by the apparent diffusion coefficient (ADC) (90). Coolen et al. postulated that the "pointillism sign" on diffusion-weighted sequences could be a way to distinguish between benign and

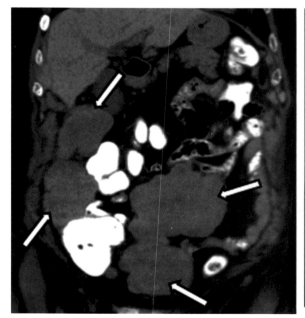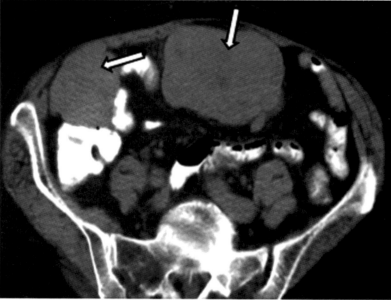

Figure 3.26 Peritoneal metastases from invasive thymoma. Axial and coronal images from CT of the abdomen and pelvis with oral contrast demonstrate heterogeneous soft-tissue masses in the peritoneal cavity that were consistent with peritoneal metastases from invasive thymoma (white arrows).

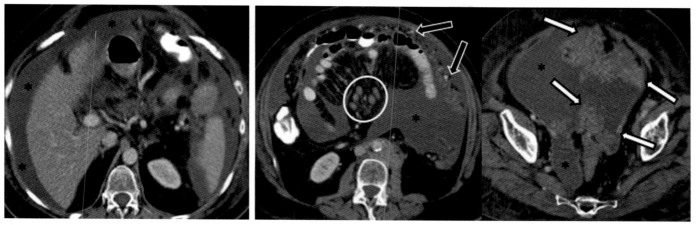

Figure 3.27 Peritoneal lymphomatosis. Axial images from CT abdomen and pelvis with oral and intravenous contrast demonstrate moderate-volume ascites in the peritoneal space (*). There is enhancement, nodular thickening, and confluent tumor infiltration of the peritoneum (white arrows) and omentum (black arrows) in keeping with peritoneal lymphomatosis. Mesenteric lymphadenopathy is also present (encircled).

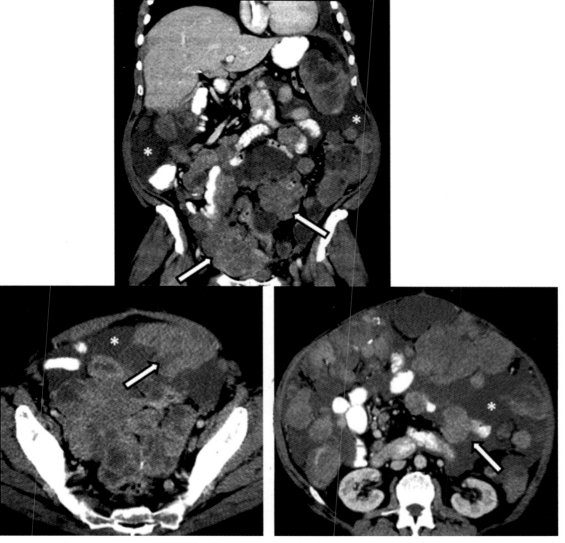

Figure 3.28 Peritoneal sarcomatosis. Coronal and axial CT images of the abdomen and pelvis with oral and intravenous contrast show innumerable enhancing peritoneal nodules and masses (white arrows) in this patient with peritoneal sarcomatosis. There is also ascites (*).

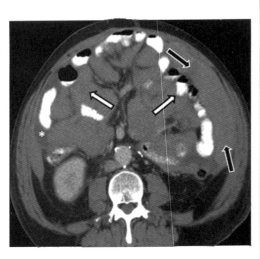 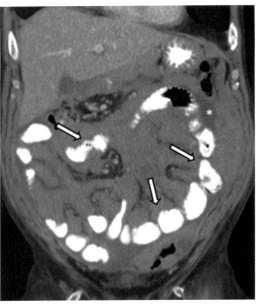

Figure 3.29 Peritoneal lymphomatosis. Axial and coronal CT images with oral and intravenous contrast demonstrate extensive peritoneal (white arrows) and omental (black arrows) tumor consistent with peritoneal lymphomatosis in this patient with diffuse large B-cell lymphoma. The tumor infiltrates the mesentery (white arrows) and encases the small bowel without obstruction. Note associated small-volume ascites (*). There is sparing of the retroperitoneal compartment posteriorly.

malignant pleural diseases (82,91). They studied 31 patients suspected of having pleural malignancy. Using histopathology results from pleural biopsy as the reference standard for malignant pleural disease, they found that the sensitivity, specificity, and accuracy of PET/CT and DWI/MR using an ADC threshold of 1.52×10^{-3} mm^2/s to distinguish benign from malignant etiology was 100 percent, 35 percent, and 65 percent and 71 percent, 100 percent and 87 percent, respectively. ADC could have relevance in determining the histopathologic subtype of MPM (92). Both quantitative and qualitative DWI has potential for assessment of peritoneal malignancy. Combined with contrast-enhanced MRI, restricted diffusion improves the detection of tumor involvement with reported sensitivity and specificity of 90 percent and 95 percent (89,97).

Dynamic contrast-enhanced (DCE) MR provides an assessment of tissue perfusion by observing and quantifying the flow of contrast to the tissue and its subsequent clearance. Pharmacokinetic analysis can be performed on DCE-MR images to elucidate biologic properties of the microcirculation. Giesel et al. studied the kinetic parameters of amplitude (amp), redistribution rate constant ($k$ep) and elimination rate constant ($k$el) in 19 patients with MPM undergoing chemotherapy, to ascertain any differences between benign and malignant tissue and compare kinetic parameters with clinical outcomes. They found that pathologic and normal tissue could be differentiated by amp and $k$el ($p \leq 0.001$) (93). Patients with clinical response showed lower median redistribution rate constant ($k$ep) while those with higher values had less-favorable responses to therapy. This is logical given that neoangiogenesis is essential for tumor growth and prior research has shown that increased tumor vascularity is a poor prognostic sign (94). This is felt to be related to the finding that increased vascular density in tumors is associated with increased levels of pro-neovascularization factors such as VEGF (95), which are substantial potentiators of microvascular permeability that may be reflected on functional imaging as high $k$ep (96). DCE-MRI also has potential applications for peritoneal malignancy; for example, the detection of ovarian metastatic disease (89,97). MR proton spectroscopy uses the detection of choline metabolites as a tumor biomarker for imaging. It can be used to characterize ovarian cancer (98).

Given the aforementioned advantages of excellent soft-tissue contrast provided by MR in the local tumor staging of MPM and the limitations of PET CT in this role, it is likely that the relatively new combination of PET MR could lead to significant improvements in preoperative staging especially as well as post-treatment surveillance for recurrent tumor.

Quantitative imaging, including volumetry, is becoming increasingly important in oncology and is already well-established in the preoperative assessment of hepatic tumors to ensure sufficient residual liver volume following resection (99,100). Given the challenges of assessing MPM disease burden on planar imaging due to its circumferential growth pattern, the use of volumetric measurement parameters could provide improved reliability and reproducibility for restaging after systemic therapy. Frauenfelder et al. compared volumetry to modified RECIST assessment of disease and found that interobserver agreement, interrater reliability for tumor response classification and number of patients classified equally were much higher with volumetric measurement; general kappa 0.9, 0.99 reliability as compared to general kappa 0.33, 0.55 reliability by RECIST criteria (101). Volumetric assessment has also been shown to have prognostic implications and can be used to stratify patients undergoing surgery (56). Nowak et al. looked at TGV quantified by PET-CT and found that baseline TGV was predictive of survival in patients with epithelioid or biphasic MPM and more predictive than TNM staging. They concluded that the volume and glucose metabolism of MPM may be more important prognostic factors than the anatomic extent of disease, based on their findings (76).

Up until now, glucose metabolism has been the focus of almost all functional imaging of pleural and peritoneal diseases. Development of novel probes for PET imaging is an area of intense biopharmaceutical research. The radiopharmaceutical [18F] FES is an estrogen analogue that shows increased avidity at disease sites affected by advanced ovarian or endometrial cancer. In addition to detection, this biomarker allows quantitative assessment of estrogen receptors in the tumor and response following hormonal therapy (102).

References

1. Gill RR, Gerbaudo VH, Jacobson FL, Trotman-Dickenson B, Matsuoka S, Hunsaker A, et al. MR imaging of benign and malignant pleural disease. *Magn Reson Imaging Clin N Am*. 2008;16:319–39, x. Available from: www.ncbi.nlm.nih.gov/pubmed/18474335

2. Benamore RE, Warakaulle DR, Traill ZC. Imaging of pleural disease. *Imaging*. 2008;20(4):236–51.

3. Salahudeen HM, Hoey ETD, Robertson RJ, Darby MJ. CT appearances of pleural tumours. *Clin Radiol*. 2009;64(9):918–30.

4. Tirkes T, Sandrasegaran K, Patel AA, Hollar MA, Tejada JG, Tann M, et al. Peritoneal and retro peritoneal anatomy and its relevance for cross sectional imaging 1. *RadioGraphics*. 2012;32(2):437–52. Available from: www.ncbi.nlm.nih.gov/pubmed/22411941

5. Jeffrey RB. Imaging of the peritoneal cavity. *Curr Opin Radiol*. 1991;3(3):471–73. Available from: www.ncbi.nlm.nih.gov/pubmed/1859782

6. Liang C, Shuang L, Wei L, Bolduc J-P, Deslauriers J. Correlative anatomy of the pleura and pleural spaces. *Thorac Surg Clin*. 2011;21(2):177–82, vii–viii. Available from: www.ncbi.nlm.nih.gov/pubmed/21477767

7. Frola C, Cantoni S, Turtulici I, Leoni C, Loria F, Gaeta M, et al. Transudative vs exudative pleural effusions: differentiation using Gd-DTPA-enhanced MRI. *Eur Radiol*. 1997;7:860–64.

8. Porcel JM, Pardina M, Bielsa S. Imaging of pleural effusions: a pictorial review. *Curr Respir Care Rep*. 2014;3(2):42–44. Available from: www.embase.com/search/results?subaction=viewrecord&from=export&id=L373061048\n

http://dx.doi.org/10.1007/s13665–014–0076–2\n
http://sfx.hul.harvard.edu/sfx_local?sid=EMBASE&issn=2161332X&id=doi:10.1007/s13665–014–0076–2&atitle=Imaging+of+pleural+ef

9. Yalcin NG, Choong CKC, Eizenberg N. Anatomy and pathophysiology of the pleura and pleural space. *Thorac Surg Clin*. 2013;23(1):1–10. Available from: http://dx.doi.org/10.1016/j.thorsurg.2012.10.008

10. Light RW. Pleural diseases. *Disease-a-Month*. 1992;266–331.

11. Jones PW, Moyers JP, Rogers JT, Rodriguez RM, Lee YCG, Light RW. Ultrasound-guided thoracentesis: is it a safer method? *Chest*. 2003;123(2):418–23. Available from: www.ncbi.nlm.nih.gov/entrez/query.fcgi?db=pubmed&cmd=Retrieve&dopt=AbstractPlus&list_uids=12576360\n papers3://publication/uuid/2F7D1E6D-5288-492C-9DC7-FDD3EFB95D39

12. McLoud TC, Flower CDR. Imaging the pleura: sonography, CT, and MR imaging. *AJR Am J Roentgenol*. 1991;156:1145–53.

13. Barnes TW, Morgenthaler TI, Olson EJ, Hesley GK, Decker PA, Ryu JH. Sonographically guided thoracentesis and rate of pneumothorax. *J Clin Ultrasound*. 2005;33:442–46.

14. Kataoka H, Takada S. The role of thoracic ultrasonography for evaluation of patients with decompensated chronic heart failure. *J Am Coll Cardiol*. 2000;35(6):1638–46.

15. Koenig SJ, Narasimhan M, Mayo PH. Thoracic ultrasonography for the pulmonary specialist. *Chest*. 2011;140(5):1332–41.

16. Agmy GM, Wafy S, Hussein A. Transthoracic Doppler chest ultrasonography: the current situation. *Chest*. 2010;138(4):818A. Available from: http://chestjournal.chestpubs.org/cgi/content/meeting_abstract/138/4_MeetingAbstracts/818A?sid=c142777c-59dd-4533-9d92-f0b4ba559563\n http://ovidsp.ovid.com/ovidweb.cgi?T=JS&PAGE=reference&D=emed9&NEWS=N&AN=70362075

17. Yilmaz U, Polat G, Sahin N, Soy O, Gülay U. CT in differential diagnosis of benign and malignant pleural disease. *Monaldi Arch Chest Dis*. 2005;63(1):17–22. Available from: www.ncbi.nlm.nih.gov/pubmed/16035560

18. Baysal T, Bulut T, Gökirmak M, Kalkan S, Dusak A, Dogan M. Diffusion-weighted MR imaging of pleural fluid: differentiation of transudative vs exudative pleural effusions. *European Radiology*. 2004;14(5):890–96. Available from: www.ncbi.nlm.nih.gov/pubmed/12904883

19. Heelan RT, Rusch VW, Begg CB, Panicek DM, Caravelli JF, Eisen C. Staging of malignant pleural mesothelioma: comparison of CT and MR imaging. *AJR Am J Roentgenol*. 1999;172:1039–47.

20. Gupta NC, Rogers JS, Graeber GM, Gregory JL, Waheed U, Mullet D, et al. Clinical role of F-18 fluorodeoxyglucose positron emission tomography imaging in patients with lung cancer and suspected malignant pleural effusion. *Chest*. 2002;122:1918–24.

21. Pannu HK, Bristow RE, Frederick J. Multidetector CT of peritoneal carcinomatosis from ovarian cancer. *Radiographics*. 2003;23(3):687–701.

22. Gore RM, Newmark GM, Thakrar KH, Mehta UK, Berlin JW. Pathways of abdominal tumour spread: the role of the subperitoneal space. *Cancer*

Imaging. 2009;9:112–20. Available from: www.pubmedcentral.nih.gov/articlerender.fcgi?artid=2821589&tool=pmcentrez&rendertype=abstract

23. Lynch KC, Oliveira CR, Matheson JS, Mitchell MA, O'Brien RT. Detection of pneumothorax and pleural effusion with horizontal beam radiography. *Vet Radiol Ultrasound.* 2012;53(1):38–43.

24. Wilkerson RG, Stone MB. Sensitivity of bedside ultrasound and supine anteroposterior chest radiographs for the identification of pneumothorax after blunt trauma. *Acad Emerg Med.* 2010;17:11–17.

25. Diacon AH, Theron J, Bolliger CT. Transthoracic ultrasound for the pulmonologist. *Curr Opin Pulm Med.* 2005;11(4):307–12.

26. Ko JM, Park HJ, Kim CH. Pulmonary changes of pleural tuberculosis: up-to-date CT imaging. *Chest.* 2014;138(4):1604–11. Available from: www.ncbi.nlm.nih.gov/pubmed/25086249

27. Baumann MH, Nolan R, Petrini M, Lee YCG, Light RW, Schneider E. Pleural tuberculosis in the United States: incidence and drug resistance. *Chest.* 2007;131:1125–32.

28. Mimidis K, Ritis K, Kartalis G. Peritoneal tuberculosis. *Ann Gastroenterol.* 2005;18(3):325–29.

29. Ti JP, Al-Aradi A, Conlon PJ, Lee MJ, Morrin MM. Imaging features of encapsulating peritoneal sclerosis in continuous ambulatory peritoneal dialysis patients. *AJR Am J Roentgenol.* 2010;195(1):W50–54.

30. Hillerdal G. Mesothelioma: cases associated with non-occupational and low dose exposures. *Occup Environ Med.* 1999;56:505–13.

31. Fletcher AC, Engholm G, Englund A. The risk of lung cancer from asbestos among Swedish construction workers: self-reported exposure and a job exposure matrix compared. *Int J Epidemiol.* 1993;22(Suppl 2):S29–35. Available from: www.ncbi.nlm.nih.gov/pubmed/8132389

32. Fortier M, Mayo JR, Swensen SJ, Munk PL, Vellet DA, Müller NL. MR imaging of chest wall lesions. *Radiographics.* 1994;14(3):597–606.

33. Inaoka T, Takahashi K, Miyokawa N, Ohsaki Y, Aburano T. Solitary fibrous tumor of the pleura: apparent diffusion coefficient (ADC) value and ADC map

to predict malignant transformation. *J Magn Reson Imaging.* 2007;26(1):155–58. Available from: www.ncbi.nlm.nih.gov/pubmed/17659560

34. Tateishi U, Gladish GW, Kusumoto M, Hasegawa T, Yokoyama R, Tsuchiya R, et al. Chest wall tumors: radiologic findings and pathologic correlation. *Radiographics.* 2003;23(6):1477–90. Available from: http://radiographics.rsna.org/content/23/6/1477.abstract\n http://radiographics.rsna.org/content/23/6/1477.full\n http://radiographics.rsna.org/content/23/6/1477.full.pdf

35. Jeung MY, Gangi A, Gasser B, Vasilescu C, Massard G, Wihlm JM, et al. Imaging of chest wall disorders. *Radiographics.* 1999;19(3):617–37.

36. Lee TJ, Collins J. MR imaging evaluation of disorders of the chest wall. *Magn Reson Imag Clin N Am.* 2008;16(2):355–79.

37. Yang H, Testa JR, Carbone M. Mesothelioma epidemiology, carcinogenesis, and pathogenesis. *Curr Treat Options Oncol.* 2008;9(2–3):147–57.

38. Weill H, Hughes JM, Churg A. Changing trends in US mesothelioma incidence. *Occup Environ Med.* 2005;62:270.

39. Price B, Ware A. Mesothelioma trends in the United States: an update based on Surveillance, Epidemiology, and End Results Program data for 1973 through 2003. *Am J Epidemiol.* 2004;159(2):107–12. Available from: www.ncbi.nlm.nih.gov/pubmed/14718210\n http://aje.oxfordjournals.org/content/159/2/107.full.pdf#page=1&view=FitH

40. Price B, Ware A. Time trend of mesothelioma incidence in the United States and projection of future cases: an update based on SEER data for 1973 through 2005. *Crit Rev Toxicol.* 2009;39(7):576–88.

41. Peto J, Decarli A, La Vecchia C, Levi F, Negri E. The European mesothelioma epidemic. *Br J Cancer.* 1999;79(3–4):666–72.

42. Tarrés J, Albertí C, Martínez-Artés X, Abós-Herràndiz R, Rosell-Murphy M, García-Allas I, et al. Pleural mesothelioma in relation to meteorological conditions and residential distance from an industrial source of asbestos. *Occup Environ Med.*

2013;70(8):588–90. Available from: www.ncbi.nlm.nih.gov/pubmed/23695414

43. Awad AHA. Environmental study in subway metro stations in Cairo, Egypt. *J Occup Health.* 2002;44:112–18.

44. Gill RR. Imaging of mesothelioma. *Recent Results Cancer Res.* 2011;189:27–43.

45. Bueno R, Reblando J, Glickman J, Jaklitsch MT, Lukanich JM, Sugarbaker DJ. Pleural biopsy: a reliable method for determining the diagnosis but not subtype in mesothelioma. *Ann Thorac Surg.* 2004;78:1774–76.

46. Yildirim H, Metintas M, Entok E, Ak G, Ak I, Dundar E, et al. Clinical value of fluorodeoxyglucose-positron emission tomography/computed tomography in differentiation of malignant mesothelioma from asbestos-related benign pleural disease: an observational pilot study. *J Thorac Oncol.* 2009;4(12):1480–84.

47. Wang ZJ, Reddy GP, Gotway MB, Higgins CB, Jablons DM, Ramaswamy M, et al. Malignant pleural mesothelioma: evaluation with CT, MR imaging, and PET. *Radiographics.* 2004;24:105–19. Available from: www.ncbi.nlm.nih.gov/pubmed/14730040

48. Kawashima A, Libshitz HI. Malignant pleural mesothelioma: CT manifestations in 50 cases. *AJR Am J Roentgenol.* 1990;155:965–69.

49. Erasmus JJ, Truong MT, Smythe WR, Munden RF, Marom EM, Rice DC, et al. Integrated computed tomography-positron emission tomography in patients with potentially resectable malignant pleural mesothelioma: staging implications. *J Thorac Cardiovasc Surg.* 2005;129(6):1364–70. Available from: www.ncbi.nlm.nih.gov/pubmed/15942579

50. Gill RR, Gerbaudo VH, Sugarbaker DJ, Hatabu H. Current trends in radiologic management of malignant pleural mesothelioma. *Semin Thorac Cardiovasc Surg.* 2009;21:111–20.

51. Abdel Rahman ARM, Gaafar RM, Baki HA, El Hosieny HM, Aboulkasem F, Farahat EG, et al. Prevalence and pattern of lymph node metastasis in malignant pleural mesothelioma. *Ann Thorac Surg.* 2008;86(2):391–95. Available from: www.ncbi.nlm.nih.gov/pubmed/18640302

52. Antman KH, Corson JM. Benign and malignant pleural mesothelioma. *Clin Chest Med.* 1985;6:127–40.

53. Sugarbaker DJ, Mentzer SJ, DeCamp M, Lynch TJ, Strauss GM. Extrapleural pneumonectomy in the setting of a multimodality approach to malignant mesothelioma. *Chest.* 1993;103(4 Suppl):377S–81S. Available from: www.ncbi.nlm.nih.gov/pubmed/8462329

54. Pilling JE, Stewart DJ, Martin-Ucar AE, Muller S, Byrne KJO, Waller DA. The case for routine cervical mediastinoscopy prior to radical surgery for malignant pleural mesothelioma. *Eur J Cardiothor Surg.* 2004;25:497–501.

55. Patz EF, Rusch VW, Heelan R. The proposed new international TNM staging system for malignant pleural mesothelioma: application to imaging. *AJR Am J Roentgenol.* 1996;166:323–27.

56. Gill RR, Richards WG, Yeap BY, Matsuoka S, Wolf AS, Gerbaudo VH, et al. Epithelial malignant pleural mesothelioma after extrapleural pneumonectomy: stratification of survival with CT-derived tumor volume. *AJR Am J Roentgenol.* 2012;198(2):359–63. Available from: www.ncbi.nlm.nih.gov/pubmed/22268178

57. Flores RM, Pass HI, Seshan VE, Dycoco J, Zakowski M, Carbone M, et al. Extrapleural pneumonectomy versus pleurectomy/decortication in the surgical management of malignant pleural mesothelioma: results in 663 patients. *J Thorac Cardiovasc Surg.* 2008;135(3):620–6, 626.e1–3. Available from: www.ncbi.nlm.nih.gov/pubmed/18329481

58. Rusch VW, Giroux D, Kennedy C, Ruffini E, Cangir AK, Rice D, et al. Initial analysis of the international association for the study of lung cancer mesothelioma database. *J Thorac Oncol.* 2012;7(11):1631–39. Available from: www.ncbi.nlm.nih.gov/pubmed/23070243

59. Aziz T, Jilaihawi A, Prakash D. The management of malignant pleural mesothelioma; single centre experience in 10 years. *Eur J Cardiothorac Surg.* 2002;22:298–305. Available from: www.ncbi.nlm.nih.gov/pubmed/12142203

60. Richards WG, Godleski JJ, Yeap BY, Corson JM. Proposed adjustments to pathologic staging of epithelial malignant pleural mesothelioma based on analysis of 354 cases. *Cancer.* 2010;1510–17.

61. Van Meerbeeck JP, Scherpereel A, Surmont VF, Baas P. Malignant pleural mesothelioma: the standard of care and challenges for future management. *Crit Rev Oncol.* 2011;78(2):92–111. Available from: http://sfxhosted .exlibrisgroup.com/hinc?sid=OVID: medline&id=pmid: 20466560&id=doi:10.1016/j.critrevonc .2010.04.004&issn = 1040–8428&isbn = &volume = 78&issue = 2&spage = 92&pages = 92–111&date = 2011&title = Critical+Reviews+in+Oncology-Hematology&atitle = Malignant+pleur

62. Flores RM, Akhurst T, Gonen M, Zakowski M, Dycoco J, Larson SM, et al. Positron emission tomography predicts survival in malignant pleural mesothelioma. *J Thorac Cardiovasc Surg.* 2006;132(4):763–68.

63. Nakas A, Black E, Entwisle J, Muller S, Waller DA. Surgical assessment of malignant pleural mesothelioma: have we reached a critical stage? *Eur J Cardio-Thoracic Surg.* 2010;37(6):1457–63. Available from: http://dx.doi.org/10.1016/j.ejcts.2009 .12.039

64. Rusch VW, Giroux D. Do we need a revised staging system for malignant pleural mesothelioma? Analysis of the IASLC database. *Ann Cardiothorac Surg.* 2012;1(4):438–48. Available from: www.pubmedcentral.nih.gov/ articlerender.fcgi?artid=3741785& tool=pmcentrez&rendertype=abstract

65. Sugarbaker DJ, Strauss GM, Lynch TJ, Richards W, Mentzer SJ, Lee TH, et al. Node status has prognostic significance in the multimodality therapy of diffuse, malignant mesothelioma. *J Clin Oncol.* 1172;11(6):1172–78. Available from: http://ovidsp.ovid.com/ovidweb.cgi? T=JS&CSC=Y&NEWS=N&PAGE= fulltext&D=med3&AN=8501504

66. Rusch V, Baldini EH, Bueno R, De Perrot M, Flores R, Hasegawa S, et al. The role of surgical cytoreduction in the treatment of malignant pleural mesothelioma: meeting summary of the International Mesothelioma Interest Group Congress, September 11–14, 2012, Boston, Mass. *J Thorac Cardiovasc Surg.* 2013;145(4):909–10. Available from: www.ncbi.nlm.nih.gov/ pubmed/23415687

67. Schouwink JH, Kool LS, Rutgers EJ, Zoetmulder FAN, van Zandwijk N, v d Vijver MJ, et al. The value of chest computer tomography and cervical mediastinoscopy in the preoperative assessment of patients with malignant pleural mesothelioma. *Ann Thorac Surg.* 2003;75(6):1715–18; discussion 1718–19. Available from: www.ncbi .nlm.nih.gov/pubmed/12822605

68. Abdel Razek AAK, Soliman NY, Elkhamary S, Alsharaway MK, Tawfik A. Role of diffusion-weighted MR imaging in cervical lymphadenopathy. *Eur Radiol.* 2006;16(7):1468–77.

69. Kent M, Rice D, Flores R. Diagnosis, staging, and surgical treatment of malignant pleural mesothelioma. *Curr Treat Options Oncol.* 2008;9(2–3):158–70. Available from: www.ncbi.nlm.nih.gov/entrez/query .fcgi?cmd=Retrieve&db=PubMed& dopt=Citation&list_uids=18758965

70. Jänne PA, Baldini EH. Patterns of failure following surgical resection for malignant pleural mesothelioma. *Thorac Surg Clin.* 2004;14:567–73.

71. Baldini EH, Recht A, Strauss GM, DeCamp MM, Swanson SJ, Liptay MJ, et al. Patterns of failure after trimodality therapy for malignant pleural mesothelioma. *Ann Thorac Surg.* 1997;63(2):334–38. Available from: www.ncbi.nlm.nih.gov/pubmed/ 9033296

72. Byrne MJ. Modified RECIST criteria for assessment of response in malignant pleural mesothelioma. *Ann Oncol.* 2004;15(2):257–60. Available from: http://annonc.oupjournals.org/cgi/doi/ 10.1093/annonc/mdh059

73. Armato SG. Computerized analysis of mesothelioma on CT scans. *Lung Cancer.* 2005;49(Suppl 1):S41–44.

74. Armato SG, Ogarek JL, Starkey A, Vogelzang NJ, Kindler HL, Kocherginsky M, et al. Variability in mesothelioma tumor response classification. *AJR Am J Roentgenol.* 2006;186(4):1000–06.

75. Kaira K, Serizawa M, Koh Y, Takahashi T, Hanaoka H, Oriuchi N, et al. Relationship between 18F-FDG uptake on positron emission tomography and molecular biology in malignant pleural mesothelioma. *Eur J Cancer.* 2012;48:1244–54.

76. Nowak AK, Francis RJ, Phillips MJ, Millward MJ, Van Der Schaaf AA,

Boucek J, et al. A novel prognostic model for malignant mesothelioma incorporating quantitative FDG-PET imaging with clinical parameters. *Clin Cancer Res.* 2010;16(8):2409–17.

77. Pickhardt PJ, Bhalla S. Primary neoplasms of peritoneal and sub-peritoneal origin: CT findings. *Radiographics.* 2005;25(4):983–95.

78. Kebapci M, Yalcin OT, Dundar E, Ozalp SS, Kaya T. Computed tomography findings of primary serous papillary carcinoma of the peritoneum in women. *Eur J Gynaecol Oncol.* 2003;24(6):552–56. Available from: http://ovidsp.ovid.com/ovidweb.cgi? T=JS&CSC=Y&NEWS=N&PAGE= fulltext&D=emed6&AN=2003484592\n http://oxfordsfx.hosted.exlibrisgroup .com/oxford?sid=OVID:embase& id=pmid:&id=doi:&issn=0392–2936& isbn=&volume=24&issue=6&spage= 552&pages=552–556& date=2003&title=Euro

79. Bonomo L, Feragalli B, Sacco R, Merlino B, Storto ML. Malignant pleural disease. *Eur J Radiol.* 2000;34:98–118.

80. Low RN, Sigeti JS. MR imaging of peritoneal disease: comparison of contrast-enhanced fast multiplanar spoiled gradient-recalled and spin-echo imaging. *AJR Am J Roentgenol.* 1994;163(5):1131–40. Available from: www.ncbi.nlm.nih.gov/pubmed/ 7976889

81. Heelan RT, Demas BE, Caravelli JF, Martini N, Bains MS, McCormack PM, et al. Superior sulcus tumors: CT and MR imaging. *Radiology.* 1989;170:637–41.

82. Coolen J, De Keyzer F, Nafteux P, De Wever W, Dooms C, Vansteenkiste J, et al. Malignant pleural disease: diagnosis by using diffusion-weighted and dynamic contrast-enhanced MR imaging – initial experience. *Radiology.* 2012;263(3):884–92.

83. Healy JC. Detection of peritoneal metastases. *Cancer Imaging.* 2001;1(2):4–12. Available from: www .ncbi.nlm.nih.gov/pubmed/18203670

84. Patel CM, Sahdev A, Reznek RH. CT, MRI and PET imaging in peritoneal malignancy. *Cancer Imaging.* 2011;11(1):123–39.

85. Oei TN, Jagannathan JP, Ramaiya N, Ros PR. Peritoneal sarcomatosis versus peritoneal carcinomatosis: imaging findings at MDCT. *AJR Am J Roentgenol.* 2010;195(3):229–35.

86. Cabral FC, Krajewski KM, Kim KW, Ramaiya NH, Jagannathan JP. Peritoneal lymphomatosis: CT and PET/CT findings and how to differentiate between carcinomatosis and sarcomatosis. *Cancer Imaging.* 2013;13:162–70. Available from: www .ncbi.nlm.nih.gov/pubmed/23598428

87. Diop D, Fontarensky M, Montoriol P, Da Ines D. CT imaging of peritoneal carcinomatosis and its mimics. *Diagn Interv Imaging.* 2014;95(9):861–72. Available from: www.ncbi.nlm.nih.gov/ pubmed/24631039

88. Kwee TC, Takahara T, Ochiai R, Nievelstein R a J, Luijten PR. Diffusion-weighted whole-body imaging with background body signal suppression (DWIBS): features and potential applications in oncology. *Eur Radiol.* 2008;18(9):1937–52.

89. Sala E, Priest AN, Kataoka M, Graves MJ, McLean MA, Joubert I, et al. Apparent diffusion coefficient and vascular signal fraction measurements with magnetic resonance imaging: feasibility in metastatic ovarian cancer at 3 Tesla: technical development. *Eur Radiol.* 2010;20(2):491–96. Available from: www.ncbi.nlm.nih.gov/pubmed/ 19657643

90. Bammer R, Holdsworth SJ, Veldhuis WB, Skare ST. New methods in diffusion-weighted and diffusion tensor imaging. *Magn Reson Imaging Clin N Am.* 2009;17(2):175–204. Available from: http://dx.doi.org/10.1016/j.mric .2009.01.011

91. Armato SG, Labby ZE, Coolen J, Klabatsa A, Feigen M, Persigehl T, et al. Imaging in pleural mesothelioma: a review of the 11th International Conference of the International Mesothelioma Interest Group. *Lung Cancer.* 2013;82(2):190–96.

92. Gill RR, Umeoka S, Mamata H, Tilleman TR, Stanwell P, Woodhams R, et al. Diffusion-weighted MRI of malignant pleural mesothelioma: preliminary assessment of apparent diffusion coefficient in histologic subtypes. *AJR Am J Roentgenol.* 2010;195(2):W125–30. Available from: www.ncbi.nlm.nih.gov/pubmed/ 20651171

93. Giesel FL, Choyke PL, Mehndiratta A, Zechmann CM, von Tengg-Kobligk H, Kayser K, et al. Pharmacokinetic analysis of malignant pleural mesothelioma – initial results of tumor microcirculation and its correlation to microvessel density (CD-34). *Acad Radiol.* 2008;15(5):563–70. Available from: www.ncbi.nlm.nih.gov/pubmed/ 18423312

94. Jeswani T, Padhani AR. Imaging tumour angiogenesis. *Cancer Imaging.* 2005;5:131–38. Available from: www .pubmedcentral.nih.gov/articlerender .fcgi?artid=1665235&tool=pmcentrez& rendertype=abstract

95. Goel HL, Mercurio AM. VEGF targets the tumour cell. *Nat Rev Cancer.* 2013;13(12):871–82. Available from: www.pubmedcentral.nih.gov/ articlerender.fcgi?artid=4011842& tool=pmcentrez&rendertype=abstract

96. Giesel FL, Bischoff H, Von Tengg-Kobligk H, Weber MA, Zechmann CM, Kauczor HU, et al. Dynamic contrast-enhanced MRI of malignant pleural mesothelioma: a feasibility study of noninvasive assessment, therapeutic follow-up, and possible predictor of improved outcome. *Chest.* 2006;129(6): 1570–76.

97. Priest A, Sala E, Graves M, Joubert I, McLean M, Griffin N, et al. ADC and perfusion signal fraction measurements: feasibility in ovarian cancer at 3 Tesla. *Proceedings 16th Scientific Meeting, International Society for Magnetic Resonance in Medicine.* 2008. p. 3846. Available from: /MyPathway2008/3846

98. Sala E, Kataoka MY, Priest AN, Gill AB, McLean MA, Joubert I, et al. Advanced ovarian cancer: multiparametric MR imaging demonstrates response- and metastasis-specific effects. *Radiology.* 2012;263(1):149–59.

99. Lemke A-J, Brinkmann MJ, Schott T, Niehues SM, Settmacher U, Neuhaus P, et al. Living donor right liver lobes: preoperative CT volumetric measurement for calculation of intraoperative weight and volume. *Radiology.* 2006;240(3):736–42.

100. Dello SAWG, Stoot JHMB, van Stiphout RSA, Bloemen JG, Wigmore SJ, Dejong CHC, et al. Prospective volumetric assessment of the liver on a personal computer by nonradiologists prior to partial hepatectomy. *World J Surg.* 2011;35(2):386–92. Available

from: www.pubmedcentral.nih.gov/
articlerender.fcgi?artid=3017311&
tool=pmcentrez&rendertype=abstract

101. Frauenfelder T, Tutic M, Weder W,
Götti RP, Stahel RA, Seifert B, et al.
Volumetry: an alternative to assess
therapy response for malignant pleural
mesothelioma? *Eur Respir J.*
2011;38(1):162–68.

102. Yoshida Y, Kurokawa T, Sawamura Y,
Shinagawa A, Okazawa H, Fujibayashi
Y, et al. The positron emission
tomography with F18 17beta-estradiol
has the potential to benefit diagnosis
and treatment of endometrial cancer.
Gynecol Oncol. 2007;104(3):764–66.
Available from: www.ncbi.nlm.nih.gov/
pubmed/17156828

Processing of Pleural and Peritoneal Pathologic Specimens for the Diagnosis of Malignant Mesothelioma

Françoise Galateau-Sallé

The pleura is the most frequent location (90 percent) of malignant mesothelioma, a rare cancer of the serous membranes, followed by the peritoneum (10 percent), the pericardium, and the testis vaginalis (< 1 percent) (French National Mesothelioma Surveillance Program) (1–13). The diagnosis of this unusual neoplasm is based purely on histopathologic evaluation and can be difficult, as malignant mesothelioma can exhibit protean morphologic features that can mimic benign processes, carcinomas of the lung and other origin and other neoplasms.

Various diagnostic and reporting evidence-based criteria have been proposed by various international groups of experts and adherence to them is very important for a correct diagnosis of malignant mesothelioma (1–4). In addition to diagnosis, histological subtyping of these tumors is considered as a very important prognostic and predictive factor and is a major feature considered during the management of patients with the disease.

Evaluation of adequate pathologic specimens and optimal handling of these specimens is essential to provide accurate diagnoses of malignant mesothelioma. Novel technologies such as next-generation sequencing, fluorescent *in-situ* hybridization (FISH) and others offer promise as aids in the diagnosis and the selection of targeted therapies, but it is very important to integrate the results obtained with these techniques with the time-tested information provided by the pathologic features.

Routine practice has changed during the past decade and there is a trend to use cytology specimens and/or small biopsy procedures for the initial diagnosis of pleural and peritoneal mesotheliomas. The diagnosis of mesothelioma in these small tumor samples requires the routine use of ancillary techniques such as immunohistochemistry and molecular analysis to be able to provide accurate diagnoses and prognostic and predictive information that can help thoracic surgeons, oncologists and radiation oncologists manage mesothelioma patients in an individualized manner. Diagnostic and other recommendations have been recently upgraded in the 2015 WHO classification for pleural tumors (1,2) and in the guidelines and recent recommendations by the International Mesothelioma Panel (3), the College of American Pathologists (4), the Royal College of Pathologists from Australasia and the United Kingdom (5,6), the US and Canadian Academy of pathologists, the European Respiratory Society (7), and the ICCG (International Collaborative Cancer Group) for the diagnosis of mesothelioma of

the pleura, peritoneum, and other rare locations (8–10). Diagnostic challenges and controversies have also been extensively reported by the Australian group in 2013 (11,12). The majority of the guidelines and recommendations for diagnosis and processing serosal tumors have been published for pleural lesions, but very few are established for the other locations (1–13).

This chapter is devoted to give an overview of the recommendations for pathological diagnosis of malignant mesothelioma, and to provide guidance for processing pleural and peritoneal biopsies.

The Use of Cytological Samples and Cellblocks for the Diagnosis of Pleural and Peritoneal Malignant Mesothelioma

Pleural Effusion Cytology

Pleural effusion is often present as an early clinical manifestation in patients with malignant mesothelioma and metastatic diseases to the pleura as well as in many benign processes. It is important to correlate the findings on cytological samples with those in concurrent small biopsies samples because these specimens are frequently sent to the pathology laboratory as combined specimens and the findings in one sample can help interpret those in the other specimens for an accurate diagnosis of mesothelioma. Cytology diagnosis is extensively reported in more detail in Chapter 5.

Pleural fluid examination is rapid and cost-effective and offers the initial simple procedure used for diagnosis (14–16). However, it has been controversial whether an initial diagnosis of malignant mesothelioma can be rendered on pleural fluid cytological specimens. Multiple studies have questioned the value of this method as the sensitivity and specificity of pleural fluid evaluation was quite low in comparison with the results obtained from tissue biopsy samples (please see Chapter 5). Several reasons can explain this discrepancy:

- Malignant mesothelial cells are present in pleural fluid in 80 percent of the cases of epithelioid-type mesothelioma, but sarcomatoid mesotheliomas rarely shed tumor cells into the fluid, resulting in false negative results.
- Malignant mesothelial cells may present with an extremely bland morphology, while reactive mesothelial cells may

exhibit atypical cytological features. Therefore, the diagnosis between malignant mesothelioma and benign atypical reactive processes can be extremely challenging based on cytomorphology alone, presenting a major risk for diagnostic error. Adipose tissue invasion, an important diagnostic feature for malignant mesothelioma in biopsy specimens, cannot be evaluated on cytological samples (17).

- Finally, pleural effusion is extremely frequent in patients older than 50 years old with many benign and metastatic lesions that are far more frequent than malignant mesothelioma. Approximately 42–77 percent of exudative pleuritis (18) are of neoplastic origin and 50 percent of patients with a metastatic disease develop pleural effusions (19). For example, Chailleux et al. (20) showed that pleural effusions showing carcinoma cells are observed in 40.7 percent of the cases with pleural effusions. In 69.5 percent of these cases the histology is adenocarcinoma, frequently mimicking a mesothelioma. Breast and lung represents one-fourth of neoplastic pleural effusion, followed by ovaries in 17 percent, and stomach in less than 10 percent (3). A series of 766 patients selected from 1998 to 2004 from MESOPATH National Reference Center showed a clear predominance of bronchopulmonary carcinoma in 63 percent, breast metastasis in 15 percent, followed by renal or urothelial origin in 7 percent of the cases (not published). Surprisingly, out of the 15 percent of mammary carcinoma origin, 25 percent were observed in males. These statistical results are probably due to selection bias in our center, but are important to take into consideration because breast metastases are great mimickers of malignant mesothelioma in neoplastic pleural effusion and this is not a first-choice diagnostic consideration in male patients. Mesothelioma is considerably less frequent in our experience, depending on the geographical zone of asbestos exposure or the location of the referral center. About 5–10 percent of metastatic pleural effusion remains of unknown origin.

This preamble underscores the need to use ancillary techniques such as immunohistochemistry for the diagnosis of mesothelioma on pleural effusion specimens. Immunohistochemistry includes the use of a panel of two positive markers (e.g., calretinin, WT-1 or CK5/6, and/or EMA clone E29) and two negative markers (e.g., TTF-1, Ber-EP4 or ER α, CDX2, PAX-8, RCC, others) as recommended by the 2015 WHO book to avoid misdiagnosis of a metastasis (1). Fluorescent *in-situ* hybridization (FISH) analysis for the presence of p16 homozygous deletion is also very helpful to distinguish benign from malignant mesothelial cells, particularly in sarcomatous lesions.

Ascites Effusion Cytology

It has been reported that in 52–54 percent of cases of peritoneal carcinomatosis, ascites effusion is the initial symptom of abdominal malignancy, but there are only rare reports on the accuracy of cytology for the diagnosis of malignant ascites (1). The diagnostic sensitivity in these specimens is 50–60 percent, but it has also been reported that up to 97 percent of patients with peritoneal carcinomatosis have positive cytology, making it a highly sensitive test for the diagnosis of a peritoneal carcinomatosis (21,22). Metastatic cancer from ovarian, pancreatic, and gastric cancers are present more frequently in these specimens. The sensitivity of effusion cytology for the diagnosis of peritoneal mesothelioma is very low due to the rarity of the disease.

Older studies have reported that ascites effusion specimens yield lower than 30 percent accuracies for the diagnosis of malignant mesothelioma, but modern laboratory techniques such as immunohistochemistry and FISH have recently improved the diagnostic yield, as described in Chapter 5.

Diagnosis of Malignant Mesothelioma on Small Biopsy Samples: International Diagnostic Guidelines and Recommendations

Pleural biopsy has been proposed as the diagnostic Gold Standard for the correct management of patients harboring this dramatic disease. Several guidelines have been recently published and updated to guide pathologists when they have to deal with a diagnosis of malignant mesothelioma (1–8). For example, multiple evidence-based recommendations have been recently updated in the 2016 International Collaboration on Cancer Reporting (ICCR) data set for malignant mesothelioma of the pleura and peritoneum (8). Other recommendations and guidelines for the international community of pathologists have also been published; by the College of American Pathologists (CAP) as well as by the International Mesothelioma Interest Group (IMIG) and are summarized in the WHO 2015 book on classification of pleural tumors (1). Other guidelines have been published in different countries, such as those reported by the Royal College of Pathologists (RCPath) in the United Kingdom, the Australian group (10), the National French Institute of Cancer (INCA data set), the TASK Force from the European Respiratory Society (7), the ESMO guidelines for clinical practice (8), the American committee on Cancer (AJCC), and the International Association for the Study of Lung Cancer (IASLC) guidelines for surgical resection and for the assessment of pTNM staging (Tables 4.1 and 4.2).

The ICCR recommendations have supported the opinion that "the type of the biopsy selected may affect the accuracy of the final diagnosis" (Figure 4.1a) and emphasize the concept that "the approach of diagnosis using biopsy is dependent on the clinical presentation, the age of the patient and his comorbidities." It is also dependent of imaging characteristics, of the expertise of the multidisciplinary team including the clinician, the surgeon, the radiologist, and the pathologist.

Table 4.1 Mesothelioma staging: T component (AJCC/UICC/IASLC)

Staging T Descriptors

TX Primary tumor cannot be assessed

T0 No evidence of primary tumor

T1 Tumor limited to the ipsilateral parietal pleura with or without involvement of
– visceral pleura
– mediastinal pleura
– diaphragmatic pleura

T2 Tumor involving each of the ipsilateral pleural surfaces with at least one of the following features:
– involvement of diaphragmatic muscle
– extension of tumor from visceral pleura into the underlying pulmonary parenchyma

T3 Describes locally advanced but potentially resectable tumor involving all the ipsilateral pleural surfaces with at least one of the following features:
– involvement of the endothoracic fascia
– extension into the mediastinal fat
– solitary, completely resectable focus of tumor extending into the soft tissues of the chest wall
– nontransmural involvement of the pericardium

T4 Describes locally advanced technically unresectable tumor extending beyond T3

Nowak, A, et al., The IASLC Mesothelioma Staging Project: Proposals for Revisions of the T Descriptors in the Forthcoming Eighth Edition of the TNM Classification for Pleural Mesothelioma. *Journal of Thoracic Oncology.* 11(12):2089–99, December 2016.

Specimen Characteristics and Technical Details for the Processing of Biopsies in Patients with Suspected Malignant Mesothelioma

Biopsy Techniques for the Diagnosis of Malignant Mesothelioma

Small Biopsy Samples

Maskell et al. (14) noted in a large 2013 review the lack of randomized trials evaluating which type of pleural biopsy offers

Table 4.2 Proposal for staging regional lymph IASLC

Nodes (N) Definition

NX	Regional lymph nodes cannot be assessed
N0	No regional lymph node metastases
N1	Metastases in the ipsilateral bronchopulmonary, hilar, or mediastinal (including the internal mammary, peridiaphragmatic, pericardial fat pad, or intercostal lymph nodes) lymph nodes
N2	Metastases in the contralateral bronchopulmonary, hilar, or mediastinal lymph nodes or ipsilateral or contralateral supraclavicular lymph nodes

AJCC/UICC, American Joint Committee on Cancer/Union for International Cancer Control.
Rice, D., et al., The IASLC Mesothelioma Staging Project: Proposals for Revisions of the N Descriptors in the Forthcoming Eighth Edition of the TNM Classification for Pleural Mesothelioma. *Journal of Thoracic Oncology.* 11(12):2100–11, December 2016.

the optimal diagnostic method for malignant mesothelioma, and on the fact that there have been no significant technical improvements in needle biopsy techniques in over 40 years. The standard technique uses closed pleural biopsy samples include Abram's (guillotine), Cope (hook) and Van Silverman (puncture) needles without image guidance as an initial source of diagnostic test.

Blind "Closed Needle" Pleural Biopsy

Abrams or Cope needles were routinely used before 2000 (Figure 4.1a), because this procedure was considered less-invasive and less-expensive than open pleural biopsy (23–26). Specimens are usually smaller than 0.2 cm and commonly include muscle, exudate, fibrous tissue, or very minimal area of adipose tissue. These biopsy materials are frequently suboptimal for a diagnosis of mesothelioma and do not allow extensive immunohistochemical or molecular analysis. Indeed, since 2005, it is well known that blind percutaneous biopsies are not recommended in patients with suspected mesothelioma or other malignancies because of the lower than 50 percent sensitivity of the procedure for a diagnosis of malignancy. Moreover, a negative biopsy result does not exclude a diagnosis of granulomatous disease and other conditions (27). For example, fewer than 30 percent of malignant mesotheliomas can be diagnosed with this method (28,29).

Blind closed biopsies are more likely to be useful for the diagnosis of tuberculosis (30). The diagnostic yield for this diagnosis has been reported by Kirsch et al. to be less than 60 percent, but can reach 87 percent when histology is associated with microbiological culture, and nearly 100 percent when more than six biopsies are evaluated by a pathologist (31). Finally, when adding closed pleural biopsy to ADA and lymphocyte count, diagnostic accuracy approaches that of thoracoscopy (32). Figure 4.1b shows a comparison of different specimens obtained by various procedures.

Percutaneous Approaches (CT and Ultrasound-guided Pleural Biopsy)

The use of percutaneous transthoracic biopsy has currently increased and this technique is usually performed by radiologists under computerized tomography (CT) or ultrasound (US) guidance. A core of tissue of 1 mm wide and 1 cm long can be obtained and processed like any other biopsy samples received in a surgical pathology laboratory. These preferred diagnostic modalities are considered to have a greater diagnostic sensitivity compared with blind closed pleural biopsy. Maskell et al. (33) conducted a trial including 50 patients and showed that the sensitivity for malignant pleural effusion was significantly higher for CT-guided transthoracic needle biopsies than with blind Abram's biopsies (CT-guided 87 percent versus 47 percent for Abram's biopsy). The specificity, predictive positive value, and predictive negative value in this series were, respectively, 100 percent, 100 percent, and 80 percent for CT-guided biopsies with the corresponding values for Abram's needle biopsies of 100 percent, 100 percent, and 44 percent, respectively. It was noticed that both procedures were specific

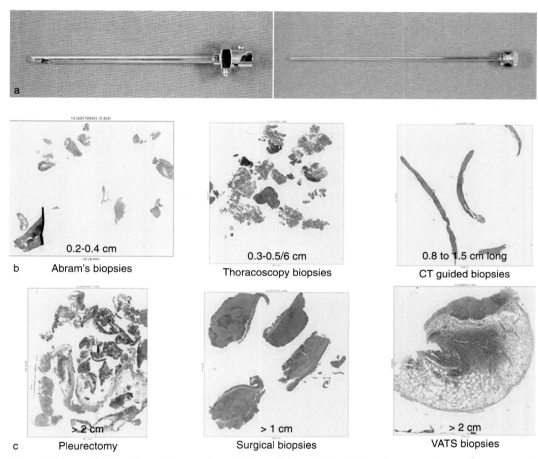

Figure 4.1 Examples of needle used for transthoracic biopsy of pleural lesions. (a) Transthoracic needle core biopsies provide small specimens of variable size according to the needle used. (b) The figure shows examples of specimens obtained with different needles and compares them with (c) specimens obtained with open biopsies, pleurectomy specimens, and video thoracoscopic surgery biopsies.

when a lesion could be adequately sampled. Interestingly, the CT-guided cutting-needle biopsy was also efficient in patients presenting pleural thickening with fluid present and also in patients with pleural thickening of less than 5 mm of maximum thickness (33–35). Moreover, the cumulative yield of ultrasonography and ultrasound needle biopsy guidance (US-guided thoracocenthesis) can reach a sensitivity of 97 percent comparable to thoracoscopy in suitable patients (36). It may considerably improve the diagnosis of pleural aspiration alone, particularly in patients showing pleural nodularity, pleural thickening, or pleural-based mass tumors. Finally, thoracoscopy is still considered the Gold Standard for investigating malignant pleural diseases. However, this technique is not available everywhere and is not suitable for patients with contraindications for pleuroscopy. Abram's biopsies are indicated for the diagnosis of tuberculous pleuritis, particularly in resource-poor clinical settings (Figure 4.1a) (37).

The core specimen generated by these techniques vary according to the size of the needle used (18, 19, 20G) and are usually larger than 1 cm long and 0.1 cm thickness. The fine-needle (22-gauge) biopsies yield sufficient materials to pre-pare cell suspensions for cytology while the use of an 18-gauge biopsy yields a thin core tissue biopsy more suitable for histology. It is possible to perform 1–3 biopsy specimens and to cryopreserve one fresh sample for further molecular analysis and/or for microbiological evaluation and cultures. In cases of a clinical suspicion of lymphoma, specialized assay could be performed and a fresh sample could be preserved in cell culture solution for CMF that allows a diagnosis of lymphocytic clone favoring a diagnosis of lymphoma that remains to be certified on FFPE block with the additional correct immunostaining for a more specific diagnosis. From our experience the combined presence of a malignant mesothelioma and a malignant lymphoma is not exceptional and the latter may be difficult to differentiate from a florid reactive lymphocytic infiltrate.

To avoid drying artifacts, the material obtained from aspiration contained in the needle can be immediately rinsed in 4 percent buffered formalin fixative solution and processed in the laboratory as a small biopsy specimen. It is also recommended to immediately agitate the sample placed in the solution to avoid crush artifacts. It allows the collection of sufficient material for processing immunohistochemistry and molecular analysis.

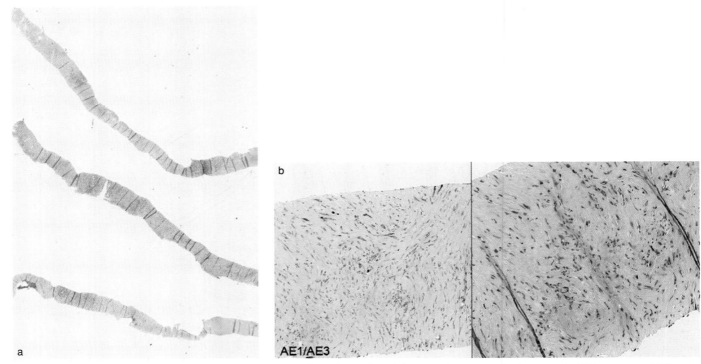

Figure 4.2 (a) Percutaneous transthoracic needle core biopsy is usually performed by radiologists under computerized tomography (CT) or ultrasound (US) guidance and provides the type of specimens shown in the figure. (b) Transthoracic needle core biopsy often provides sufficient tissue samples to perform immunostains. The tumor shown on H&E stained preparation on the right panel exhibits keratin AE1/AE3 immunoreactivity, shown on the left panel.

In order to ensure a complete immunohistochemical analysis at least two positive and two negative markers for the diagnosis of mesothelioma are generally used and it is recommended to prepare extra unstained sections at the time of initial sectioning to save materials. These materials can be needed if additional ancillary techniques (e.g., FISH analysis, RNAseq, other molecular techniques) are necessary for diagnosis or for inclusion in trials (additional biomarkers; BAP1, mesothelin, other mutations) (1–3).

In 2008, Attanoos et al. (38) reported the experience in a single center rendering a 100 percent definitive diagnosis over more than seven years on first biopsy using CT-guided biopsies compared to a 9 percent diagnosis using blind biopsies. Additionally, the MESOPATH experience from a large cohort of 4998 cases retrieved from 1998 to 2014 showed that the number of cases excluded for inadequate material in suspected cases of mesothelioma was 14 percent with blinded biopsies compared to 11 percent with US-guided biopsies, 9 percent with CT-guided biopsies, and 2 percent with biopsy under thoracoscopy, $p < 0.001$ (unpublished data) (Figure 4.2a,b).

Finally, according to the ICCR recommendations the number of biopsy specimens should be counted and their size clearly noted in the report. At the microscopic level, on the H&E, the different histological layers of the pleura should be described and evaluated and if no adipose tissue is visualized on the parietal pleura, it should be reported to alert the clinician of the risk of inadequate material for a definitive diagnosis. In this situa-tion, serial sections in the absence of invasion in the initial sections should be recommended before the material is considered inadequate.

Thoracoscopy Biopsy

Thoracoscopy biopsy is the gold standard procedure for mesothelioma diagnosis. In the study performed by Boutin et al. (39,40), the overall diagnostic sensitivity was as high as 90 percent. The sensitivity for malignancy was 88 percent and the specificity 96 percent. Morbidity was considered low (< 1 percent) and related to the development of pleural empyema, pleuro-cutaneous fistulae, and transcutaneous tumor seeding. The increasing sensitivity of imaging in the diagnosis of malignant mesothelioma continue to give a pivotal dual role to medical thoracoscopy. First, thoracosopy allows the visualization of the entire pleural cavity when possible (Figure 4.3), and to select the exact sites of the biopsies, second to treat the patient with talc pleurodesis or local chemotherapy. When the biopsies are taken under direct vision they are larger in size and of better quality. In most centers with experienced operators the procedure is very well tolerated by patients. The greater the number of biopsy specimens the greater likelihood of achieving a correct diagnosis, allowing serial recuts for immuno-histochemistry and molecular analysis. However, even after performing all these diagnostic modalities the diagnosis may remain unclear. Some patients will require a surgical procedure because the tumor may elicit a marked local fibrous tissue

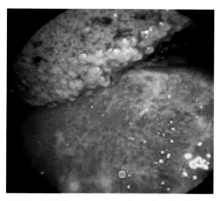

Figure 4.3 Thoracoscopy allows for visualization of the multiple tumor nodules shown in the figure.

response and the tumor may be missed on small biopsy samples. Thoracoscopy is probably mandatory for the diagnosis of desmoplastic mesothelioma and early mesothelial lesions.

Other disadvantages of small versus large biopsies have been reported by Greillier et al. (41), on a series of 95 patients that included 75 cases treated with extrapleural pneumonectomy (EPP), nine treated with pleuropneumonectomy and 11 others undergoing pleurectomies. Although thoracoscopy is considered as the Gold Standard for the diagnosis of pleural mesothelioma, this study reported that the procedure was inadequate for the diagnosis of the biphasic subtype of the tumor. This mesothelioma subtype is considered by these and other authors as a negative prognostic factor and a contraindication for surgery. In their analysis they found that 12 patients who were initially diagnosed with epithelioid malignant mesothelioma (13.8 percent) were diagnosed with the biphasic subtype after surgical workup. Their results were similar to those reported by Bueno et al. (42), who found a misclassification rate of 20 percent in their series of > 300 patients undergoing preoperative open pleural biopsies. The subtype analysis at pleural biopsy was proved correct in 80 percent (226/282). Most patients (174/192) with epithelioid type at final diagnosis were diagnosed correctly at pleural biopsy. However, 44 percent (45/103) with pathologic diagnosis of non-epithelioid type at resection were initially misdiagnosed with the epithelioid type. They reported a sensitivity of pleural biopsy for epithelioid MPM was 97 percent with a specificity of 56 percent.

Video-assisted Thoracoscopy Biopsy

Video-assisted thoracoscopic surgery (VATS) is indicated when a large biopsy sample is necessary and in cases with contraindications for thoracoscopic biopsies. New advances in the practice of VATS have changed the indication of pleural biopsy by conventional surgical procedure. The morbidity and the mortality of this procedure is low and allows for short hospitalizations compared to surgical standard thoracotomy. The major indications for VATS are when the clinical presentation or previous biopsy results suggest the need to distinguish an organizing pleuritis from sarcomatoid or desmoplastic mesothelioma or in

cases of superficial mesothelial proliferations when a diagnosis of mesothelioma vs. atypical mesothelial proliferation needs to be validated. The large amount of biopsy specimens obtained with this procedure, measuring at least 2–3 cm wide and 0.5–1 cm thick, provide a higher diagnostic confidence (Figure 4.4a) and in a greater percentage of cases permits the visualization of adipose tissue invasion, a very important diagnostic feature for desmoplastic and other variants of malignant mesothelioma (Figure 4.4b). Keratin immunostains of the tumor can facilitate the detection of adipose tissue invasion (Figure 4.4c). When visceral pleura are present it is possible to evaluate lung parenchyma invasion, diffuse lymphangitic involvement, or to reach ipsilateral nodes for staging. Moreover, Kao et al. (43) reported that the determination of histological type from a diagnostic biopsy is difficult due to sampling error, with a high risk of missing heterogeneity of the tumor. An adequate specimen obtained from surgical biopsy increases the accuracy of subtype classification, and heterogeneity evaluation compared with radiological-guided biopsies.

Before sample processing begins, it is important in resected specimens to find out from the clinician the type of procedure used and the details of gross observation made by the operator. Fresh tissue samples should be collected for microbiological analysis depending on the clinical suspicion of infection. One to six tumor samples combined with the same number of normal tissue samples are snap-frozen for cryopreservation for molecular analysis (WES, RNAseq, etc.). In cases with small biopsies the specimens should be sampled entirely to avoid missing a tiny focal lesion. The remainder of the biopsy tissue is immediately fixed in formalin. The volume of fixative should be correct for the biopsy volume specimen (ratio of 10:1 volume formalin: tumor specimen).

Surgical Biopsy – Decortication – Pleuropneumonectomy and Extrapleural Pneumonectomy

The specimens sent to the pathology laboratory are dependent on the procedure used as already mentioned, and could be a decortication of pleura, giving numerous long and fine sample biopsies of 3–6 cm long and less than 0.1 cm thick. In the case of open pleural space it is easier for the surgeon to select the nodule for pathological examination (44). If the space is obliterated, interface biopsies will be useful to find tumor infiltration into fat or muscle for assessment of florid reactive pleural fibrosis from desmoplastic or sarcomatoid mesothelioma. This can be a large piece of thickened pleura showing focally granulations or nodules. The gross appearance should be evaluated and precisely reported. Due to the heterogeneity of mesothelioma in the same patient, extensive sampling should be performed and include each different gross aspect. It is important for future molecular analysis to snap-freeze a sample combined with a mirror paraffin-embedded block, and when possible, pieces of normal tissue should also be snap-frozen, with the FFPE block mated with the tumor sample (WES analysis, etc.). When a hyaline fibrous plaque is present, it is recommended to sample at the edge of the hyaline fibrous plaque, because when the tumor

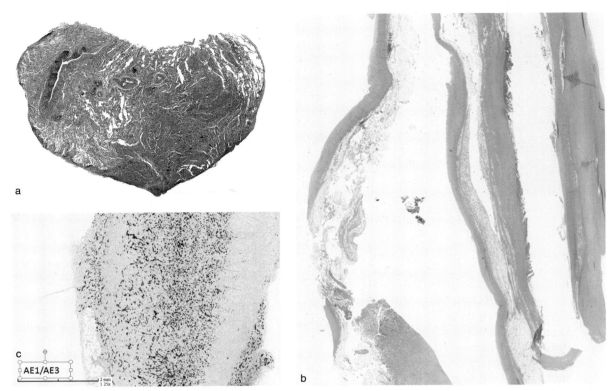

Figure 4.4 (a) Video-assisted thoracoscopy (VATS) allows for the collection of much larger biopsy samples than the previously described procedures, as shown in this photomicrograph. (b) VATS also allows for the performance of decortication and pleurectomies, yielding multiple samples of pleural tissue, as shown in the photomicrograph, that can be evaluated for the presence of mesothelioma and other lesions. (c) Immunostain for keratin AE1/AE3 highlights the presence of adipose tissue invasion by a mesothelioma.

is present it is always at the bottom edge of the hyaline fibrous plaque and not on the surface or inside the plaque. This might facilitate the detection of early mesothelioma lesion. The time of fixation should be adapted to the volume of the sample and it is more efficient to perform macroscopic analysis on a fresh sample. It is not recommended to assess the margin status of surgical biopsy specimens because by definition the surgical biopsy procedure is limited and the margin status is represented by the entire pleura (8) (Figure 4.5).

Pleuropneumonectomy and extra-pleural pneumonectomy: the gross characteristics of malignant mesothelioma are dependent on the stage of disease progression at the time of surgery

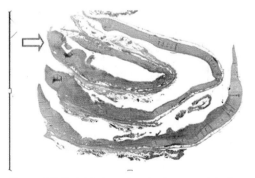

Figure 4.5 Parietal pleura showing tumor nodules (arrow).

(Figure 4.6). Typically, the tumor encases the lung as a rind and diffusely grows along the interlobar septa, finally compressing the lung. The anterior to posterior and apical to inferior dimensions and estimation of the size of the tumor should be evaluated. The gross dissection and sampling should respond to several points important for the management of the patient. First, sample for evaluation of the thickness of the tumor for correlation with advanced radiological techniques; second, the extent and depth of the tumor for p TNM staging according to the 8th edition of the AJCC/UICC/IASLC staging (see Tables 4.1 and 4.2); finally, it is recommended to extensively sample the parietal, visceral, and diaphragmatic pleura due to the heterogeneity of the tumor and frequent heterogeneous expression of biomarkers for the adequate management of the patient. Moreover, it is advised for optimal gross examination to section from a fixed lung which is easier to slice thinly with a sharp knife (45). The gross examination of the cut surface is usually white gray and firm. The gross description may be difficult to appreciate in the case of the dense diffuse fibrotic process of a desmoplastic mesothelioma. In extra-pleural pneumonectomy the margin is identified by the surgeon who controls a dissection beneath the endothoracic fascia (8,46,47).

The extent of invasion is an important part of the p TNM staging and is represented by the invasion of adipose tissue for the parietal pleura or by invasion of lung parenchyma on the

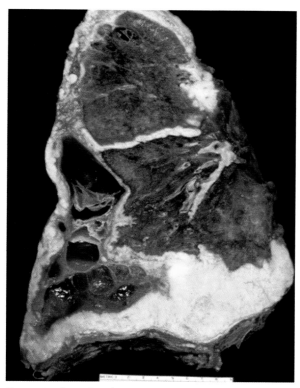

Figure 4.6 Extra-pleural pneumonectomy specimen showing extensive pleural invasion by a mesothelioma that encases the lung with a thick, gray rind. The tumor invades the major and minor fissures and shows areas of necrosis and hemorrhage.

visceral pleura, which is the hallmark for separating benign mesothelial processes from malignant. The exact p TNM should be reported in the conclusion of the reports according to the 8th UICC and AJCC and to the last IASLC edition, which will be a useful tool for prognostic research and for a better selection of treatment for the patient in the near future (48–51) (see Tables 4.1 and 4.2). Other cases are diagnosed only at necropsy for medicolegal purpose.

Reporting and Minimal Required Elements

As previously reported, above and according to the recommendations from the ICCR (8), the clinical information is essential and should be summarized on the report. It is important to describe clinical history, the radiologic growth pattern, comorbidities, and a previous history of cancer, which are all important item guides for further analysis of the specimen. Neoadjuvant therapy should be noticed in the general information as the pathologist will have to appreciate tumor regression for evaluating the response to chemotherapy. When a previous history of cancer is present a review of prior archival material and an order for ancillary techniques, such as additional organ-specific antibodies by immunohistochemistry or molecular tests to exclude a carcinomatous metastasis and avoid misdiagnosis with a metastasis of sarcoma, might be requested. A context of asbestos exposure is not relevant for the diag-

nosis of the samples because it should not influence the final diagnosis. The size and type of specimen submitted should be described: FNA cytology or cell block, CT-guided/not CT-guided biopsy, core needle biopsy, surgical resection (surgical biopsy, wedge, radical pleurectomy, decortication, pneumonectomy/EPP, debulking or others), and the type of tissue preservation (snap-frozen for further molecular analysis) or FFPE; the type of tissue fixation (additionally, if the tissue has been processed with decalcification solution, the type of solution should be documented and the reagent used).

The macroscopic tumor site is essential for pathologic staging and should be reported (8) as well as the size of the specimen and the number of FFPE blocks realized and, if possible, the indices linked to number of the block related to a specific growth pattern in order to further facilitate selection of the block for macrodissection of the tumoral spot of interest. The pathologist needs to perform the evaluation of the percentage of viable tumor before extraction of DNA for molecular analysis. The histology tumor type should be described according to the 2015 WHO classification (4th edition) and classified as epithelioid/biphasic/sarcomatoid. The various histologic patterns are important to describe in the report, primarily to avoid diagnostic confusion with a non-mesothelioma diagnosis, but additionally because of their prognostic implication. These include various patterns such as papillary, trabecular, tubulopapillary, acinar, solid, micropapillary and pleomorphic for epithelioid type, the latter associated with a worse prognosis. They should be included as mesothelioma of epithelioid type as part of the ultimate diagnosis. The lymphohistiocytoid unusual variant is important to identify and to describe, because this variant could be a good candidate for immunotherapy. For sarcomatoid mesothelioma, the histologic variants including heterologous elements (osteosarcomatous, chondrosarcomatous, rhabdomyosarcomatous) are important to report to avoid misdiagnosis and for prognostic purpose. Grade and Ki67 index have been reported to have clinical prognostic significance, and it would perhaps be sensible to describe these items in the near future for predicting survival within the various clinicopathologic categories (52,53).

Pre-analytical and Analytical Steps Recommended for Immunohistochemistry and Molecular Tests

In agreement with the recommended standard for reporting results and interpretation of a biopsy sample with a suspicion of mesothelioma, it is recommended to take attention to the pre-analytical and the analytical processing step. The data set for routine practice is available on the ICCR website: www .iccr-cancer.org.

Immunohistochemistry

The pre-analytical and analytical phases of processing are of the utmost importance for the performance of ancillary techniques used in the diagnosis of malignant mesothelioma. Engel et al. (54) identified the diverse sources of pre-analytical variations in specimen fixation and processing that can impair the accuracy of the diagnosis and cause false negative results. Fifteen pre-analytical variables were able to impact on protein detection. The most important were the delay, type and duration of fixation (55,56). It is well known that under-fixation is as noxious as over-fixation for protein detection and a minimum of 6 hours and a maximum of 48–72 hours is recommended for a uniform and reproducible immunostaining on a small biopsy specimen. Guidelines for specific practice are made by the Clinical Laboratory Standard Institute (57) for a good practice of immunohistochemistry when clinicians need results in emergency for the management of the patient and the basic time could not be respected. The fixative time is dependent on the type of tissue (adipose tissue needs a longer time than other tissue) and the size of the sample. Among the published reports there is a general agreement to select 4 percent neutral-buffered formalin at a solution pH 5–7 compared to unbuffered formalin for an optimal immunostaining for most antigens. From experience, the temperature of the fixative is important. It is also recommended not to preserve the formalin-fixed sample in a cold area or in the fridge at a temperature of less than 4°C before sending it to the pathology laboratory to avoid under fixation. The biopsy specimen should be submersed in a sufficient volume of fixative with a ratio of at least 10:1. Other non-aldehyde fixatives and alcoholic fixatives may alter tissue antigenicity and DNA integrity and are not recommended; they also can alter morphology by producing artifacts. Acidic fixatives such as Bouin's fluid, AFA, and those based on hard metal salts should be avoided to preserve DNA integrity. Moreover, guidelines and recommendations stress the fact that paraffin with a melting point of 55–58°C during 0.5 to 4.5 hours, 15 minutes to 3 hours per stage with two to three stages is an optimal option for immunohistochemistry. The last point of good practice concerns paraffin block storage, and the guidelines insist on the fact that paraffin-embedded blocks will benefit from being preserved indefinitely at least in an air-conditioned room or a room at 4°C for a stable immunostaining.

Evaluation of Immunostains

Mesothelioma is a great mimicker of benign and malignant tumors from diverse origins and requires immunohistochemical analysis with at least two positive (calretinin + WT-1 or CK5/6, EMA membranous) and two negative markers (Ber-EP4, CEA moab, MOC31, etc.) together with organ-specific markers (ER α, TTF-1) depending on the morphology for epithelioid malignant mesothelioma and two Pan CKS of different molecular weights in case of spindle-cell proliferations, together with p40 for a definitive diagnosis of sarcomatoid malignant mesothelioma. Immunohistochemistry is extremely valuable for separating most metastatic adenocarcinoma and for suggestion of the primary. This has been extensively covered

in the new WHO classification 2015 (1,2). The clone of the antibodies (e.g., EMA clone E29 for membranous staining, or TTF1 clone 8G7G3/1 is more specific and less sensitive, while clone SP142 is less specific and more sensitive with a risk of misdiagnosis). The type of expression of the biomarker (membranous vs. cytoplasmic, nuclear vs. cytoplasmic) has to be qualitatively evaluated and reported. In case of negative expression a positive control should be evaluated and reported.

Molecular Analysis

Pre-analytical standards for molecular testing are as strict as those described above. Guidance has also been recently published for diagnosis requesting molecular analysis and the pathology department should ensure that the processing is strictly followed step by step. The three major molecular alterations observed in mesothelioma are the homozygous deletion of the *CDKN2A* gene (encoding the p16 protein), and the mutations of BRCA1 associated protein-1 (*BAP1* gene) and neurofibromin type 2 (*NF2* gene). Loss of BAP-1 is evaluated by immunohistochemistry and present in 45–100 percent, mostly of epithelioid type (56) and is a very useful marker for the separation of benign versus malignant proliferation in the context of strong clinical and radiological features for malignancy (58). The presence of a homozygous deletion of *CDKN2A* (p16) by FISH is also observed in 45–100 percent and nearly 100 percent in the sarcomatoid type (17). This biomarker is correlated with a poorer prognosis in mesothelioma, and a useful marker in the separation of benign noninvasive cellular spindle cell processes (benign organizing pleuritis) versus sarcomatous and desmoplastic mesotheliomas which can be morphologically very difficult. Deletion of p16 (*CDKN2A*) by FISH testing seems to be a reliable marker of malignancy in mesothelial proliferations, and more recently it has been reported that, in this setting, loss of *BAP1* by immunohistochemistry is only seen in malignant mesotheliomas (59). Churg et al. showed that together, *BAP1* IHC and p16 FISH are 58 percent sensitive for detecting malignancy in comparison with previous reported combinations in the literature of p53, EMA, *IMP3*, and *GLUT1* that showed reasonably high specificity (96–98 percent) but poor to extremely poor sensitivity. Finally, combined *BAP1* IHC/p16 FISH testing is a highly specific method of diagnosing malignant mesotheliomas when tissue invasion by mesothelial cells cannot be demonstrated (60). *NF2* is not currently used in routine practice. Singhi et al. recently showed that dual-color FISH using *CDKN2A* and *NF2* locus-specific probes and *BAP1* immunohistochemistry identified homozygous *CDKN2A* deletions ($n = 25$, 29 percent), hemizygous *NF2* loss ($n = 30$, 35 percent), and/or loss of *BAP1* protein expression ($n = 49$, 57 percent) in 68 of 86 (79 percent) peritoneal mesotheliomas (61). Moreover, Churg et al. showed that it was not a useful biomarker in the separation of benign versus malignant superficial proliferation by immunohistochemistry in the therapeutic management of the patient (62).

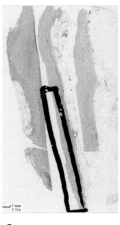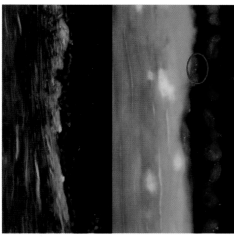

Figure 4.7 (a) Fluorescent *in-situ* hybridization (FISH) for the detection of homozygous deletion of *CDKN2A* (p16) is a very useful and accurate test to distinguish mesothelioma from reactive mesothelial proliferations. As shown in the left panel of this photograph, it is important to select the areas suspicious for tumor on H&E-stained slides so that the test can be performed in adjacent slides, shown in the other two panels of the photograph. (b) FISH shows the presence of homozygous deletion of *CDKN2A* (p16). The majority of the cells shown in the photomicrograph lack the green signal and only exhibit the background red signal used to identify cells.

FISH Analysis: Probes

To detect homozygous deletions of *CDKN2A*, the most widely used methods are dual-colour FISH analysis for the *CDKN2A* locus (9p21) and the centromere of the chromosome 9 (CEP-9), using the ZytoVision probe (ZytoLight SPEC CDKN2A/CEN 9 Dual Color Probe, # Z-2063–200), or the Abbott Molecular probe (Vysis LSI CDKN2A SpectrumOrange/Vysis CEP 9 SpectrumGreen Probes, # 04N61–020).

FISH analysis may also be of great help in making the correct diagnosis in the case of a spindle-cell unclassified tumor mimicking sarcomatoid mesothelioma looking for SS18, FOXO1, EWSR1 translocation, or MDM2 and CDK4 amplification favoring sarcoma.

FISH Analysis Requirements

Pre-analytical standards are requested and of utmost importance for FISH analysis. The small biopsy should be rapidly placed in neutral 4 percent buffered formaldehyde and fixation should be controlled by the pathologist. Once again, the time of cold ischemia should be less than 1 h between excision and fixation and the time of fixation should not exceed 72 h to avoid DNA degradation. It is recommended to definitively avoid Bouin's fluid and acidic fixative as it results in false negative or non-interpretable results by lack of hybridization. It is for this reason that acidic decalcification of bone (for example, cases of bone metastasis by desmoplastic mesothelioma when bone biopsy is the only material available and pan CK are not expressed) usually fail to hybridize and may give false results. It is necessary to perform fresh serial recuts for FISH analysis from the FFPE block stored in the correct conditions protected from light, humidity, and high temperature (63). For small sample biopsies it is recommended to perform serial recuts at one time including one H&E stained slide and

5–10 unstained slides of 3–5 μm thickness for immunohistochemistry followed by one H&E for evaluation of residual tumor on the slides. When unstained slides are sent for consultation it is frequently necessary to customize the protocol for optimizing the result. The tissue permeabilization is also an important variable to control under pepsin digestion at 37°C and is variable, depending on the type of the tissue analyzed (fibrotic versus non-fibrotic tissue). The next important step to control is the deposit of the probe, on the slide to avoid inversion of the probe, and finally the washing post-hybridization and the final coloration with DAPI for visualization of the nuclei for counting.

Evaluation of the Tumor Samples and Assessment of the Hybridized Tumor Sample

The pathologist should first evaluate the sample and mark the area of the section at the exact site of the neoplastic area or the hot spot with the highest cellularity density selected for FISH analysis or for later microdissection and DNA extraction. It is also important to take into consideration the tumor heterogeneity in selecting various areas. A selected area of up to 60 percent of positive tumor cells is considered to be accurate for molecular analysis, but depends on the size of the sample. The discrimination between mesothelioma and metastasis should have been previously established as described above on the morphologic and immunohistochemical characteristics of the tumor.

The selection for the content of neoplastic cells is highly dependent on the presence or absence of the molecular abnormality or for defining the limit of the detection. A minimum of 100 cells is needed for the evaluation of the status of *CDKN2A* by FISH analysis by two independent observers (Figure 4.7a, b). More than 80 percent of nuclei should be hybridized. The number of nuclei with no copy and those with one copy should be strictly counted, recorded on a score sheet and reported. It is important to avoid misinterpretation of isolated signal and misdiagnosis of homozygous deletion due to cross-section of nuclei generating missing signals on the slide. Moreover, the quality of the morphology and the intensity of DAPI staining is of great value for a rigorous assessment of the size of the neoplastic nuclei and correct counting. From our experience a cut-off value of 20 percent of nuclei with no *CDKN2A* copy is considered a positive result for the presence of a homozygous deletion. In some cases, a clonal disposition of the nuclei showing a homozygous deletion can confirm this interpretation. In cases of less than one copy observed in less than 20 percent of the nuclei the result is evaluated as negative for homozygous deletion. Heterozygous deletion is not a strict criterion for malignancy. To avoid technical bias and false results, a two-step assessment with one trained technician and one molecular biologist or pathologist is recommended. The criteria for validating the FISH technique for quality assessment is based on internal laboratory validation and, when possible, external control. Both semi-automated or manual analyses are available and depend on site organization. In an equivocal case an aCGH array procedure should be performed.

Tissue-based NGS and WES, RNA seq

Tissue-based next-generation sequencing (NGS) applicable in routine analysis is a very early emerging technique in the mesothelioma field. This is a new technology enabling the analysis of nucleic acid sequencing mostly for research purposes. However, whole exome DNA sequencing (WES) and whole transcriptome RNA sequencing allow the detection of new diagnostic mutations (63). With more therapies coming online every year and immune checkpoint modulation, the use of these technologies is a real opportunity (64). Pre-analytical factors that might affect the performance of NGS are common with those previously described for FISH analysis and again it is important to provide high-quality DNA from FFPE samples to strictly observe international guidelines during the pre-analytical phase (65–67). It is of the utmost importance to continue to consider that an expert review by a pathologist with a morphomolecular approach is needed to avoid low or no tumor concentration or non-mesothelioma area and misinterpretation. The era of personalized medicine is approaching and requires both histological-based tissue diagnoses together with molecular pathology mutational analysis of the tumor.

References

1. WHO (World Health Organization). *WHO classification of tumours of the lung, pleura, thymus and heart.* 4th ed. Travis WD, Brambilla E, Burke AP, Marx A, Nicholson AG, editors. Lyon: IARC Press; 2015.

2. Galateau-Sallé F, Churg A, Roggli V, Travis WD. The 2015 WHO classification of tumors of the pleura: advances since the 2004 classification. *J Thoracic Oncol.* 2016;11(2):142–54.

3. Husain AN, Colby T, Ordonez N, Krausz T, Attanoos R, Beasley MB, et al. Guidelines for Pathologic Diagnosis of Malignant Mesothelioma: 2012 Update of the Consensus Statement from the International Mesothelioma Interest Group. *Arch Pathol Lab Med.* 2013;137(5):647–67.

4. CAP (College of American Pathologists). Cancer protocols and checklists. 2015. Available from: www.cap.org/cancer-reporting-tools/cancer-reportingtemplates?afrLoop=5315966824823314#

5. RCPA (Royal College of Pathologists of Australasia). Structured pathology reporting of cancer protocols. 2010–2015. Available from: www.rcpa.edu.au/Library/Practising-Pathology/Structured-Pathology-Reporting-of-Cancer/Cancer-Protocols.

6. RCP (Royal College of Pathologists). Datasets and tissue pathways. 2015. Available from: www.rcpath.org/index.asp?PageID=254.

7. Scherpereel A, Astoul P, Baas P, Berghmans T, Clayson H, de Vuyst P, et al. Guidelines of the European Respiratory Society and the European Society of Thoracic Surgeons for the management of malignant pleural mesothelioma. *Eur Respir J.* 2010;35(3):479–95.

8. Churg A, Attanoos R, Borczuck A, Chirieac LR, Galateau-Sallé F, Gibbs A, et al. Dataset for reporting of malignant mesothelioma of the pleura and peritoneum: recommendations from the International Collaboration on Cancer Reporting (ICCR). *Arch Pathol Lab Med.* 2016; 140(10):1104–10.

9. Stahel RA, Weder W, Felip E, ESMO Guidelines Working Group. Malignant pleural mesothelioma: ESMO clinical recommendations for diagnosis, treatment and follow-up. *Ann Oncol.* 2008;19(Suppl 2):ii43–44.

10. van Zandwijk N, Clarke C, Henderson D, Musk AW, Fong K, Nowak A, et al. Guidelines for the diagnosis and treatment of malignant pleural mesothelioma. *J Thorac Dis.* 2013; 5(6):E254–307.

11. Henderson WD, Reid G, Kao SC, van Zandwijk N, Klebe S. Challenges and controversies in the diagnosis of malignant mesothelioma: Part 1. Cytology-only diagnosis, biopsies, immunohistochemistry, discrimination between mesothelioma and reactive mesothelial hyperplasia and biomarkers. *J Clin Pathol.* 2013; 66(10):847–53.

12. Henderson WD, Reid G, Kao SC, van Zandwijk N, Klebe S. Challenges and controversies in the diagnosis of malignant mesothelioma: Part 2. Malignant mesothelioma subtypes, pleural synovial sarcoma, molecular and prognostic aspects of mesothelioma, *BAP1*, aquaporin-1 and microRNA. *J Clin Pathol.* 2013; 66(10):854–61.

13. Goldberg M, Imbernon E, Rolland P, Gilg Soit Ilg A, Savès M, de Quillacq A, et al. The French National Mesothelioma Surveillance Program. *Occup Environ Med.* 2006;63(6): 390–95.

14. Maskell NA, Butland RJ; Pleural Diseases Group, Standards of Care Committee, British Thoracic Society. BTS guidelines for the investigation of a unilateral pleural effusion in adults. *Thorax.* 2003;58(Suppl 2):ii8–17.

15. Du Rand I, Maskell N. Introduction and methods: British Thoracic Society pleural disease guideline 2010. *Thorax.* 2010;65(Suppl 2):ii1–eii3.

16. Roberts ME, Neville E, Berrisford RG, Antunes G, Ali NJ, BTS Pleural Disease Guideline Group. Management of a malignant pleural effusion: BritishThoracic Society pleural disease guideline 2010. *Thorax.* 2010;65(Suppl 2):ii32–eii40.

17. Churg A, Sheffield BS, Galateau-Sallé F. New markers for separating benign from malignant mesothelial proliferations: are we there yet? *Arch Pathol Lab Med.* 2015;140(4):318–21.

18. ATS. *Am J Respir Crit Care Med.* 2000;162:19872001. Available from: www.atsjournals.org

19. Egan AM, McPhillips D, Sarkar S, Breen DP. Malignant pleural effusion. *Q J Med.* 2014;107(3):179–84.

20. Cellerin L, Marcq M, Sagan C, Chailleux E. Pleurésies malignes révélatrices d'un cancer: comparaison des étiologies avec les pleurésies métastatiques. *Rev Mal Respir.* 2008;25(9):1104–09.

21. Karoo RO, Lloyd TD, Garcea G, Redway HD, Robertson GS. How valuable is ascetic cytology in the detection and management of malignancy. *Postgrad Med.* 2003;79:292–94.

22. Motherby H, Nadjari B, Friegel P, Kohaus J, Bocking A. Diagnostic accuracy of effusion cytology. *Diagn Cytopathol.* 1999;20(6):350–57.

23. Abrams LD. A pleural-biopsy punch. *Lancet.* 1958;1:30–31.

24. Von Hoff DD, LiVolsi V. Diagnostic reliability of needle biopsy of the parietal pleura. A review of 272 biopsies. *Am J Clin Pathol.* 1975;64(2):200–03.

25. Cagle PT, Allen TC. Pathology of the pleura: what the pulmonologists need to know. *Respirology.* 2011;16(3): 430–38. doi: 10.1111/j.1440–1843. 2011.01957.x.

26. Cope C. New pleural biopsy needle. *JAMA* 1958;167:1107–08.

27. Tomlinson JR. Invasive procedures in the diagnosis of pleural disease. *Semin Respir Med.* 1987;9:30–60.

28. Nance KV, Shermer RW, Askin FB. Diagnostic efficacy of pleural biopsy as compared with that of pleural fluid examination. *Mod Pathol.* 1991;4: 320–24.

29. Loddenkemper R, Boutin C. Thoracoscopy: present diagnostic and therapeutic indications. *Eur Respir J.* 1993;6:1544–55.

30. Diacon AH, Van de Wal BW, Wyser C, Smedema JP, Bezuidenhout J, Bolliger CT, et al. Diagnostic tools in tuberculous pleurisy: a direct comparative study. *Eur Respir J.* 2003;22:589–91.

31. Kirsch CM, Kroe DM, Azzi RL, Jensen WA, Kagawa FT, Wehner JH. The optimal number of pleural biopsy specimens for a diagnosis of tuberculous pleurisy. *Chest.* 1997;112(3):702–06.

32. Light RW. Update on tuberculous pleural effusion. *Respirology.* 2010;15(3):451–58.

33. Maskell NA, Gleeson FV, Davies RJ. Standard pleural biopsy versus CT-guided cutting-needle biopsy for diagnosis of malignant disease in pleural effusions: a randomised controlled trial. *Lancet.* 2003;361(9366):1326–30. PubMed PMID: 12711467.

34. Dixon G, de Fonseka D, Maskell N. Pleural controversies: image guided biopsy vs. thoracoscopy for undiagnosed pleural effusions? *J Thorac Dis.* 2015;7(6):1041–51.

35. Bibby AC, Maskell NA. Pleural biopsies in undiagnosed pleural effusions; Abrams vs image-guided vs thoracoscopic biopsies. *Curr Opin Pulm Med.* 2016;22(4):392–98.

36. Yang PC, Kuo SH, Luh KT. Ultrasonography and ultrasound guided needle biopsy of chest diseases: indications, techniques, diagnostic yields and complications. *J Med Ultrasound.* 1993;1:53–63.

37. Walker SP, Morley AJ, Stadon L, De Fonseka D, Arnold DA, Medford AR, et al. Nonmalignant pleural effusions: a prospective study of 356 consecutive unselected patients. *Chest.* 2017; 151(5):1099–105. PubMed PMID: 28025056.

38. Attanoos RL, Gibbs AR. The comparative accuracy of different pleural biopsy techniques in the diagnosis of malignant mesothelioma. *Histopathology.* 2008;53(3):340–44. doi: 10.1111/j.1365–2559.2008.03099.x. Epub 2008 Jul 18.)

39. Boutin C, Astoul P. Diagnostic thoracoscopy. *Clin Chest Med.* 1998;19(2):295–309.

40. Boutin C, Schlesser M, Frenay C, Astoul P. Malignant pleural mesothelioa. *Eur Respir J.* 1998;12:972–81.

41. Greillier L, Cavailles A, Fraticelli A, Scherpereel A, Barlesi F, Tassi G, et al. Accuracy of pleural biopsy using thoracoscopy for the diagnosis of histologic subtype in patients with malignant pleural mesothelioma. *Cancer.* 2007;110(10):2248–52.

42. Bueno R, Reblando J, Glickman J, Jaklitsch MT, Lukanich JM, Sugarbaker DJ. Pleural biopsy: a reliable method for determining the diagnosis but not subtype in mesothelioma. *Ann Thorac Surg.* 2004; 78(5):1774–76.

43. Kao SC, Yan TD, Lee K, Burn J, Henderson DW, Klebe S, et al. Accuracy of diagnostic biopsy for the histological subtype of malignant pleural mesothelioma. *J Thorac Oncol.* 2011;6(3):602–05.

44. Rubin JW, Finney NR, Borders BM, Chauvin EJ. Intrathoracic biopsies, pulmonary wedge excision, and management of pleural disease: is video-assisted closed chest surgery the approach of choice? *Am Surg.* 1994;60(11):860–63.

45. Litzky LA, Gal A. Lung specimen handling and practical considerations. In: Hasleton P, Fiedler DB, editors. *Spencer Pathology of the Lung*, sixth edition, chapter 2. Cambridge: Cambridge University Press; 2013.

46. Opitz I. Management of malignant pleural mesothelioma – the European experience. *J Thorac Dis.* 2014;6(Suppl 2):S238–52.

47. D'Amico TA, Rocco G. The biomolecular era for thoracic surgeons: the example of the ESTS Biology Club. *J Thorac Dis.* 2014;6(Suppl 2):S265–71.

48. Nowak AK, Chansky K, Rice DC, Pass HI, Kindler HL, Shemanski L, et al. The IASLC Mesothelioma Staging Project: proposals for revisions of the T descriptors in the forthcoming eighth edition of the TNM Classification for Pleural Mesothelioma. *J Thorac Oncol.* 2016;11(12):2089–99.

49. Rice D, Chansky K, Nowak A, Pass H, Kindler H, Shemanski L, et al. The IASLC Mesothelioma Staging Project: proposals for the M descriptors and for revision of the TNM stage groupings in

the forthcoming (eighth) edition of the TNM Classification for Mesothelioma. *J Thorac Oncol.* 2016;11(12):2100–11.

50. Rusch VW, Chansky K, Kindler HL, Nowak AK, Pass HI, Rice DC, et al. The IASLC Mesothelioma Staging Project: proposals for revisions of the N descriptors in the forthcoming eighth edition of the TNM classification for pleural mesothelioma. *J Thorac Oncol.* 2016;11(12):2112–19.

51. Pass H, Giroux D, Kennedy C, Ruffini E, Cangir AK, Rice D, et al. The IASLC Mesothelioma Staging Project: improving staging of a rare disease through international participation. *J Thorac Oncol.* 2016;11(12):2082–88.

52. Pillai K, Pourgholami MH, Chua TC, Morris DL. Prognostic significance of Ki67 expression in malignant peritoneal mesothelioma. *Am J Clin Oncol.* 2015;38(4):388–94.

53. Engel KB, Moore H. Effects of pre analytical variables on the detection of proteins by immunohistochemistry in formalin fixed paraffin embedded tissue. *Archiv Pathol Lab Med.* 2011;135:537–43.

54. Khoury T. Delay to formalin fixation alters morphology and immunohistochemistry for breast carcinoma. *Appl Immunohistochem Mol Morphol.* 2012;20(6):531–42. PubMed PMID: 22495358.

55. Khoury T, Sait S, Hwang H, Chandrasekhar R, Wilding G, Tan D, et al. Delay to formalin fixation effect on breast biomarkers. *Mod Pathol.* 2009;22(11):1457–67. PubMed PMID: 19734848.

56. Lightfoote MM, Ball DJ, Hannon WH, Ridderhoh JC, Vogt RF. *Quality assurance for design control and implementation of immunohistochemistry assays; approved guideline.* 2nd edition. Wayne, PA: Clinical and Laboratory Standards Institute (CLSI); 2010.

57. Righi L, Duregon E, Vatrano S, Izzo S, Giorcelli J, Rondón-Lagos M, et al. BRCA1-associated protein 1 (Bap1) immunohistochemical expression as a diagnostic tool in malignant pleural mesothelioma classification: a large retrospective study. *J Thorac Oncol.* 2016;11(11):2006–17.

58. Hwang HC, Pyott S, Rodriguez S, Cindric A, Carr A, Michelsen C, et al. *BAP1* immunohistochemistry and p16 FISH in the diagnosis of sarcomatous and desmoplastic mesotheliomas. *Am J Surg Pathol.* 2016;40(5):714–18.

59. Sheffield BS, Hwang HC, Lee AF, Thompson K, Rodriguez S, Tse CH, et al. *BAP1* immunohistochemistry and p16 FISH to separate benign from malignant mesothelial proliferations. *Am J Surg Pathol.* 2015;39(7):977–82.

60. Singhi AD, Krasinskas AM, Chourdy HA, Bartlett DL, Pingpank JF, Zeh HJ, et al. The prognostic significance of *BAP1*, *NF2*, and *CDKN2A* in malignant peritoneal mesothelioma. *Mod Pathol.* 2016;29(1):14–24.

61. Sheffield BS, Lorette J, Shen Y, Marra MA, Churg A. Immunohistochemistry for NF2, LATS1/2, and YAP/TAZ fails to separate benign from malignant mesothelial proliferations. *Arch Pathol Lab Med.* 2016;140(5):391.

62. Grillo F, Pigozzi S, Ceriolo P, Calamaro P, Fiocca R, Mastracci L. Factors affecting immunoreactivity in long-term storage of formalin-fixed paraffin-embedded tissue sections. *Histochem Cell Biol.* 2015;144(1): 93–99.

63. Bueno R, Stawiski EW, Goldstein LD, Durinck S, De Rienzo A, Modrusan Z, et al. Comprehensive genomic analysis of malignant pleural mesothelioma identifies recurrent mutations, gene fusions and splicing alterations. *Nat Genet.* 2016;48(4):407–16.

64. Hynes SO, Pang B, James JA, Maxwell P, Salto-Tellez M. Tissue-based next generation sequencing: application in a universal healthcare system. *Br J Cancer.* 2017;116(5):553–60. PubMed PMID: 28103613

65. Cree IA, Deans Z, Ligtenberg MJ, Normanno N, Edsjö A, Rouleau E, et al. Guidance for laboratories performing molecular pathology for cancer patients. *J Clin Pathol.* 2014;67(11):923–31.

66. Deans ZC, Costa JL, Cree I, Dequeker E, Edsjö A, Henderson S, et al. Integration of next-generation sequencing in clinical diagnostic molecular pathology laboratories for analysis of solid tumours; an expert opinion on behalf of IQN Path ASBL. *Virchows Arch.* 2017;470(1):5–20.

67. Aziz N, Zhao Q, Bry L, Driscoll DK, Funke B, Gibson JS, et al. College of American Pathologists' laboratory standards for next-generation sequencing clinical tests. *Arch Pathol Lab Med.* 2015;139(4):481–93.

Chapter 5

Cytology of Pleural and Peritoneal Lesions

Shikha Bose

Cytologic examination of fluid obtained from serous cavities (pleural, peritoneal, and pericardial) is one of the commonest specimen types submitted to a hospital-based cytology laboratory. Accumulation of fluid in the serous cavities is always abnormal. The common indication for cytologic examination is to rule out malignancy, either primary or metastatic, although effusions may be tapped to provide symptomatic relief. Obtaining samples is a relatively simple procedure, but diagnosis of malignancy is challenging. Interpretation is hindered by similarities between benign conditions and malignancies that are limited not only to the morphology of the cells but which also extend to immunohistochemical and molecular features. This chapter outlines the algorithms for reaching an accurate diagnosis and the common pitfalls encountered so as to limit false positive and negative diagnoses, as either may carry grave consequences for the patient.

Laboratory Requirements

Proper cytopreparation of the fluid sample is of paramount importance. Effusion samples should preferably be sent fresh to the laboratory as soon as possible. Anticoagulants or heparin should be added to prevent clotting, because clots frequently trap neoplastic cells and limit the utilization of the sample. A minimum of 5 ml is recommended. The sample should be refrigerated at 4°C until processed (1). When long transportation times are anticipated an equal volume of 50 percent ethanol should be added to the sample for preservation.

Cytologic processing involves concentration of the cellular material by centrifugation at 1000g or more for 10 min and preparing smears from the cell pellet. Should the sample be hemorrhagic, hemolysis may be attempted prior to slide preparation. Both wet-fixed and air-dried smears are examined. The air-dried smear may be used as a rapid screen for triaging for lymphoma studies or preparation of a cell block for immunologic studies. Two to five milliliters of the cell-free supernatant may also be stored at –20°C for subsequent biomarker analysis. Thin-layer preparations are reported to yield similar to better results (2,3).

Benign Cellular Constituents

Mesothelial Cells

Effusions contain detached mesothelial cells present singly or in clusters. Individual cells vary in size from 12 to 20 μm, and have round to oval single or multiple nuclei with small nucleoli. Cytoplasm is abundant with a characteristic perinuclear condensation (Figure 5.1a). A characteristic feature noted in clusters of mesothelial cells is "windows." This is a clear space present between cells and represents the long surface microvilli of mesothelial cells (Figure 5.1b). In cavity washings and percutaneous fine-needle aspiration biopsies mesothelial cells are present as cohesive sheets of monolayered cells or as balls of cells with variable central cores of collagen (Figure 5.2). Long-standing effusions show degenerative changes in mesothelial cells in the form of intracytoplasmic vacuoles that may be confused with histiocytes or adenocarcinoma (Figure 5.3).

Inflammatory Cells

Macrophages and leukocytes may be present in varying numbers. Macrophages or histiocytes may be present singly or in loosely cohesive clusters. Molding, windows, tight groups, or papillae are not observed. They may be prominent in cancers and chronic inflammatory conditions like tuberculosis and embolism. Phagocytosed debris, hemosiderin, and red blood cells may frequently be present in the cytoplasm.

A few lymphocytes may be present in effusions; however, they are prominent in long-standing effusions of congestive heart failure and renal failure. T lymphocytes predominate in inflammatory processes and when associated with metastatic tumors. A prominent population of B lymphocytes is suggestive of lymphoma.

Eosinophils in effusions are a non-specific finding, although they may be associated with infections and hypersensitivity reactions. Frequently peripheral blood eosinophilia is concurrent in a third to half the cases. Neutrophils suggest an acute inflammation, although their presence in bloody effusions may be an artifact of the blood contamination. Differential diagnostic considerations are summarized in Table 5.1.

Psammoma Bodies

These are rounded, laminated calcifications formed from papillary structures and are seen in benign and malignant. conditions (Figure 5.4, Table 5.2). They are more commonly associated with benign conditions. A malignancy may be suspected when they are present in large numbers and rimmed by atypical cells.

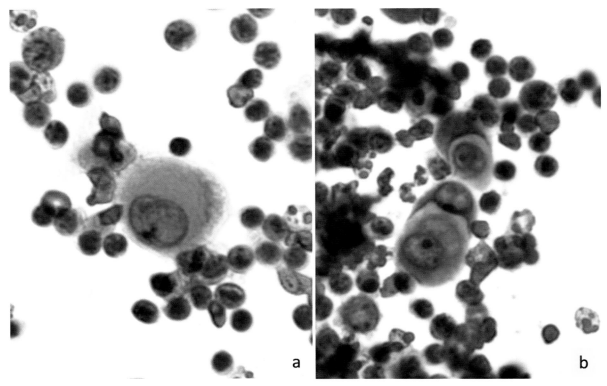

Figure 5.1 Benign mesothelial cells. (a) Showing perinuclear cytoplasmic condensation; (b) windows (Papanicolaou stain, ×60).

Causes of Effusions

Neoplastic: Common conditions include carcinoma, melanoma, lymphoma, and mesothelioma.

Non-neoplastic: Common conditions include congestive heart failure, nephrotic syndrome, pulmonary infections, pulmonary infarcts, and collagen vascular diseases, e.g., rheumatoid pleuritis and trauma.

Evaluation of Effusions

The approach to evaluating effusion fluid cytology can be addressed as answers to three important questions:

1. Are the cells malignant?
2. If malignant, is it a primary or metastatic tumor?
3. If metastatic, what is the primary site?

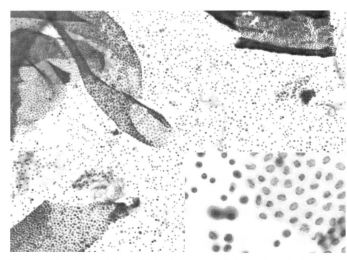

Figure 5.2 Pelvic washings with benign mesothelial cells. Cohesive flat sheets are a characteristic finding. ×10. **Inset**: Sheets are made up of benign mesothelial cells. ×40.

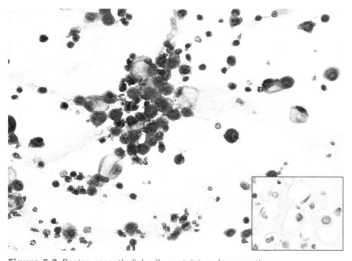

Figure 5.3 Benign mesothelial cells containing degenerative intracytoplasmic vacuoles. Note lack of typical signet-ring cell features, i.e., lack of nuclear indentation and tapering of nuclear ends demonstrated in Figure 5.9. **Inset**: Vacuolated cells were negative for Ber-EP4 immunostaining performed on the cell block section. ×40.

Table 5.1 Diagnostic considerations of increased numbers of hematopoietic cells

Cell type	Differential diagnosis
Histiocytes	Cancer
	Chronic inflammation, e.g., tuberculosis
	Embolism
Lymphocytes	Congestive heart failure, renal failure, cirrhosis
	Chronic inflammation, e.g., TB, SLE, rheumatoid disease, sarcoid
	Lymphoma
Eosinophils	Idiopathic
	Trauma leading to air in cavity
	Hypersensitivity
	Peripheral eosinophilia
Neutrophils	Acute infection
	Embolism, infarction

Diagnostic Challenges

1. Reactive mesothelial cells vs. malignant mesothelial cells.
2. Reactive mesothelial cells vs. metastatic malignant cells.
3. Malignant mesothelioma vs. metastatic carcinoma.
4. Determination of the primary site of a metastatic malignancy.
5. Differential diagnosis of an effusion containing prominent lymphoid population.

Are the Cells Malignant?

Determining if the effusion contains malignant cells is the most important consideration and requires diagnostic conservatism. The presence of malignant cells is a poor prognostic sign and could result in either withholding of or intensification of therapy regimens. Diagnosis should be made on well-preserved material. It is common to find degenerative changes in long-standing effusions that may limit diagnosis. Examination of a re-accumulated sample in these instances may yield better preserved material.

Accumulated fluid may be a transudate or exudate.

Transudates are effusions with low specific gravity (< 1.01), low protein and cell content and occur due to changes in the osmotic pressure resulting in transfer of fluid from the capillary spaces to the serous cavity. Clinical conditions giving rise to such effusions include congestive heart failure, liver and kidney failure, and severe malnutrition with protein deficiency.

Exudates are fluids with high specific gravity (> 1.01), high protein and cell content. This type of effusion is seen commonly in inflammatory conditions or in malignancies involving the mesothelium. These fluids contain a rich population of cells and are difficult to evaluate. Misdiagnosis of malignancy may label the patient with advanced disease and change the therapeutic options available.

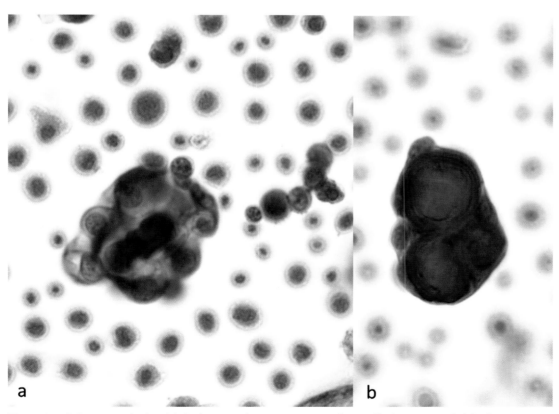

Figure 5.4a,b Psammoma bodies. Calcific deposits with concentric rings and rimmed by benign mesothelial cells. ×40.

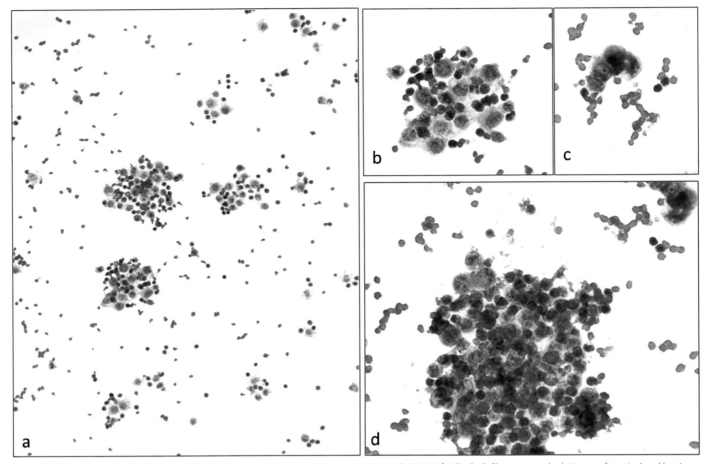

Figure 5.5 Reactive mesothelial cells. (a) Cellular smear with loosely cohesive monolayered sheets of cells. (b,d) Clusters reveal admixture of atypical and benign mesothelial cells and inflammatory cells. (c,d) Atypical mesothelial cells with enlarged nuclei containing prominent nucleoli are interspersed among benign mesothelial cells. ×40.

Cytologic features indicative of malignancy (Table 5.3a) include the presence of:

a. many aggregates and sheets of cells, particularly when present as three-dimensional clusters; and
b. cytologic atypia in the form of variable sized cells with altered nuclear cytoplasmic ratio, anisonucleosis, enlarged nuclei demonstrating irregular nuclear membranes, coarse chromatin and prominent nucleoli.

Reactive mesothelial cells are a difficult differential diagnosis. They may demonstrate cytologic atypia and architectural formations similar to malignant cells (Table 5.3b). The

Table 5.2 Diagnostic considerations of psammoma bodies

	Differential diagnosis
Benign conditions	Mesothelial hyperplasia Endosalpingiosis
Malignant conditions	Serous papillary ovarian cancer Other cancers, e.g., breast, lung, pancreas, colon, endometrium Mesothelioma

Table 5.3a Characteristics of malignant cells

Atypical cells
  Large cells: mesothelioma, carcinoma, sarcoma, melanoma
  Small cells: lymphomas, small cell tumors, breast
  Medium cells: gastric, breast, lung, pancreatic, and prostate
  carcinomas

Foreign population of cells
Well-formed, cohesive three-dimensional structures, papillae, glands
Intracellular epithelial mucin

Table 5.3b Mimics of benign mesothelial cells

Benign formations of mesothelial cells	**Mimics**
2–3-dimensional clusters	Adenocarcinoma
Papillae	Papillary adenocarcinoma
Single files	Breast carcinoma
Cell in cell	Squamous cell carcinoma
Signet rings	Signet-ring carcinoma
Single cells	Carcinoma, lymphoma

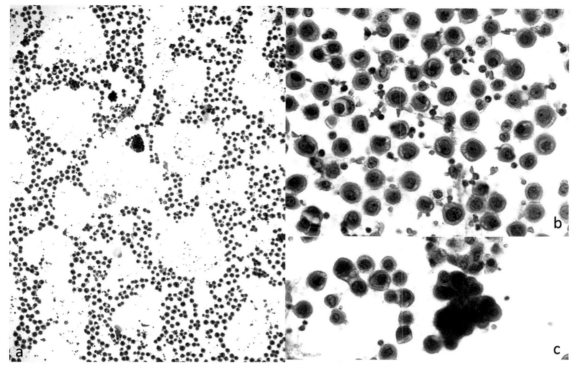

Figure 5.6 Reactive mesothelial cells. This pleural effusion from a 62-year-old male with long-standing congestive heart failure showed cellular smear with many atypical mesothelial cells and few small cohesive three-dimensional clusters raising a concern for mesothelioma (a,b). Correlation with clinical history was diagnostic. (c) Note the knobby outer border of the cluster that is characteristic of mesothelial cells. ×40.

presence of few atypical cells demonstrating a gradation of changes from benign to atypical, and the presence of flat sheets lacking the three-dimensional clustering commonly noted in malignant cells are helpful distinguishing features (Figures 5.5 and 5.6).

If Malignant – Is It a Primary or Metastatic Tumor?

Metastatic malignancy, particularly adenocarcinoma from various origins, is the most commonly encountered malignancy in effusions. Other tumors encountered include small cell carcinomas, squamous cell carcinomas, lymphomas, melanomas, and sarcomas (Tables 5.4a–c).

Table 5.4a Common primary sites for metastatic malignancies in adult females

Pleural fluid	Peritoneal fluid
Breast	Ovary
Lung	Breast
Ovary	GI tract Colon, stomach, pancreas
Gastrointestinal tract: Stomach, esophagus, colon	Lung
Lymphoma	Lymphoma

Table 5.4b Common primary sites for metastatic malignancies in adult males

Pleural fluid	Peritoneal fluid
Lung	GI tract Colon, pancreas, stomach
Gastrointestinal tract: Esophagus, stomach, colon	Lymphoma
Lymphoma	Melanoma

Metastatic Carcinoma

Adenocarcinoma

Adenocarcinomas will demonstrate all of the cytologic features of malignancy. In addition, identification of a "foreign cell population" in the effusion distinct from the present morphologically benign mesothelial cells is of diagnostic importance. Malignant cells tend to cluster as tightly cohesive three-dimensional structures with smooth community borders (Figures 5.7 and 5.8). Intracytoplasmic mucin, present as a single large vacuole or multiple small vacuoles, is also frequently

Table 5.4c Common primary sites for metastatic malignancies in children

Hematologic – leukemias
Small cell tumors – neuroblastoma, Wilms' tumor

Figure 5.7 Metastatic adenocarcinoma, Müllerian origin. The patient, a 65-year-old woman with bilateral ovarian masses, presented with ascites and left-sided pleural effusion. Smears were very cellular and showed many tightly cohesive clusters of malignant cells. Note the smooth outer community borders.

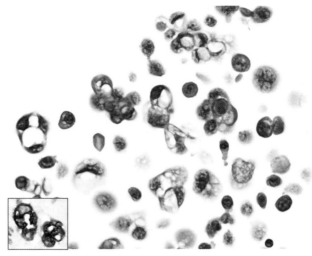

Figure 5.9 Metastatic adenocarcinoma, ovarian origin, showing "signet-ring cells." Note indented nuclei with tapered ends. **Inset**: Positivity for glandular markers was confirmatory. Ber-EP4 immunostain. ×40.

noted. Such signet-ring cells characteristically contain peripherally situated nuclei indented by the vacuoles. The nuclei have sharp irregular edges and pointed ends as opposed to signet-ring type of degenerative changes frequently noted in benign mesothelial cells, which demonstrate benign nuclear features

and lack mucin (Figure 5.9). It is not uncommon for adenocarcinoma to present as single cells lacking significant atypia in effusions (4), a feature commonly noted with metastatic lobular breast carcinomas. These carcinomas are difficult to diagnose and careful evaluation is necessary including confirmation

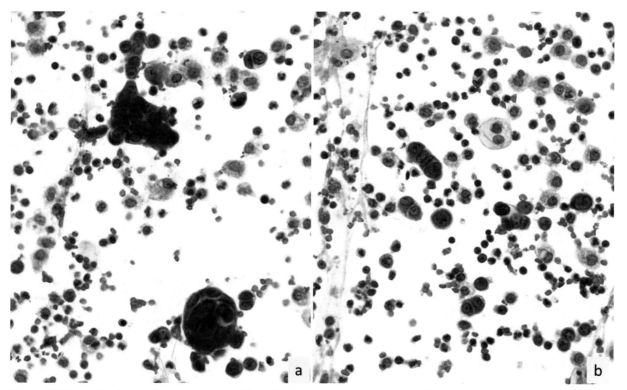

Figure 5.8 Metastatic adenocarcinoma, breast origin. Pleural fluid from a 56-year-old woman with history of breast cancer 4 years ago showing diagnostic features of metastatic carcinoma. (a) Malignant epithelial cells and benign mesothelial cells are seen. Malignant cells are present as tightly cohesive clusters with smooth outer borders. (b) Note the single-file arrangement characteristic of breast carcinoma.

Table 5.5 Immunohistochemical markers for differentiation of malignant/reactive mesothelial cells from metastatic adenocarcinoma cells

	Immunomarker
Mesothelial cells – benign or malignant	Calretinin, Wilms' tumor gene product (WT-1), podoplanin (D2–40), mesothelin, cytokeratin 5 or cytokeratin 5/6, HBME-1
Glandular cells	Claudin-4, Ber-EP4, MOC-31, CEA, CD15, B72.3, BG8

Table 5.6 Examples of lineage-specific immunohistochemical stains for determination of origin of malignancy

Tumor	Immunomarker
Mesothelium	Calretinin, WT-1, D2–40, CK5/6
Lung (adenocarcinoma)	TTF-1, Napsin-A
Lung (squamous cell carcinoma)	p63, CK5/6, p40
Breast	ER, PR, GATA-3, GCDFP, Mammaglobin
Prostate	PSA, PAP, PSMA
Ovary	ER, WT-1, PAX-8
Colorectal	CDX-2, CK20
Bladder	Uroplakin III, S100p, GATA3, p63
Kidney	RCC, PAX-8, S100A1
Neuroendocrine	Synaptophysin, chromogranin A, TTF-1, CDX-2 (GI NE tumors)
Melanoma	S-100, melan A, HMB-45, tyrosinase

by immunohistochemistry utilizing glandular and mesothelial markers (Figure 5.10, Table 5.5). Adenocarcinomas originating from various primary sites demonstrate overlapping morphology features and are difficult to diagnose morphologically. Some specific features reported include long, single-file arrangement of malignant cells with small intracytoplasmic vacuoles in metastatic breast cancer, and large pleomorphic malignant cells with large vacuoles distending the cytoplasm in metastatic ovarian carcinoma. It is important to note that these features are not specific and the diagnosis of the primary site requires careful correlation with clinical and radiologic features and utilization of immunohistochemistry and other ancillary molecular studies (Table 5.6).

Squamous Cell Carcinoma

These carcinomas rarely shed into effusions. Pleural effusions on rare occasions will contain metastatic squamous cell carcinomas of lung origin. Cytologic features include the presence of squamous pearls, keratinized cells, epithelioid cells with dense cytoplasm, spindle-shaped and tadpole-shaped cells (Figure 5.11).

Small Cell Carcinomas

It is unusual for small cell lung carcinomas (SCLCs) to present primarily as effusions. Morphologically they resemble large, immature lymphoid cells, but differ from them in their tendency to form tissue aggregates. Nuclear features are characteristic with the "salt and pepper" chromatin pattern, nuclear molding and stacking. Demonstration of neuroendocrine markers is diagnostic (Figure 5.12).

Desmoplastic small round cell tumor is a rare aggressive sarcoma that typically involves pelvic and abdominal organs of young (less than 40 years old) males, who usually present at advanced stage with poor prognosis. It is rarely diagnosed in effusions. Cytomorphology is characterized by undifferentiated small blue cell indistinguishable from other neuroendocrine

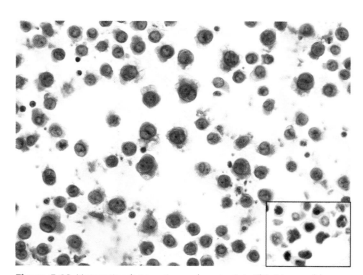

Figure 5.10 Metastatic adenocarcinoma, breast origin. This 54-year-old woman had a remote history of breast carcinoma. Smears revealed mostly single small cells with mild anisocytosis. A dual population was not readily apparent. **Inset**: Immunostains confirmed metastatic adenocarcinoma. Most cells were positive for estrogen receptor. ×40.

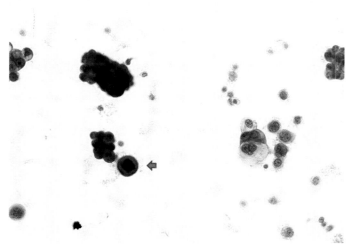

Figure 5.11 Metastatic squamous cell carcinoma, lung origin. Few atypical keratinized cells were present (blue arrow), which suggested a squamous differentiation. The remaining predominant population of cells comprised clusters of epithelioid cells, some with vacuolated cytoplasm, a feature that may be noted in exfoliated squamous cells or cells from adenosquamous carcinomas. ×40.

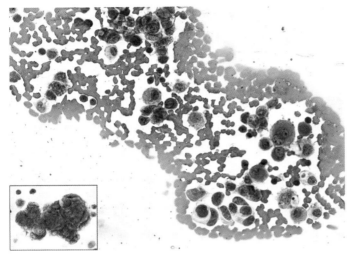

Figure 5.12 Metastatic neuroendocrine carcinoma. Malignant cells are easily discernible from the benign mesothelial cells. Note the characteristic hyperchromatic nuclei with salt and pepper chromatin, nuclear molding and scant cytoplasm. **Inset**: Malignant cells were positive for synaptophysin. ×40.

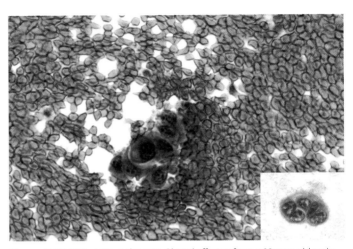

Figure 5.13 Metastatic melanoma. Pleural effusion from a 92-year-old male with a history of treated scalp melanoma. Cellularity was low. Large atypical epithelioid cells with prominent nucleoli were present. Intranuclear cytoplasmic inclusions nor melanin pigment was identified. **Inset**: Malignant cells were positive for S100 but negative for other melanoma markers (HMB-45, Melan A). ×60.

tumors. Cohesive spheroidal groupings with a peripheral layer of flattened cells may also be noted (5). They are associated with specific chromosomal translocations t(11;22)(p13;q12) involving *EWSR1* and *WT1* genes that can be detected by molecular studies. Immunohistochemically, the tumor cells express cytokeratins and EMA (> 90 percent of cases), desmin (90 percent of cases), and variable neural markers (chromogranin, synaptophysin, and CD 56) (6).

Renal Cell Carcinoma

Clear cell carcinoma may present in effusions with cells containing clear cytoplasm or cytoplasm with multiple tiny vacuoles and nuclei with prominent nucleoli.

Melanoma

Malignant melanoma recurrences may rarely present with effusion as a primary finding. Melanomas are notorious for their ability to mimic a variety of neoplasms. Malignant cells often are epithelioid, present mostly as single large cells with eccentric nuclei containing prominent nucleoli and intranuclear cytoplasmic invaginations (Figure 5.13). The presence of melanin pigment is diagnostic, but should be differentiated from the more commonly encountered hemosiderin pigment.

Sarcoma

Sarcomas are rarely seen in effusions. When present, a history of the underlying sarcoma is available. They are easily diagnosed as malignant, although subtyping is rarely possible on morphology alone. Cytomorphology is characterized by sparse cellularity, cells with bizarre, large shapes present mostly singly (7) (Figure 5.14).

Primary – Malignant Mesothelioma

Malignant mesothelioma is an uncommon neoplasm with a poor prognosis. As such its diagnosis carries grave clinical and legal consequences. Until recently, effusion cytology was considered of limited usefulness for the diagnosis of mesothelioma (8). This was because the diagnosis of mesothelioma from small tissue biopsies relied heavily on the unequivocal presence of stromal invasion into fat and/or skeletal muscle. Recently, however, the International Mesothelioma Interest Group stated that the cytologic diagnosis of mesothelioma supported by ancillary tests was as reliable as a histologic diagnosis. This has also been endorsed by the International Academy of Cytopathology and the Papanicolaou Society of Pathoogy (9–11). They provided practical guidelines for the cytologic diagnosis of epithelioid and mixed mesotheliomas and recommended that cytology be considered as an accepted method for the diagnosis of mesothelioma. It is important to remember that sarcomatoid and desmoplastic mesotheliomas rarely shed diagnostic cells into the effusion and therefore cannot be diagnosed by cytology. Additionally, a proportion of epithelioid mesotheliomas is morphologically bland and lacks discernible cytologic features of malignancy. These cases would therefore constitute the inherent limitation of cytology and are responsible for the false negative diagnoses. The sensitivity of cytodiagnosis of malignant mesothelioma is reported to vary widely, from 32 to 76 percent (12–15) and is felt to be largely dependent on the experience of the cytopathologist. With the availability of ancillary studies, it is felt that when all of the cytological criteria for epithelioid malignant mesothelioma are fulfilled in an effusion fluid specimen, a diagnosis of malignant mesothelioma may be made at a high level of specificity. This should always be fully supported by careful clinical–pathologic and radiologic correlation to exclude other neoplasms that may mimic mesothelioma

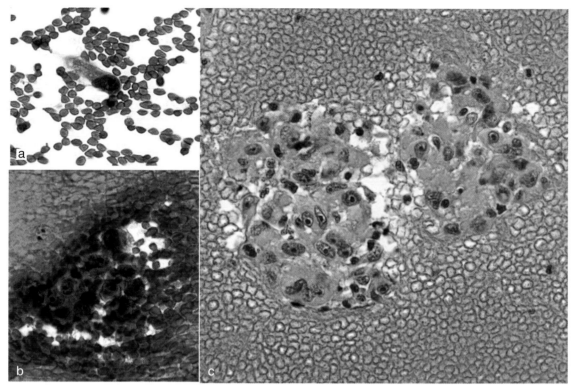

Figure 5.14 Metastatic sarcoma. Fifty-nine-year-old male with a history of pleomorphic undifferentiated sarcoma of the right thigh. Pleural effusion revealed (a) bizarre single spindle cell, an uncommon finding in effusions where cells tend to round up and are commonly seen as epithelioid cell clusters (b). (c) Cell block section showing similar findings. ×40.

(12,16). It has been determined that a positive pleural cytology is a reliable indicator of visceral pleural invasion (17).

The International Mesothelioma Interest Group (8) recommends that one of the following criteria be fulfilled for the diagnosis of mesothelioma:

- Indisputable malignant cells on cytomorphological criteria which demonstrate a mesothelial phenotype, which should be verified by ancillary techniques (Figure 5.15)
- Cytomorphological features which are not unequivocally malignant, but ancillary techniques confirm malignancy and a mesothelial phenotype.

Cytologic features indicative of a mesothelial phenotype are based upon the presence of:

1. Monotonous population of atypical cells present singly, in sheets, or as papillary clusters (Figure 5.16)
2. Cell clusters with knobby or scalloped borders (Figure 5.15a)
3. Smaller groups of cells revealing windows or slit-like spaces, cell-within-cell arrangements known commonly as "cell cannibalism" or cellular clasping and pinching
4. Individual cells with differential staining of the central and peripheral cytoplasm, a peripherally situated brush border identified on well-fixed specimens and macronucleoli.

(Note that the latter two characteristics are those of normal mesothelial cells. Thus, a highly cellular effusion with tissue fragments of mesothelial-appearing cells either bland or atypical should raise the suspicion for mesothelioma.)

Ancillary Studies

Mesothelioma vs. Adenocarcinoma

In order to establish a diagnosis of malignant mesothelioma, it is imperative to confirm the mesothelial origin of the malignant cells and to differentiate them from the more common metastatic adenocarcinomas. A panel of four immunostains are recommended – two to confirm mesothelial origin, and two to rule out metastatic adenocarcinoma (10). These stains are ideally performed on cell blocks prepared from the effusions and are similar to those used for histopathologic diagnosis. Many markers are available (Table 5.5) and can effectively distinguish mesotheliomas from metastatic adenocarcinoma with high sensitivity and specificity. Calretinin is considered to be the most useful and specific marker for mesotheliomas, provided cells show labeling of nuclei and cytoplasm (12). It is important to know that immunostains have certain cross-reactivities, e.g., calretinin is expressed in 15 percent of a subset of high-grade, *BRAC1*-associated breast carcinomas

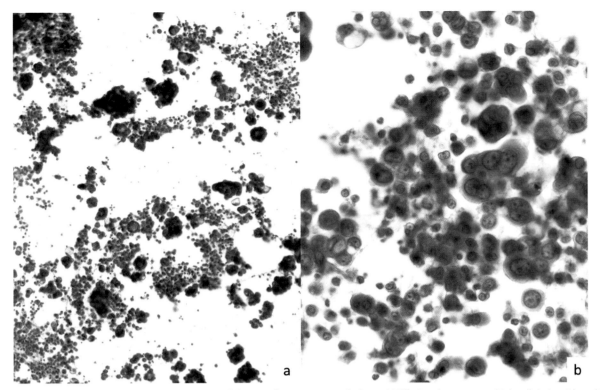

Figure 5.15 Malignant mesothelioma. Patient with history of recurrent mesothelioma. (a) Effusion demonstrates high cellularity with multiple three-dimensional clusters of epithelioid cells showing knobby outer borders. (b) Higher magnification reveals atypical cells. Immunostains demonstrated mesothelial immunophenotype (calretinin and Wilms' tumor-1 protein positivity). ×40.

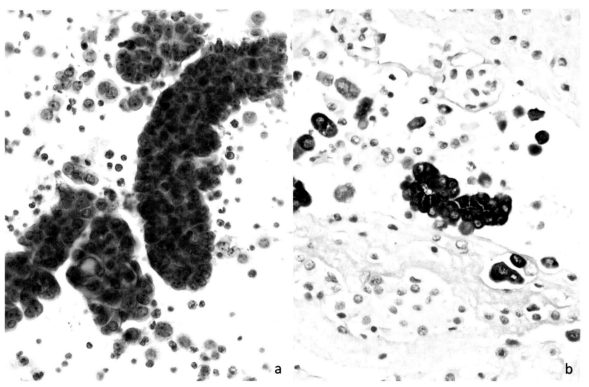

Figure 5.16 Malignant mesothelioma. Effusion with many three-dimensional clusters of atypical epithelioid cells. Some of the clusters demonstrate smooth outer borders. Immunostains show positivity for calretinin confirming mesothelial origin. ×40.

Table 5.7 Diagnostic panel for the differential diagnosis of malignant epithelioid cells in pleural effusions

Males	Females
Calretinin	Calretinin
TTF-1	TTF-1
PSA	ER
CDX-2	CA125

Panels provide 100 percent specificity and 50 percent and 77 percent sensitivity in male and female patients, respectively.

(18,19), while WT-1 is also expressed in ovarian carcinomas (20). Recently, claudin-4, a tight-junction-associated protein that is expressed in most epithelial cells and not in mesothelial cells, has been shown to distinguish adenocarcinoma from malignant mesothelioma with high sensitivity and specificity (21,22). Panels of immunostains are best selected based upon the differential diagnosis in individual cases derived from careful consideration of the clinical and radiologic information. In patients lacking a definitive history, broad panels may be used. Westfall et al. (23) developed such a panel using evidence-based methodology for pleural effusions with malignant epithelioid tumors (Table 5.7). The panel provides 100 percent specificity and 77 percent and 50 percent sensitivity for accurate diagnosis in female and male patients with malignant pleural effusions.

Reactive Mesothelial Cells vs. Adenocarcinoma

Reactive benign mesothelial cells in most instances show similar immunoreactivity as malignant mesothelial cells; hence, they may be differentiated from metastatic adenocarcinomas using panels similar to those used for differentiating malignant mesothelioma from metastatic adenocarcinoma.

Determination of Origin of Adenocarcinoma

A multitude of lineage-specific immunomarkers are now available that may be used for confirmation of the origin of metastatic malignancy (Table 5.6). The choice of the markers is left to individual laboratories and their familiarity/experience with the markers. Pancreatico-biliary carcinomas pose the greatest difficulty because they lack specific markers. Diagnosis is often made by exclusion of other tumor sites. In many cases a diagnosis just of metastatic carcinoma may be sufficient for patient care.

Reactive Mesothelial Cells vs. Malignant Mesothelioma

Differentiating reactive mesothelial cells from malignant mesothelioma is the most challenging task in the evaluation of effusion cytology. Formation of three-dimensional cell groups of variable sizes and shapes containing knobby or berry-like contours and the presence of cell-in-cell engulfment are more often observed in mesotheliomas. In contrast, reactive mesothelial cells are usually present as flat, monolayered sheets (24). However, considerable variability exists in the morphologic diagnosis of mesothelioma, with some studies reporting sensitivity values as low as 35 percent (15). It is well known that significant cytologic atypia may be present in reactive mesothelial cells while mesotheliomas may be monomorphic and bland-appearing, in which cases demonstration of tissue invasion is diagnostic (25). In recent years several immunostains have been investigated in an effort to resolve this issue. Epithelial membrane antigen (EMA), glucose transporter-1 (Glut-1), and desmin have been found to be most useful with high sensitivities and specificities (26,27). *BAP1* (*BRCA1*-associated protein 1) is another such marker that has recently been shown to be mutated in a subset of mesotheliomas. The presence of *BAP1* is detectable in the nuclei of normal mesothelial cells with immunohistochemistry. In contrast, nuclei of mesothelioma cells lose nuclear immunoreactivity for *BAP1*. *BAP1*, however, has low sensitivity for mesotheliomas, being reported in 15–83 percent of mesotheliomas (28–30) (Table 5.8). The use of panels may improve specificity. Additionally, homozygous deletion of p16 by fluorescent *in-situ* hybridization (FISH), when present, has been shown to be diagnostic of mesothelioma (31). It is one of the most common cytogenetic abnormalities reported in mesotheliomas and most specific. Initial studies show that the test can be reproducibly performed on effusion samples (32) and may be applied for the diagnosis of mesothelioma. The absence of the deletions, however, does not exclude mesothelioma.

Table 5.8 Immunostains useful in the distinction of reactive and malignant mesothelial cells in pleural effusions

Immunostain	Reactive mesothelial cells (% positive)	Mesothelioma (% positive)	Sensitivity (%)	Specificity (%)
Desmin ≥ 20%	84	6	84	94
EMA ≥ 20%	100	9	100	91
BAP1 positive	100	33	–	–
Glut-1 ≥ 20%	12	47	47	88
P53 ≥ 10%	2	47	47	98

Malignant Lymphoma/Leukemia

Lymphomas and leukemias cause effusions late in the course of disease. A history of malignant lymphoma is usually present in most cases, the exception being primary effusion lymphoma. These patients usually have a better prognosis than those with mesotheliomas or metastatic carcinomas. Small cleaved-cell lymphomas are the most common subtype encountered in effusions. Hodgkin's disease is rarely diagnosed in effusions. In most instances a diagnosis of involvement by the lymphomatous process is all that is required because effusions may be present in patients with lymphoma/leukemia in the absence of malignant cells.

Cytomorphology is characterized by the presence of a monomorphic population of single atypical cells. True tissue aggregates are not formed. Morphology varies based upon the subtype of lymphoma, the B-cell immunophenotype being the most common (33). The differential diagnosis includes inflammatory effusions with prominent lymphocytic infiltrate. Distinguishing features are the presence of a polymorphous population of lymphocytes, frequently trapped in a fibrinous exudate that is polyclonal with a predominance of T lymphocytes. Small-cell lymphomas are the most difficult to distinguish from reactive lymphocytic proliferations. Flow cytometry is easily performed on effusions not only for confirmation of the diagnosis of lymphoma but also its subtyping (34). Although intermediate and large-cell lymphomas are easily diagnosed as malignant, distinguishing them from carcinomas or melanomas may be problematic. In such cases a panel of immunostains including CD45 for lymphoma, pankeratin for carcinoma and melanoma-specific markers may be used (Figure 5.17).

Primary Effusion Lymphoma

Primary effusion lymphoma (PEL) is a human herpes virus 8 (HHV-8)-positive large B-cell neoplasm that presents as a pleural, peritoneal, or pericardial effusion with no detectable tumor elsewhere (Figure 5.17). They are rare lymphomas occurring mostly in immune-deficient individuals either due to human immunodeficiency virus infection or other conditions, such as solid-organ transplant recipients. PEL is an aggressive neoplasm with a poor prognosis (35,36). The cells show diverse morphologies, ranging from immunoblastic or plasmablastic

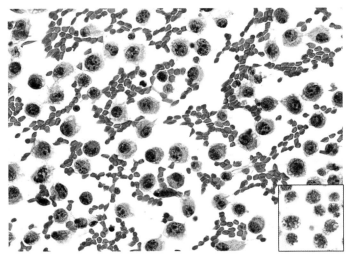

Figure 5.17 Primary effusion lymphoma (PEL). Clinical history is characteristically that of a young patient with AIDS presenting with pleural effusion. Large abnormal single cells with moderate cytoplasm raise the possibilities of PEL, Ki-1 lymphoma, and metastatic carcinoma. Immunostains are helpful for diagnosis. **Inset**: Positivity for HHV-8 is diagnostic for PEL. ×40.

to anaplastic. They have a distinct immunophenotype characterized by expression of CD45, lymphocyte activation antigens, and plasma cell-associated antigens (CD30, CD38, CD71, and CD138) and lack of B-cell markers (CD19 and CD79a). Diagnosis of PEL requires the demonstration of a B-cell genotype and HHV-8. In most cases, PEL cells also harbor the Epstein–Barr virus (EBV) genome (37–39).

PELs should be differentiated from HHV-8-negative, EBV-positive, body cavity-based lymphomas in immunocompetent patients with long-standing chronic diseases like tuberculous pleuritis, chronic liver disease, and various other conditions. Despite their morphological similarity, these lymphomas show high expression of B-cell markers (40,41). Correct diagnosis is essential to manage and predict the outcome of patients with PEL and related disorders (42).

Medico-legal Aspects

The etiologic relationship between asbestos and mesothelioma is well known and in spite of strict regulations banning the use of and the mining of asbestos, cases are still occurring and are being subjected to litigation. Cytopathologists should therefore be aware of this possibility when rendering this diagnosis.

References

1. Manosca F, Schinstine M, Fetsch PA, Sorbara L, Wilder AM, Brosky K, et al. Diagnostic effects of prolonged storage on fresh effusion samples. *Diagn Cytopathol.* 2007;35:6–11.

2. Moriarty AT, Schwartz MR, Ducatman BS, Booth CN, Haja J, Chakraborty S, et al. A liquid concept – do classic preparations of body cavity fluid perform differently than ThinPrep cases? Observations from the College of American Pathologists Interlaboratory Comparison Program in Nongynecologic Cytology. *Arch Pathol Lab Med.* 2008;132: 1716–18.

3. Hoda RS. Non-gynecologic cytology on liquid-based preparations: a morphologic review of facts and artifacts. *Diagn Cytopathol.* 2007;35:621–34.

4. Moriarty AT, Stastny J, Volk EE, Hughes JH, Miller TR, Wilbur DC. Fluids – good and bad actors: observations from the College of American Pathologists Interlaboratory Comparison Program in

Nongynecologic Cytology. *Arch Pathol Lab Med.* 2004;128:513–18.

5. Zhu H, McMeekin EM, Sturgis CD. Desmoplastic small round cell tumor, a "floating island" pattern in pleural fluid cytology: a case report and review of the literature. *Case Rep Pathol.* 2015;2015:676894.

6. Hassan I, Shyyan R, Donohue JH, Edmonson JH, Gunderson LL, Moir CR, et al. Intraabdominal desmoplastic small round cell tumors: a diagnostic and therapeutic challenge. *Cancer.* 2005;104:1264–70.

7. Abadi MA, Zakowski MF. Cytologic features of sarcomas in fluids. *Cancer.* 1998;84:71–76.

8. Husain AN, Colby TV, Ordonez NG, Allen TC, Attanoos RL, Beasley MB, et al. Guidelines for pathologic diagnosis of malignant mesothelioma: 2017 update of the consensus statement from the International Mesothelioma Interest Group. *Arch Pathol Lab Med.* 2017, Epub ahead of print.

9. Hjerpe A, Ascoli V, Bedrossian CW, Boon, ME, Creaney J, Davidson B, et al. Guidelines for the cytopathologic diagnosis of epithelioid and mixed-type malignant mesothelioma. Complementary statement from the International Mesothelioma Interest Group, also endorsed by the International Academy of Cytology and the Papanicolaou Society of Cytopathology. *Acta Cytol.* 2015;59:2–16.

10. Hjerpe A, Ascoli V, Bedrossian CW, Boon, ME, Creaney J, Davidson B, et al. Guidelines for the Cytopathologic Diagnosis of Epithelioid and Mixed-Type Malignant Mesothelioma: a secondary publication. *Cytopathology.* 2015;26:142–56.

11. Hjerpe A, Ascoli V, Bedrossian CW, Boon, ME, Creaney J, Davidson B, et al. Guidelines for the cytopathologic diagnosis of epithelioid and mixed-type malignant mesothelioma: Complementary Statement from the International Mesothelioma Interest Group, Also Endorsed by the International Academy of Cytology and the Papanicolaou Society of Cytopathology. *Diagn Cytopathol.* 2015;43:563–76.

12. Henderson DW, Reid G, Kao SC, Kao SC, van Zandwijk N, Klebe S. Challenges and controversies in the diagnosis of mesothelioma: Part 1.

Cytology-only diagnosis, biopsies, immunohistochemistry, discrimination between mesothelioma and reactive mesothelial hyperplasia, and biomarkers. *J Clin Pathol.* 2013;66: 847–53.

13. Paintal A, Raparia K, Zakowski MF, Nayar R. The diagnosis of malignant mesothelioma in effusion cytology: a reappraisal and results of a multi-institution survey. *Cancer Cytopathol.* 2013;121:703–07.

14. Rakha EA, Patil S, Abdulla K, Abdulkader M, Chaudry Z, Soomro IN. The sensitivity of cytologic evaluation of pleural fluid in the diagnosis of malignant mesothelioma. *Diagn Cytopathol.* 2010;38:874–79.

15. Renshaw AA, Dean BR, Antman KH, Antman KH, Sugarbaker DJ. The role of cytologic evaluation of pleural fluid in the diagnosis of malignant mesothelioma. *Chest.* 1997;111:106–09.

16. Bedrossian CW. An update on pleuro-pulmonary cytopathology: Part I: Cytological diagnosis of mesothelioma and molecular cytology of lung cancer with an historical perspective. *Diagn Cytopathol.* 2015;43:513–26.

17. Pinelli V, Laroumagne S, Sakr L, Marchetti GP, Tassi GF, Astoul P. Pleural fluid cytological yield and visceral pleural invasion in patients with epithelioid malignant pleural mesothelioma. *J Thorac Oncol.* 2012;7:595–98.

18. Taliano RJ, Lu S, Singh K, Mangray S, Tavares R, Noble L, et al. Calretinin expression in high-grade invasive ductal carcinoma of the breast is associated with basal-like subtype and unfavorable prognosis. *Hum Pathol.* 2013;44:2743–50.

19. Duhig EE, Kalpakos L, Yang IA, Clarke BE. Mesothelial markers in high-grade breast carcinoma. *Histopathology.* 2011;59:957–64.

20. Hecht JL, Lee BH, Pinkus JL, Pinkus GS. The value of Wilms tumor susceptibility gene 1 in cytologic preparations as a marker for malignant mesothelioma. *Cancer.* 2002;96:105–09.

21. Jo VY, Cibas ES, Pinkus GS. Claudin-4 immunohistochemistry is highly effective in distinguishing adenocarcinoma from malignant mesothelioma in effusion cytology. *Cancer Cytopathol.* 2014;122:299–306.

22. Afshar-Moghaddam N, Heidarpour M, Dashti S. Diagnostic value of claudin-4 marker in pleural and peritoneal effusion cytology: does it differentiate between metastatic adenocarcinoma and reactive mesothelial cells? *Adv Biomed Res.* 2014;3:161.

23. Westfall DE, Fan X, Marchevsky AM. Evidence-based guidelines to optimize the selection of antibody panels in cytopathology: pleural effusions with malignant epithelioid cells. *Diagn Cytopathol.* 2010;38:9–14.

24. Cakir E, Demirag F, Aydin M, Unsal E. Cytopathologic differential diagnosis of malignant mesothelioma, adenocarcinoma and reactive mesothelial cells: a logistic regression analysis. *Diagn Cytopathol.* 2009;37:4–10.

25. Churg A, Colby TV, Cagle P, Corson J, Gibbs AR, Gilks B, et al. The separation of benign and malignant mesothelial proliferations. *Am J Surg Pathol.* 2000;24:1183–200.

26. Hasteh F, Lin GY, Weidner N, Michael CW. The use of immunohistochemistry to distinguish reactive mesothelial cells from malignant mesothelioma in cytologic effusions. *Cancer Cytopathol.* 2010;118:90–96.

27. Kuperman M, Florence RR, Pantanowitz L, Visintainer PF, Cibas ES, Otis CN. Distinguishing benign from malignant mesothelial cells in effusions by Glut-1, EMA, and Desmin expression: an evidence-based approach. *Diagn Cytopathol.* 2013;41:131–40.

28. Hwang HC, Sheffield BS, Rodriguez S, Thompson K, Tse CH, Gown AM, et al. Utility of BAP1 immunohistochemistry and p16 (CDKN2A) FISH in the diagnosis of malignant mesothelioma in effusion cytology specimens. *Am J Surg Pathol.* 2016;40:120–26.

29. Sheffield BS, Hwang HC, Lee AF, Thompson K, Rodriguez S, Tse CH, et al. BAP1 immunohistochemistry and p16 FISH to separate benign from malignant mesothelial proliferations. *Am J Surg Pathol.* 2015;39:977–82.

30. Churg A, Sheffield BS, Galateau-Sallé F. New markers for separating benign from malignant mesothelial proliferations: are we there yet? *Arch Pathol Lab Med.* 2016;140:318–21.

31. Ito T, Hamasaki M, Matsumoto S, Hiroshima K, Tsujimura T, Kawai T,

et al. p16/CDKN2A FISH in differentiation of diffuse malignant peritoneal mesothelioma from mesothelial hyperplasia and epithelial ovarian cancer. *Am J Clin Pathol.* 2015;143:830–38.

32. Hida T, Matsumoto S, Hamasaki M, Kawahara K, Tsujimura T, Hiroshima K, et al. Deletion status of p16 in effusion smear preparation correlates with that of underlying malignant pleural mesothelioma tissue. *Cancer Sci.* 2015;106:1635–41.

33. Das DK, Al-Juwaiser A, George SS, Francis IM, Sathar SS, Sheikh ZA, et al. Cytomorphological and immunocytochemical study of non-Hodgkin's lymphoma in pleural effusion and ascitic fluid. *Cytopathology.* 2007;18:157–67.

34. Bangerter M, Hildebrand A, Griesshammer M. Combined cytomorphologic and immunophenotypic analysis in the diagnostic workup of lymphomatous effusions. *Acta Cytol.* 2001;45:307–12.

35. Pinzone MR, Berretta M, Cacopardo B, Nunnari G. Epstein–Barr virus- and Kaposi sarcoma-associated herpesvirus-related malignancies in the setting of human immunodeficiency virus infection. *Semin Oncol.* 2015;42:258–71.

36. Jones D, Ballestas ME, Kaye KM, Gulizia JM, Winters GL, Fletcher J, et al. Primary-effusion lymphoma and Kaposi's sarcoma in a cardiac-transplant recipient. *N Engl J Med.* 1998;339:444–49.

37. Cesarman E, Nador RG, Aozasa K, Delsol G, Said JW, Knowles DM. Kaposi's sarcoma-associated herpesvirus in non-AIDS related lymphomas occurring in body cavities. *Am J Pathol.* 1996;149:53–57.

38. Nador RG, Cesarman E, Chadburn A, Dawson DB, Ansari MQ, Said J, et al. Primary effusion lymphoma: a distinct clinicopathologic entity associated with the Kaposi's sarcoma-associated herpes virus. *Blood.* 1996;88:645–56.

39. Matolcsy A, Nádor RG, Cesarman E, Knowles DM. Immunoglobulin VH gene mutational analysis suggests that primary effusion lymphomas derive from different stages of B cell maturation. *Am J Pathol.* 1998;153:1609–14.

40. Wu W, Youm W, Rezk SA, Zhao X. Human herpesvirus 8-unrelated primary effusion lymphoma-like lymphoma: report of a rare case and review of 54 cases in the literature. *Am J Clin Pathol.* 2013;140:258–73.

41. Xiao J, Selvaggi SM, Leith CP, Fitzgerald SA, Stewart J 3rd. Kaposi sarcoma herpesvirus/human herpesvirus-8-negative effusion-based lymphoma: report of 3 cases and review of the literature. *Cancer Cytopathol.* 2013;121:661–69.

42. Klepfish A, Zuckermann B, Schattner A. Primary effusion lymphoma in the absence of HIV infection–clinical presentation and management. *Q J Med.* 2015;108:481–88.

Chapter 6

Surgical Pathology of Non-neoplastic Conditions of the Pleura, Pericardium, and Peritoneum

A. Valeria Arrossi and Fadi W. Abdul-Karim

The serosal membranes can be involved with a large variety of non-neoplastic conditions listed in Table 6.1. As this volume is primarily intended to review in detail the pathology of malignant mesothelioma and other neoplasms involving the pleura, peritoneum, and other serosal membranes, this chapter will only provide a brief description of the pathology of the spectrum of non-neoplastic conditions than can involve the serosal membranes.

Acute and Chronic Serositis

The serosal membranes, visceral and parietal linings of the pericardial, pleural, and peritoneal cavities share similar histologic and anatomic compartments. As described in more detail in Chapter 1, a surface layer of endothelioid polygonal mesothelial cells covers a thin layer of fibroconnective tissue, normally less than a few millimeters thick. The submesothelial stroma varies from loose fibrous tissue to dense fibroelastotic tissue and the architectural organization of this collagenous and elastic association varies according to site.

Serosal membranes can become inflamed as a result of underlying pulmonary disorders, such as infectious pneumonia, infarcts, abscesses, systemic disorders such as collagen vascular diseases, uremia, diffuse systemic infections or other etiologies listed in Table 6.2. These conditions may result in serositis that, irrespective of cavity, manifests with similar histopathologic features. Serositis are usually classified by their clinical course and pathologic features into acute and chronic and by their location as pleuritis, peritonitis, and pericarditis.

Acute serositis or fibrinous serositis is characterized by the presence of extensive fibrinous exudates, marked congestion, neovascularization, variable infiltration by neutrophils and eosinophils and reactive mesothelial hyperplasia that may occasionally exhibit nuclear atypia, mitoses and rarely atypical mitoses (Figure 6.1). As the process becomes chronic, the neutrophilic infiltrates are progressively replaced by mononuclear cells, and fibrosis (Figure 6.2). Within the fibrotic pleura the proliferating reactive mesothelial cells exhibit a zonation effect, which is described in more detail in the section on reactive and atypical mesothelial hyperplasia (Figure 6.3).

Table 6.1 Non-neoplastic conditions of the serosal membranes

A. Acute and chronic serositis
  Pleuritis
  Pericarditis
  Peritonitis
  Others

B. Other non-neoplastic lesions of the pleura
  Pneumothorax
  Reactive and atypical reactive mesothelial hyperplasia
  Parietal pleural plaques
  Rounded atelectasis
  Amyloidosis

C. Other non-neoplastic lesions of the pericardium and peritoneum
  Mesothelial inclusion cysts
  Endometriosis and endosalpingiosis
  Deciduosis
  Trophoblastic implants
  Walthard rests
  Splenosis
  Melanosis peritonei
  Gliomatosis peritonei
  Omental–mesenteric myxoid hamartoma

D. Tumor-like conditions of the serosal membranes
  Calcifying pseudotumor
  Others

Table 6.2 Etiology of acute and chronic serositis

Infectious
  Bacterial
  Viral
  Fungi
  Parasites

Autoimmune
  Systemic lupus erythematosus
  Rheumatoid disease
  Acute rheumatism
  Endocrinopathies

Foreign body granulomatous
  Talc (Mg silicate)
  Starch (Mg oxide)
  Particulate (cellulose, plastic)

Drug-induced

Allergic
  Eosinophilic serositis
  Continuous ambulatory peritoneal dialysis (CAPD)*

Metabolic
  Uremic serositis
  Cholesterol serositis

Genetic
  Recurrent hereditary polyserositis

Physical
  Peritoneal dialysate*

* Only peritoneal surface involvement.

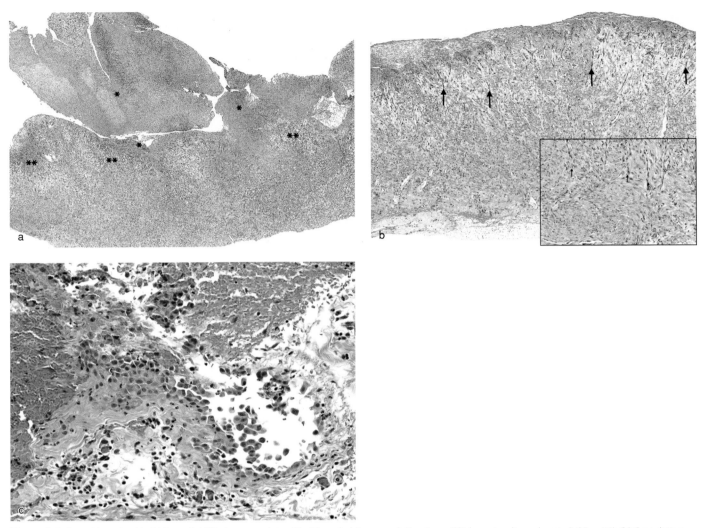

Figure 6.1 Organizing pleuritis. (a) Superficial fibrinous exudates (*) with underlying granulation tissue (**), hematoxylin and eosin (H&E, ×2.3). (b) Granulation tissue with capillaries perpendicular to the serosal surface (arrows) (H&E, ×4.6) (**Inset**: H&E, ×16.2). (c) Mesothelial hyperplasia with reactive atypia (H&E, ×20).

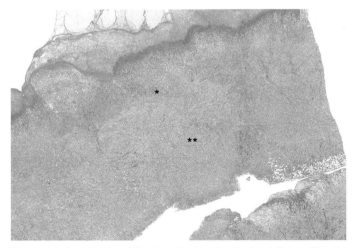

Figure 6.2 Organizing and fibrosing pleuritis. Mononuclear infiltrates (*) and fibrosis (**) replace granulation tissue (H&E, ×0.8).

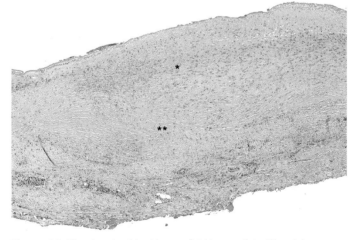

Figure 6.3 Fibrosing pleuritis with superficial hypercellular (*) and deep hypocellular (**) areas (H&E, ×4.2).

Infectious, Hemorrhagic, and Granulomatous Pleuritis

Pleuritis of infectious etiology is usually secondary to a pulmonary infection and is clinically diagnosed as a parapneumonic pleurisy. Less commonly, the other sources from the chest, such as vertebral osteomyelitis or abdominal cavity, contribute to pleural infection. The causative agent as well as the morbidity and mortality vary according to clinical background, i.e., community- or hospital-acquired pneumonia, and immune-competent or immunocompromised patient. *Streptococcus* milleri group is usually the most frequent organism isolated in community-acquired pneumonia (1), while staphylococcal infection (including methicillin-resistant *Staphylococcus aureus*), *Enterococcus* and Enterobacteriaceae are more common in hospital-acquired pneumonia (2). Anaerobic organisms such as *Fusobacterium* and *Actinomyces* sp. are present in up to 25 percent of pleural infections associated with community-acquired pneumonia (2,3). Viruses, including influenza, parainfluenza, coxsackievirus and respiratory syncytial virus, can lead to pleural disease, most commonly pleural effusions in the immunocompromised patient (4). Fungal infections may involve the pleura. In immunocompetent patients, Coccidioidomycosis, blastomycosis and histoplasmosis involve the pleural surface in up to 10 percent of cases of pulmonary infection, respectively. In these cases, the pleura shows histologic features that resemble those in the lung, with the characteristic necrotizing granulomas (Figure 6.4). Pleural aspergillosis is seen in immunocompetent patients usually associated with the presence of bronchopleural fistula, and in immunocompromised patients with invasive aspergillosis (Figure 6.5). Unusual bacterial infections include *Rickettsia*, *Coxiella*, and *Bacillus anthracis* (5). *Rickettsia* infections manifest with hemorrhagic pleuritis. The presence of serosanguineous inflammatory pleural fluid should be distinguished from hemorrhagic diatheses and neoplastic pleural involvement.

Parapneumonic effusions/pleurisy develop through three main stages. (1) The acute or exudative stage (simple parapneumonic effusion): the pleural cavity contains a serous pleural effusion with low leukocytes ($< 10,000/l$), low LDH (<1000 UI/l) and normal glucose (> 60 mg/dl) and pH (> 7.30), without isolated microorganisms. (2) Fibrinopurulent or transitional stage (complicated parapneumonic effusion/empyema): fibrinoid exudates and inflammation occur in the pleural tissue (Figure 6.1). This usually occurs in patients who are not receiving antibiotics or if the antibiotic therapy is not adequate. The pleural fluid shows numerous leukocytes, bacterial organisms and cellular debris, low glucose (< 40 mg/dl) and pH (< 7.20) and elevated LDH > 1000 UI/l. (3) The chronic or organizing stage: the pleural tissue is replaced by granulation tissue and fibrosis, which can be prominent and result in fibrothorax and entrapped lung complications (Figure 6.3).

Long-term complications of infectious pleuritis include bronchopleural fistula or empyema necessitatis (pleurocutaneous fistula).

Mycobacterial Granulomatous Pleuritis

Mycobacterium tuberculosis and other mycobacterial infections can involve the pleura in two forms: (1) self-limited pleural effusion that develops in primary disease or less frequently reactivation, and (2) rupture of a tuberculous cavity into the pleural space. Pleural exudates from these cases contain high levels of protein and numerous lymphocytes that usually enter the pleural space through a microscopic ruptured focus of lung disease.

Histopathologically, necrotizing granulomatous pleuritis occurs as a result of a hypersensitive reaction type IV to *Mycobacteria* antigens. Epithelioid granulomas show variable necrosis and may be associated with round cell inflammatory infiltrates, neovascularization, fibrosis, and reactive mesothelial hyperplasia. Acid-fast organisms are usually found with Ziehl Neelsen or Fite stains (Figure 6.6).

Other Causes of Serositis: Uremia, Cholesterolosis, and Hereditary Autoinflammatory Diseases

Uremic serositis develops in patients with severe renal insufficiency as a result of serosal irritation caused by retention of nitrogenous waste products. All serosal membranes can be affected to a similar degree, but uremic pericarditis is associated with the greatest morbidity and mortality. The pleura, pericardium, and peritoneum in uremia show the same histopathologic features of a fibrinous pleuritis. Distinctive cytoplasmic inclusions may be observed with electron microscopy studies, which have been implicated in the pathogenesis of serositis in uremic states (6).

Chylothorax and pseudochylothorax share the milky, turbid appearance characteristic of the pleural effusion as a result of its high lipid content. However, they represent separate disease processes. The pleural fluid in chylothorax contains lymphatic fluid enriched in lymphocytes and occurs as a result of chyle leak from the thoracic duct or its tributaries due to traumatic injury or non-traumatic causes, including primary and secondary lymphangiectasis (7,8). Generalized lymphangiectasis and pulmonary lymphangiectasis usually occur in children but can also develop in the adult population (7,9) (Figure 6.7). In contrast, chyliform effusion or pseudochylothorax is an unusual form of pleural effusion due to venous outflow obstruction that results in accumulation of cholesterol or lecithin–globulin complexes in patients with chronic inflammatory conditions such as tuberculosis or rheumatoid arthritis. It is usually a unilateral process and unlike chylothorax due to the accumulation of cholesterol or lecithin–globulin complexes (8,10). Patients can develop loculated effusions that require decortication, pleurectomy, pleurodesis, and/or thoracoscopic drainage. The histologic findings vary according to the underlying disease. Chronic fibrosing pleuritis with cholesterol crystals and cholesterol granulomas are commonly seen (10).

Hereditary autoinflammatory diseases can involve the serosal membranes. Familial Mediterranean fever (recurrent

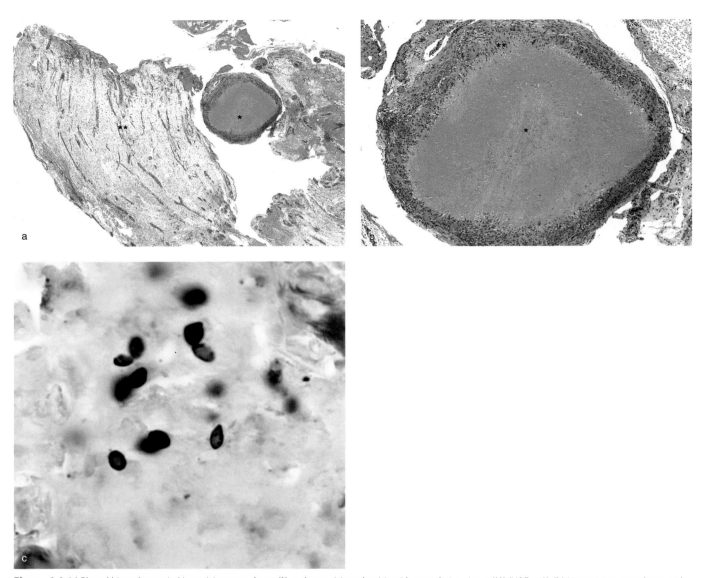

Figure 6.4 (a) Pleural histoplasmosis. Necrotizing granuloma (*) and organizing pleuritis with granulation tissue (**) (H&E, ×2). (b) Necrotizing granuloma with necrotic center (*) with peripheral palisading epithelioid histiocytes with multinucleated giant cells (**) (×7.2). (c) Pleural histoplasmosis. Fungal yeasts with narrow budding characteristic of *Histoplasma* sp. (Gomori methenamine silver, ×40).

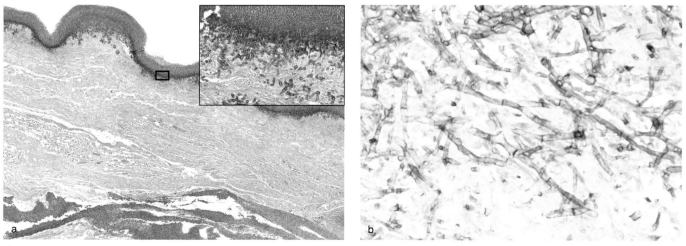

Figure 6.5 Invasive aspergillosis. (a) *Aspergillus* fungi covering necrotic pleura (H&E, ×2.6). **Inset**: Fungal hyphae (H&E, ×40). (b) Septate fungal hyphae with parallel walls and acute angle branching (Gomori methenamine silver, ×60).

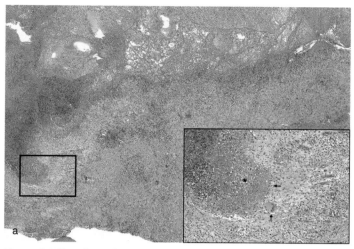

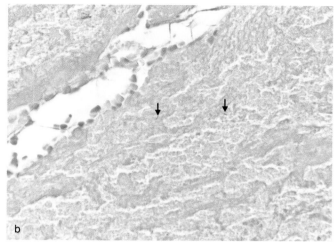

Figure 6.6 Pleural mycobacterial infection. (a) Organizing pleuritis with granulomatous inflammation (H&E, ×1.2). **Inset**: Necrotizing granuloma with epithelioid histiocytes and multinucleated giant cells (H&E, ×10). (b) Acid-fast bacilli (arrows) (Ziehl Neelsen, ×60).

hereditary polyserositis) is a genetic disorder that manifests with recurrent episodes of mostly fever, panserositis, and synovitis. The peritoneum is the most severely affected serosa and abdominal attacks and ascites are not uncommon (11). The pleura is involved in 40 percent of the cases, while the pericardium is rarely involved (12). The diagnosis of familial Mediterranean fever is clinical and tissue is seldom evaluated. In rare cases, samples are taken during episodes of acute abdominal attack which show non-specific acute fibrino-inflammatory exudates, edema, and congestion (6).

Other Non-neoplastic Lesions of the Pleura

Pneumothorax

Pneumothorax refers to the presence of air within the pleural space. It can be spontaneous, when an unexpected escape of air from the lung into the pleural space occurs, secondary to trauma or the various conditions listed in Table 6.3 (13,14).

Spontaneous primary pneumothorax occurs in healthy individuals without the presence of apparent pulmonary disorder. Spontaneous pneumothorax can be divided into primary, when there is no visible underlying lung condition, or secondary, when an underlying pulmonary disorder is present. Male sex and cigarette smoking are risk factors for the development of primary spontaneous pneumothorax. The rupture of a subpleural bleb or a bulla has been postulated as the mechanism of spontaneous pneumothorax. However, ultrastructural examination of the resected bullae in cases of spontaneous pneumothorax revealed that there is sparsity, or total absence of mesothelial cells of the exterior surface of the bulla, with the

Table 6.3 Etiologic classification of pneumothorax

Spontaneous pneumothorax
  Primary
  Secondary

Secondary in patients with previously known pulmonary disease
  Chronic obstructive pulmonary disease
  Cystic fibrosis
  Asthma
  Endometriosis (catamenial pneumothorax)
  Cannabis
  Birt–Hogg–Dubé
  Histiocytosis (Erdheim Chester, Langerhans's cell histiocytosis)
  Inherited disorders of collagen synthesis
  Lymphangioleiomyomatosis
  Sarcoidosis
  Pneumonia (*Pneumocystis jiroveci* pneumonia, tuberculosis, aspergillosis, other)
  Malignancy
  Bronchogenic carcinoma
  Metastatic carcinoma
  Trauma
    Iatrogenic
      Transthoracic or transbronchial lung biopsy
      Central venous catheterization
      Supraclavicular nerve block

Figure 6.7 Dilated lymphatic channels in the pleura in a patient with pulmonary lymphangiectasis (H&E, ×10). **Inset**: Lymphatic endothelial layer highlighted with D2–40 (podoplanin) immunostain (D2–40, ×12.8).

underlying collagen fibers consequently becoming "naked," with small pores or crevices of several microns. This observation introduced the theory of "pleural porosity" allowing air leakage into the pleural space (14,15). Furthermore, fluorescein-enhanced autofluorescence thoracoscopy studies revealed surface abnormal fluorescence even in regions that appeared normal with white light thoracoscopy, supporting the hypothesis of pleural leakage not associated with bullae or blebs (16). It is now postulated that spontaneous pneumothorax is the result of a multifactorial process, and the presence of bullae, blebs, and pleural porosity are predisposing factors that lead to spontaneous pneumothorax when combined with other contributing factors, such as but not limited to distal airway inflammation, anatomical abnormalities of the bronchial tree, ectomorphic physiognomy with more negative intrapleural pressures and apical ischaemia at the apices, low body mass index and caloric restriction, and abnormal connective tissue (14).

Patients with spontaneous pneumothorax that do not resolve after chest tube insertion or develop recurrent pneumothorax are often treated with lung wedge resections. Histopathologically, the pleura from biopsies or decortication specimens show fibrinous pleuritis with variable infiltrates by eosinophils in cases of recent pneumothorax, while fibrosis with reactive mesothelial hyperplasia and variable degrees of inflammation are seen in cases with chronic disease. Wedge biopsies from patients with recurrent pneumothorax show pleural blebs (intrapleural, unlined collections of air with histiocytic and/or multinucleated giant cell reaction), subpleural distal acinar (paraseptal) emphysema, atelectasis, collagenous fibrosis, varying degrees of chronic mononuclear inflammation, alveolar macrophages with anthracotic pigment or hemosiderin pigment, and varying degrees of chronic airway inflammation (15,17).

Two characteristic findings associated with pneumothorax are reactive eosinophilic pleuritis and pneumothorax-associated fibroblastic lesion (PAFL).

Reactive Eosinophilic Pleuritis

Reactive eosinophilic pleuritis is a non-specific inflammatory reaction commonly observed in specimens from patients with pneumothorax, in particular those that exhibit bulla and/or blebs. The pleura shows reactive hyperplastic mesothelial cells and inflammatory infiltrates consisting of numerous eosinophils, mononuclear cells, and occasional multinucleated giant cells (Figure 6.8) (18,19). Eosinophilic pleuritis may also be encountered secondary to fungal infections such as coccidioidomycosis, parasitic infections, or drug reactions (20–25).

Pneumothorax-associated Fibroblastic Lesion

PAFL is a recently described unique lesion characterized by the development of spontaneous pneumothorax in mostly male patients younger than 25 years of age. The pleura shows a pattern of temporally heterogeneous fibrosis, with dense collagenous fibrosis, and islands of young fibroblastic foci within a myxoid stroma present at the pleural–parenchymal interface or

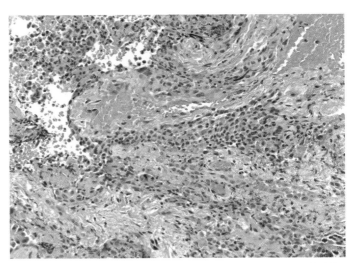

Figure 6.8 Eosinophilic pleuritis. The pleura shows hyperplastic mesothelial cells with numerous histiocytes and eosinophils (H&E, ×20).

leading edge (Figure 6.9). The lesions are often wedge-shaped with the broad base at the pleural surface, and are usually multifocal, extending varying lengths along the pleural surface with intervening normal pleura. The band of fibrosis in closest proximity to the pulmonary parenchyma often shows parallel nuclear orientation of the collagen bands and the nuclei to the border with the adjacent parenchyma. The fibrosis may extend superficially into the lung parenchyma, but usually not more than a few millimeters tracking along the alveolar or interlobular septa. Intrapleural cysts lined by reactive type II pneumocytes or reactive mesothelial cells can be observed. Given the presence of fibroblastic foci, the differential diagnoses include usual interstitial pneumonia or organizing pneumonia in the setting of chronic obstructive pulmonary disease with emphysema. The most distinguishing feature for the diagnosis of PAFL is the wedge configuration of the lesion (26,27) (Figure 6.9).

Causes of Secondary Pneumothorax

It is beyond the scope of this chapter to discuss in detail the various causes of secondary pneumothorax listed in Table 6.3. Pathologic findings of Birt–Hogg–Dubé syndrome (28), bronchogenic carcinoma, Erdheim Chester disease, or cannabis smoking (27) may rarely and unexpectedly be encountered in pleural or lung specimens resected from patients with spontaneous or secondary pneumothorax.

Catamenial Pneumothorax

Catamenial pneumothorax refers to the occurrence of spontaneous pneumothorax in association with menstruation in patients with pleural and/or diaphragmatic endometriosis (29–31). Pleural endometriosis can involve either the parietal or visceral pleura with a nodular, nodulocystic or cystic pattern (31). The pleura or subpleural connective tissue shows the classical findings of endometriosis: endometrial proliferative glands, endometrial stroma, and hemosiderin-laden macrophages, associated with inflammatory cells. The ectopic

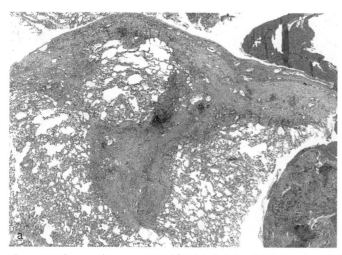
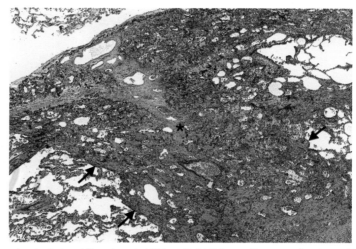

Figure 6.9 Pneumothorax-associated fibroblastic lesion. (a) Wedge-shaped pleural and subpleural fibroelastosis (H&E, ×1.3). (b) Collagen fibrosis is yellow (asterisk) and fibroblastic foci are green/blue (arrows) with Movat stains (Movat, ×3.3).

endometrial glands may show müllerian metaplastic changes and the stroma may have a pseudodecidualized or edematous appearance. Stromal spindle cells without glandular elements may also be seen, and sometimes may be focal, sometimes requiring deeper levels to achieve the diagnosis (30,31). The mesothelial lining shows reactive changes, or may be absent and replaced by fibrin. Differential diagnoses include metastatic adenocarcinoma, mesothelial hyperplasia, and mesothelioma (Figure 6.10) (30).

Reactive and Atypical Reactive Mesothelial Hyperplasia

The mesothelial cells covering the serosal membranes are flat, usually inconspicuous and normally not seen by light microscopy. The mesothelial cells lay over the submesothelial layer, rich in fibroblasts, collagen, and elastin. Regardless of the injurious factor, the mesothelial and submesothelial cellular elements of the serous membranes have the capacity to proliferate and become hyperplastic in reactive processes with different degrees of complexity from simple to florid. Simple hyperplasia consists of a monolayer of mesothelial cells that adopt cuboidal morphology, with uniform round nuclei. Florid hyperplasia, a more complex proliferation of mesothelial cells that may also show reactive atypia ("atypical" mesothelial hyperplasia), may occur particularly in the peritoneum in association with gynecologic diseases such as endometriosis, and may create a diagnostic challenge because the presence of tubules and/or papillary structures may be prominent and can mimic epithelioid malignant mesothelioma (32–35).

While invasion of the adjacent tissues by the mesothelial cells is the gold standard for the diagnosis of malignancy, this may not be as evident, especially in small samples. Even though the cellular atypia of proliferating cells in mesothelial hyperplasia many times contrast with the rather bland and monomorphous cells that usually characterize malignant mesotheliomas,

unless the nuclei of the mesothelial cells show definitive features of high-grade malignancy and thus the diagnosis of malignancy is evident, there are no cytomorphologic features that help in differentiating benign from malignant mesothelial proliferations. In this setting, the architectural arrangement may be the base of this distinction.

In benign epithelioid mesothelial proliferations, the papillae present are simple and usually lack complex fibrovascular cores, mainly forming micropapillae, i.e., round tufts of piled up epithelial cells (Figure 6.11). The tubules are usually small and round. Tubulo-papillary structures are not usually observed in benign mesothelial proliferations, and their presence favors a malignant process. The tubules and papillae are mostly present in the most superficial layers of the pleura and the intervening stroma is usually edematous, rich in myofibroblasts, with neo-formed vessels with plump endothelial cells and inflammatory cells, characteristic of repairing-type granulation tissue. At the deep level, entrapped tubules and papillae may be present in benign mesothelial proliferations, representing remnants of a former mesothelial surface. The entrapped epithelium may be differentiated from invasion by the rather linear pattern that parallels the serosal surface, usually accompanied by collagenous fibrosis. Entrapment of mesothelial cells occurs usually in cases of chronic pleuritis, and results from repetitive injury to the pleural surface that generates an acute reaction over repairing tissue in multiple events/layers.

In contrast, malignant epithelioid mesothelial proliferations are characterized architecturally by the presence of irregular, random arrangements of glands, tubules, papillae, sheets and tubulo-papillary structures that involve any level of the serosal surface (superficial, mid, and/or deep tissues), without the linear pattern seen in entrapped reactive mesothelial cells. Desmoplastic stroma is present in between the malignant mesothelial nests. Desmoplastic stroma is seen as dense irregular fibrosis with vessels arranged in a haphazard pattern. The so-called "expansile stromal nodules" is a useful feature for the

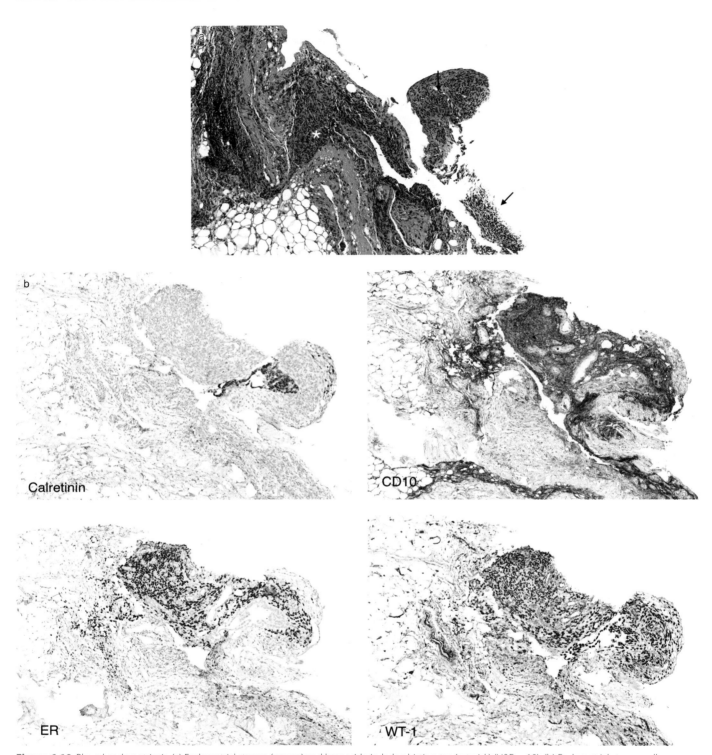

Figure 6.10 Pleural endometriosis. (a) Endometrial stroma (arrows) and hemosiderin-laden histiocytes (asterisk) (H&E, ×10). (b) Endometrial stroma cells immunoreactive to CD10, estrogen receptors and WT-1 and mesothelial cells highlighted with calretinin and WT-1 (calretinin, CD10, estrogen receptors (ER) and WT-1, ×10).

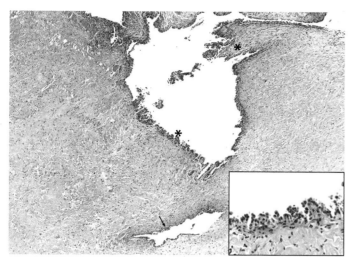

Figure 6.11 Benign mesothelial hyperplasia with entrapped mesothelial cells (arrow) and simple papillae (asterisk) (H&E, ×4). **Inset**: Mesothelial cells show moderately atypical pleomorphic nuclei (H&E, ×40).

diagnosis of malignancy and is recognized by the presence of an oval/round configuration of desmoplastic stroma and associated mesothelial cells. Involvement of the adjacent fibroadipose tissue in an expansile pattern by these nodules may be, particularly in small biopsy samples, the only indirect manifestation of invasion, without the infiltrative growth of mesothelial cells into the adjacent tissues.

The submesothelial component of the serosal membranes can also proliferate, especially in cases of organizing and fibrosing pleuritis, and can cause diagnostic difficulty in the distinction from sarcomatoid or desmoplastic mesothelioma. One of the most important features in this distinction is the so-called "zonation," which refers to a gradation or "dégradé" of the cellular density of the spindle cells throughout the thickness of the serosal membrane, showing a more cellular surface to less cellular deep tissues. Neo-formed vessels with plump endothelial

cells cross these fascicles of spindle cells perpendicularly to the serosal membrane. The vessels run from the deep tissues to the superficial layers, with a parallel arrangement, perpendicular to the serosal surface (Figure 6.1b). Inflammatory cells are usually present throughout the thickness; however, they may be inconspicuous. While immunohistochemical stains for mesothelial markers do not differentiate benign from malignant mesothelial proliferations, broad-spectrum cytokeratins are helpful as they highlight the zonation effect of the submesothelial myofibroblasts in reactive processes (Figure 6.12).

Features of malignancy in serosal spindle cell proliferations that lack unequivocal invasion include lack of zonation, and presence of stromal expansile nodules, fascicle formation, inconspicuous capillaries, haphazard or patternless arrangement of the spindle cells, and bland necrosis (Figure 6.13).

Immunohistochemistry, fluorescent *in-situ* hybridization (FISH) and molecular studies can be very helpful for the differential diagnosis between benign and malignant mesothelial proliferations. Immunohistochemistry showing the loss of BAP-1 immunoreactivity and the demonstration by FISH of p16 homozygous loss in tumor cells are the most useful tests to support malignancy. These tests are close to 100 percent specific for the diagnosis of malignancy; however, they have somewhat limited sensitivity as they mark only approximately 58 percent of cases irrespective of site and morphology, but mark 78 percent of pleural epithelioid mesotheliomas (36–45).

A more comprehensive discussion of the various markers that can assist in the distinguishing of benign atypical mesothelial proliferations from malignant mesothelioma is provided in Chapters 10 and 11 of this volume.

Parietal Pleural Plaques

Pleural plaques are discrete and localized areas of pleural thickening that are often calcified. Although pleural plaques are associated with exposure to above background levels of asbestos, they are not pathognomonic for high exposure and can develop

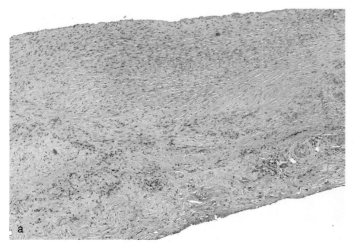
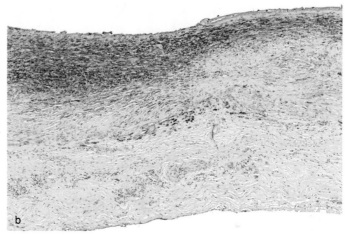

Figure 6.12 Chronic pleuritis with reactive mesothelial mesenchymal hyperplasia. (a) Zonation demonstrated by superficial hypercellular and deeper hypocellular areas (H&E, ×6.2). (b) Zonation is appreciated with keratin stains, low-molecular weight cytokeratin (CAM 5.2, ×4.2).

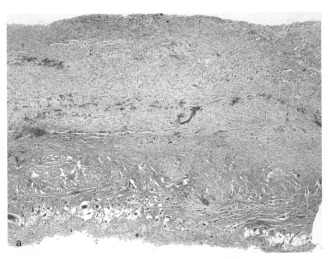 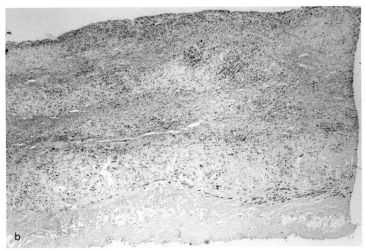

Figure 6.13 Case of malignant mesothelioma. (a) Cellular areas seem to predominate towards the surface of the thickened pleura (H&E, ×4). However, in (b), a cytokeratin stain demonstrates, in contrast to the zonation observed in Figure 6.12b, alternating hyper- and hypocellular areas even in the deep aspect of the pleural thickness (Cytokeratin AE1/AE3, ×4).

in patients with previous chronic pleuritis, trauma and other conditions (46–48). Histologically, pleural plaques are characterized by the presence of dense, sparsely cellular, hypovascular fibrosis with laminated collagen fibers with hyalinization, and a basket-weave arrangement of slit-like spaces running parallel to the pleural surface (Figure 6.14). The histomorphologic features overlap with those of pleural thickening and calcification that may occur in autoimmune diseases such as rheumatoid arthritis and scleroderma, and the distinction is usually made clinically and/or radiologically (48). Rare cases of asbestos-related pleural plaques and associated pleural vasculitides related to microscopic polyangiitis have been described (49).

Rounded Atelectasis

Rounded atelectasis is a benign inflammatory condition of the pleura that may mimic a lung mass. Like pleural plaques,

rounded atelectasis is most frequently, but not exclusively, seen in patients with above background asbestos exposure (50). It is characterized by the presence of subpleural or pleural-based opacities with characteristic imaging features on chest computed tomography.

There are two mechanisms implicated in the pathogenesis of rounded atelectasis. (1) Fluid from pleural effusion immerses in a part of the lung, which becomes atelectatic "roiled," with resulting adhesions between the apposed surfaces of visceral pleura, and subsequent expansion of the lung after the resolution of the pleural effusion. (2) The presence of diffuse fibrotic changes of the pleura that result in bronchial folding with concomitant atelectasis of the affected lung (50).

Histopathologically, the atelectatic "roiled" lung parenchyma contains entrapped pleura with fibrosis ("pleuroma") (50–53) (Figure 6.15).

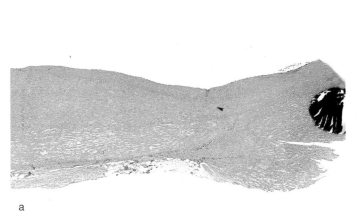 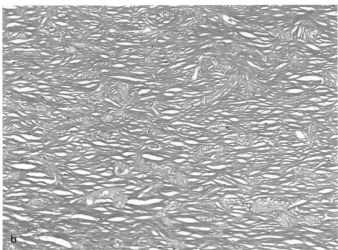

Figure 6.14 Pleural plaque. (a) Focal calcification is seen on the right side (H&E, ×2.0). (b) Acellular hyalinizing fibrosclerosis with slit-like spaces in a basket-weave pattern (H&E, ×10).

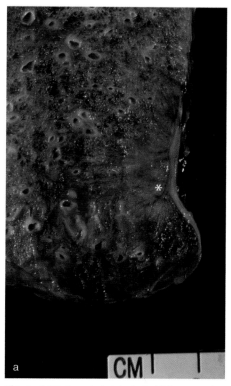
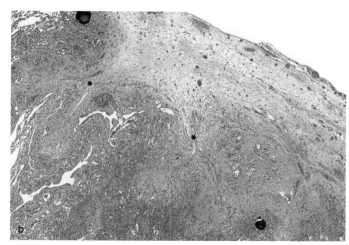

Figure 6.15 Rounded atelectasis. (a) Gross specimen showing pleural fibrosis and subpleural atelectatic lung with mass-like consolidation (asterisk). (b) Microscopic picture showing organizing pleuritis with pleural infoldings (asterisk) and atelectatic lung parenchyma (H&E, ×2.0).

Rounded atelectasis has been rarely described in patients with sarcoidosis and IgG4-related pleural disease (54,55).

Amyloidosis of Serosal Membranes

Amyloidosis can involve the serosal membranes. The pleura is affected more commonly, but peritoneum and pericardium can be affected as well, in the setting of systemic, cardiac, or pulmonary amyloidosis (56–60). Primary or secondary amyloidosis involving primarily the pleura or the peritoneum has been reported as rare case reports (61–63). The typical eosinophilic material can be seen in pleural biopsies and confirmed by Congo Red stain (Figure 6.16). Immunohistochemical stains may be helpful to further characterize the amyloid deposits into immunoglobulin light chain (AL), transthyretin (ATR), or beta-2-microglobulin (Aβ2M) amyloidosis; however, mass spectroscopy is more specific.

Other Non-neoplastic Lesions of the Pericardium and Peritoneum

Mesothelial Inclusion Cysts

Unifocal mesothelial cysts can develop in the pericardium, peritoneum, and other serosal membranes. Mesothelial cysts are usually acquired following previous inflammation, trauma, or other local events (64). Mesothelial inclusion cysts appear grossly as thin-walled, water-filled cysts without solid areas that can range in size from microcysts to several centimeters in diameter. Histopathologically the cysts have a thin wall with fibrous stroma lined by cuboidal mesothelial cells without significant cytologic atypia. The mesothelial differentiation of the epithelioid cells lining the cysts can be confirmed with immunohistochemical stains for calretinin, WT-1 and other mesothelial markers. Mesothelial cysts can also be multifocal and/or polycystic, particularly in the peritoneum. These lesions have been previously designated as the so-called "benign cystic mesothelioma" and can be associated with conditions such as appendicitis, pseudomyxoma peritonei, or ovarian carcinoma (64). The majority of multicystic peritoneal cysts are similarly lined by mesothelial cells without significant cytologic atypia. Some lesions may rarely develop mesothelial hyperplasia with focal stratification and anisocytosis of the mesothelial cells (Figure 6.17), resulting in diagnostic difficulties in the distinction from mesothelioma (65). Rarely, the cyst lining undergoes focal or extensive squamous metaplasia.

Endometriosis and Endosalpingiosis

Endometriosis, defined as the presence of endometrial glands and/or stroma outside the uterus, is most common in women of childbearing age. The peritoneum lining pelvic organs is most frequently involved, but pleura may also be affected

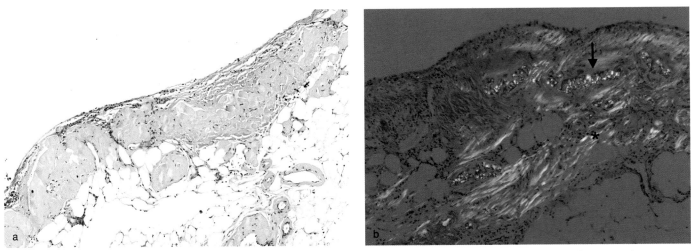

Figure 6.16 Amyloidosis. (a) Pleura thickened by deposits of extracellular waxy eosinophilic material (H&E, ×10). (b) Amyloid deposits showing apple green birefringence (asterisk). Note the white birefringence of collagen fibers (arrow) (Congo Red, ×20).

(see catamenial pneumothorax above). The pathogenesis of endometriosis is not yet completely elucidated, and different theories have been proposed, such as the presence of ectopic or displaced endometrial cells (theory of retrograde menstruation), the presence of Müllerian embryonic rests, or metaplastic change of mesenchymal stem cells towards Müllerian differentiation (celomic metaplasia) (66,67) as part of a multifactorial process that may also involve altered immunity and genetic factors (68).

The pathologic features of endometriosis may be, grossly and microscopically, quite variable. Grossly, endometriosis can present as brown–maroon areas of firmness on the peritoneal surface, fibrous adhesions, or bloody cystic lesions. Microscopically, the typical form shows endometrial glands surrounded by endometrial stroma, with accompanying hemorrhage with foamy and pigmented histiocytes; however, only one component may be present. Immunohistochemical stains are helpful to identify the endometrial epithelium with estrogen receptors and PAX-8, and the endometrial stroma with estrogen receptors and CD10. Several findings have been reported in endometriosis that may create diagnostic problems, including fibrosis, elastosis, smooth muscle metaplasia, myxoid change, decidual change, epithelial metaplastic changes, cytologic atypia, or hyperplasia (69).

Endosalpingiosis refers to the presence of fallopian tube-type ciliated epithelium-lined glands and/or cysts outside the fallopian tube, usually seen in pelvic organs including the ovaries, fallopian tube serosa, uterine serosa, myometrium, or pelvic peritoneum. Psammoma bodies and periglandular inflammatory cells may be present. Similar to endometriosis, the origin of endosalpingiosis is unclear, and implicated theories include celomic metaplasia or the extratubal growth of displaced tubal epithelium as sequela of a fallopian tube pathologic process or trauma. Metaplastic changes, such as mucinous metaplasia may occur and create diagnostic challenges in the distinction with adenocarcinoma.

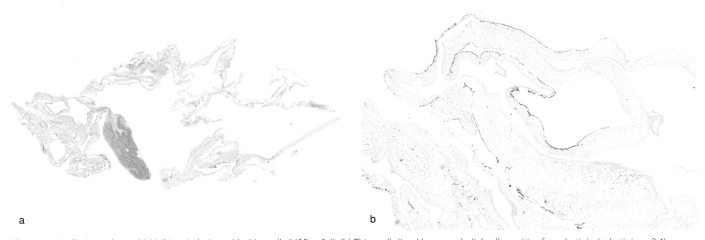

Figure 6.17 Peritoneal cyst. (a) Multicystic lesion with thin walls (H&E, ×0.4). (b) Thin walls lined by mesothelial cells positive for calretinin (calretinin, ×2.4).

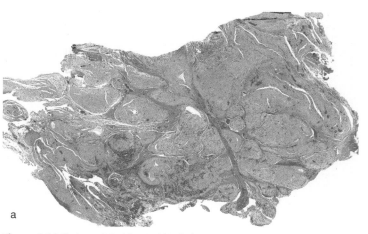
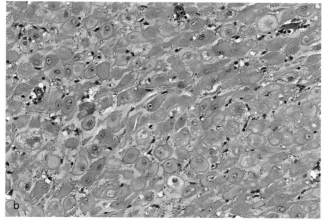

Figure 6.18 Peritoneal deciduosis. (a) Lobular arrangement of deciduoid stromal cells (H&E, ×0.5). (b) Large cells with eosinophilic cytoplasm, distinct cytoplasmic borders and round central nuclei with prominent nucleoli, similar to decidualized endometrial stroma (H&E, ×19.6).

Deciduosis

Deciduosis, or ectopic decidua, in the peritoneal cavity is a relatively common finding in pregnant women that results as a consequence of a physiologic metaplastic change of the subcelomic mesenchymal cells in response to the elevated levels of progesterone hormone levels during pregnancy. The hormone effect on pre-existing foci of endometriosis may also play a role in the development of deciduosis (70). Deciduosis is usually grossly seen in the submesothelial layer of the pelvic peritoneum as white, yellowish, or red nodules. Microscopically, deciduosis shows lobules and sheets of large cells with eosinophilic cytoplasm, distinct cytoplasmic borders, and round central nuclei with prominent nucleoli, similar to decidualized endometrial stroma (Figure 6.18). Deciduosis can mimic malignant deciduoid mesothelioma or metastatic carcinoma. Immunohistochemical stains for cytokeratins are positive in mesothelial or carcinoma proliferations and are helpful for this distinction.

Trophoblastic Implants

Rare cases of ectopic trophoblastic implants in the omentum or extratubal pelvic tissues, often associated with fibrous lesions, have been described in patients after laparoscopic salpingostomy for ectopic pregnancy (71). Patients are noted to have persistent elevation of serum human chorionic gonadotrophin hormone levels.

Walthard Rests

Walthard cell rests (Walthard cell nests) are benign epithelial clusters of transitional epithelium that develop around the fallopian tubes, broad ligaments and other pelvic areas. They are often multiple and appear grossly as small white or yellow nodules that measure up to 2 mm in size. Histopathologically Walthard cell nests are composed of solid or cystic nodules of transitional/urothelial epithelium with small cells showing

oval nuclei with prominent nuclear grooves and small nucleoli (Figure 6.19). Immunoreactivity for CK7 and involucrin can be employed to confirm the diagnosis. Walthard nests rarely may develop into parafallopian tube Brenner tumors or transitional cell carcinomas. Immunostains can be helpful in differential diagnosis as the epithelial cells of Walthard rests are negative for uroplakin while the other neoplasms can exhibit immunoreactivity with this antibody.

Splenosis

Splenosis is an acquired condition characterized by the implantation of multiple nodules of splenic tissue in the peritoneum following traumatic or iatrogenic rupture of the spleen. Splenosis is generally located in the peritoneum, omentum, or mesentery, but rare cases of splenosis has been reported in the pericardium, subcutaneous tissue, and the occipital pole of the brain (72).

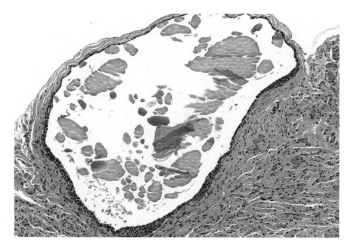

Figure 6.19 Walthard rest. Cystic nodule lined by transitional-type epithelium. This Walthard rest shows dilatation and luminal secretions (H&E, ×11.4).

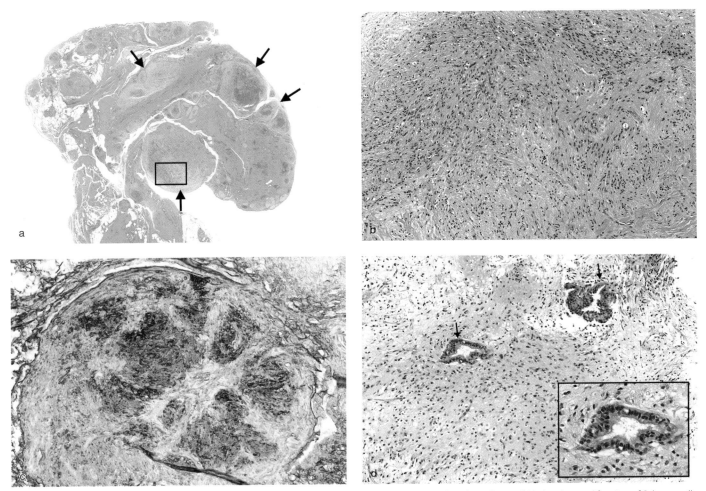

Figure 6.20 Gliomatosis peritonei. (a) Peritoneum with nodules of neural tissue (arrows) (H&E, ×1.2). (b) Selected area of (a) showing proliferation of Schwan cells within a fibrillary stroma (H&E, ×9.8). (c) The cells express GFAP (GFAP, ×20). (d) Gliomatosis peritonei associated with endosalpingiosis (H&E, ×10). **Inset**: Showing ciliated columnar epithelium (H&E, ×20).

Grossly, splenosis presents as multiple blue–red nodules that microscopically resemble splenic tissue. Splenosis need to be distinguished from congenital accessory spleens, which occur from the left dorsal mesogastrium during embryological development, are usually few in number and derive their blood supply from a branch of the splenic artery. Histopathologically, ectopic spleens exhibit a normal splenic architecture with a capsule and an organized architecture. In contrast, the ectopic splenic nodules of splenosis tend to be very numerous and are composed of unencapsulated splenic tissue.

Melanosis Peritonei

Melanosis peritonei is an extremely rare condition characterized by the presence of small pigmented nodules on the peritoneal surface and the omentum. It has been described in association with enteric duplication cysts, peritoneal cysts, and ovarian dermoid cysts. Histopathologically, melanosis peritonei is composed of pigmented melanophages usually arranged in a perivascular location.

Gliomatosis Peritonei

Gliomatosis peritonei is a rare condition characterized by the presence of peritoneal nodules composed of mature glial tissues (73) (Figure 6.20). Most cases have been associated with ovarian mature or immature teratomas and rare cases with endometriosis and ventriculo-peritoneal shunts. It has been postulated that the ectopic glial tissue results from either implantation of teratomatous tissue in the peritoneum or metaplasia of subperitoneal stem cells resulting in glial differentiation. Malignant transformation as glioblastoma multiforme arising from gliomatosis peritonei has been described. The cells of gliomatosis peritonei and glioma exhibit immunoreactivity for SOX2 and are negative for OCT4 and NANOG.

Inflammatory Myofibroblastic Tumor (Omental–Mesenteric Myxoid Hamartoma)

Omental–mesenteric myxoid hamartoma (OMH) was believed originally to be a unique and rare myxoid lesion occurring in infants, with a benign clinical behavior. Described in 1983, the term myxoid hamartoma was proposed as a descriptive term in view of its uncertain histogenesis and the presence of primitive mesenchymal cells imbedded in a myxoid stroma with delicate vascular channels. Since this first description, very few documented cases (around 10) have been reported. This reporting likely reflects the fact that, given their morphologic and behavior similarities, the lesion is considered to be a variant within the group of inflammatory myofibroblastic tumors (IMTs) (74–77). In a study of 84 extrapulmonary IMTs that included 36 cases occurring in the omentum and/or mesentery, the morphologic descriptions and clinical features described are similar to the three cases that Gonzalez et al. originally termed OMH (76,78). Similar molecular alterations have been reported in lesions thought to represent OMH and IMT, which support that the histogenesis of the two lesions is related, OMH being part of the spectrum of IMT with a distinctive presentation in the first year of life (74,79).

In general, the omentum and mesentery are the most common extrapulmonary locations for IMTs. They are usually detected in the first to second decades of life, with the majority diagnosed during infancy. The omental/mesenteric lesions are usually larger than the pulmonary counterparts and are more frequently multinodular (76). Their larger size with proximity to vital structures and multinodularity account for their increased risk of recurrence or death (76,80). Histologic transformation can rarely be observed; however, metastatic lesions were not observed (76).

Clinically, patients present with a mass, non-specific gastrointestinal symptoms, pain, or weight loss. A subset of patients develops fever and/or laboratory alterations including anemia, thrombocytosis, hypergammaglobulinemia, or elevated sedimentation rate, which usually regress after the resection of the mass (52,55). Coffin et al. described the pathologic features of the largest series of extrapulmonary IMTs with 84 cases, 36 of which were omental–mesenteric lesions. In their series, the tumor size ranged from 1 to 17 cm and there was a tendency of omental/mesenteric tumors to be multinodular. The cut surfaces are described as white/tan with a whorled, fleshy, and sometimes with myxoid appearance. Focal hemorrhage, necrosis, and calcifications can be seen in few cases. Microscopically, the lesions are composed of spindle cells proliferating with three different patterns (76) (Figure 6.21):

(1) Stellate to plump spindle cells with vesicular nuclei and eosinophilic cytoplasm growing in a myxoid/edematous background with an irregular network of blood vessels admixed with a polymorphous inflammatory infiltrate resembling granulation tissue. Mitotic activity may be brisk.

(2) Compact spindle cell proliferation that alternates with areas resembling granulation tissue similar to the first pattern. The proliferating cells have elongated nuclei with blunting of the tips and can show a fascicular or storiform arrangement, with areas of greater cellularity alternating with areas of lesser cellularity. Ganglion-like myofibroblasts with vesicular nuclei and ample eosinophilic cytoplasm are usually present, as well as foci of dense collagen deposition. Mitotic activity is variable. Plasma cells predominate in the polymorphous inflammatory infiltrate and they can be present as small aggregates, or scattered uniformly along the infiltrate.

(3) Hypocellular, dense plate-like collagen bands with sparse inflammatory infiltrates consisting of plasma cells and eosinophils.

In any of the patterns, mitotic activity varies but remains in the low rate. Dystrophic calcifications can be seen. Necrosis is uncommon.

Immunohistochemical stains are helpful for the diagnosis of IMT, as the proliferating spindle cells show a myofibroblastic phenotype, with variably staining for smooth muscle actin, muscle specific actin and desmin. Keratins and CD68 may be focally positive.

Rearrangements involving the short arm of chromosome 2 have been observed in IMT, which tend to occur in younger, male patients (81–83). Abnormalities of the ALK gene can be detected with FISH studies. Various fusion partners have been observed, including TPM3, TPM4, CLTC, and RANBP2 (82,84,85).

Expression of ALK protein is present in 50–60 percent of the cases and correlates with the presence of rearrangements of the ALK gene and constitutes an aid in the diagnosis (75,81,82,85). Three patterns of staining have been reported: diffuse cytoplasmic, granular cytoplasmic, and nuclear membrane (86) and the pattern appears to correlate with the fusion partner. Granular pattern is associated with a fusion between the clathrin heavy chain gene (CLTC) and ALK, and nuclear membrane pattern is associated with a fusion between the RANBP2 and ALK (85,86). It is speculated that the newer ALK antibody D5F3 has slightly higher sensitivity and better performance than ALK-1 to detect ALK expression in myofibroblastic tumors (87) (Figure 6.21).

IMTs are considered to have intermediate malignant potential given their tendency to recur locally and rarely metastasize. Unless the tumors show malignant transformation, there are no morphologic features that predict prognosis (76,88,89). Epithelioid inflammatory myofibroblastic sarcoma refers to a variant of IMT reported predominantly in the abdominal cavity, mostly mesentery or omentum, that shows epithelioid morphology and pursues an aggressive course with rapid local recurrences. These tumors show mostly the distinct nuclear membrane pattern of ALK staining with IHC associated with the RANBP2 fusion partner (84,85,90).

Tumor-like Conditions of the Serosal Membranes

Calcifying Fibrous Pseudotumor

Originally described in the subcutaneous and deep tissues of the extremities in children, several cases of calcifying fibrous pseudotumors (CFPTs) have been reported involving

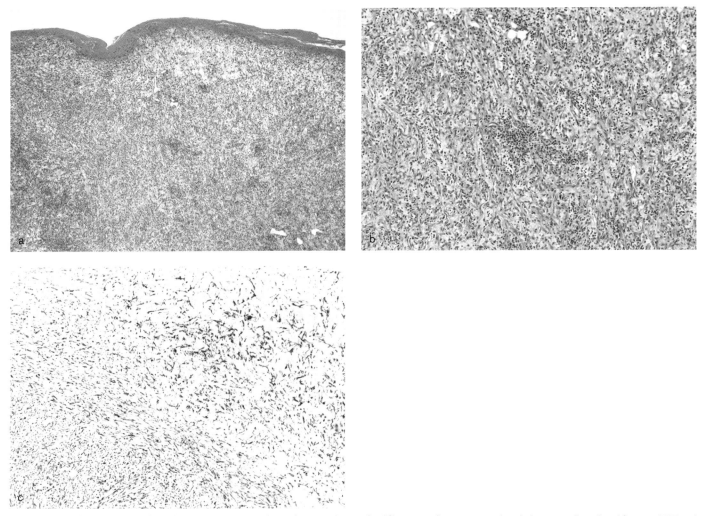

Figure 6.21 Inflammatory myofibroblastic tumor. (a) Serosal membrane with superficial fibrinous inflammation and underlying spindle cell proliferation (H&E, ×4). (b) The spindle cells are closely associated with admixed small lymphocytes (H&E, ×10). (c) ALK expression in the spindle cells (ALK D5F3, ×4).

the omentum/mesentery, peritoneum, and pleura (91–95). Although multiple lesions or recurrences may occur, CFPT are benign tumors (93).

Grossly, the lesions are usually well-circumscribed, lobulated with a white, firm, solid, somewhat whorled appearance on cut surface.

Histopathologically, calcifying fibrous pseudotumors consist of a non-encapsulated hypocellular proliferation of bland spindle cells with densely hyalinized, sclerotic stroma with varying numbers of lymphocytes and plasma cells. A characteristic feature is the presence of numerous dystrophic and psammomatous calcifications (Figure 6.22). CFPTs variably express CD34, smooth muscle actin and desmin and are negative for s-100 and ALK. Differential diagnoses include solitary fibrous tumor, old calcifying granulomas, calcified pleural plaques, chronic fibrous pleuritis, IMT, and nodular amyloidosis (93,94).

Although calcifications may be seen in solitary fibrous tumors, these lesions show a patternless pattern of dense, wire-like strands of collagen with scattered plump fibroblast-like

cells that may also adopt hemangiopericytoma-like, storiform, leiomyoma-like, or neurofibroma-like patterns, unlike the broad, band-like collagen and relatively paucicellular appearance of CFPT. An immunohistochemical stain for STAT 6 immunohistochemical stains may be helpful in this distinction, as they are positive in solitary fibrous tumors.

The dense fibrotic thickening of the pleura with calcification occurring in calcifying pleural plaques can be distinguished from CFPT by the basket-weave pattern of slit-like spaces present in the former.

IgG4-related disease may present with pleural/parenchymal masses with dense fibrous bands similar to CFPT; however, IgG4-related disease displays a more prominent plasma cell population with increased numbers of IgG4-positive plasma cells and eosinophils, and obliterative vasculitis. These lesions may also show a rather expansile infiltrative growth.

Chronic fibrous pleuritis shares the chronic inflammation and dense, hyalinized fibrous tissue with CFPT; however, chronic fibrous pleuritis usually presents with diffuse pleural

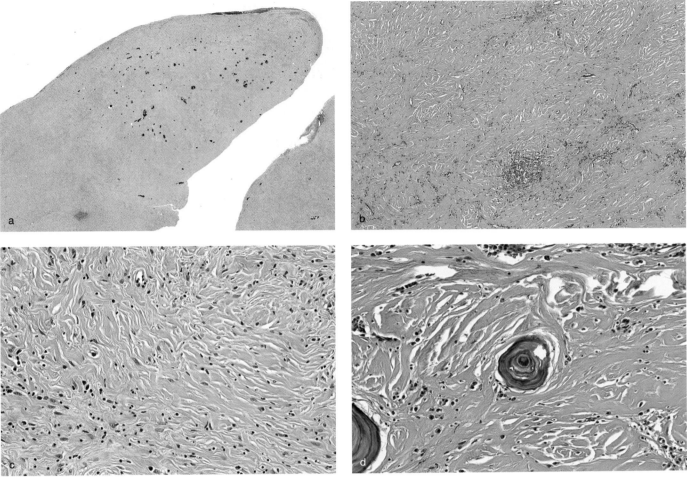

Figure 6.22 Calcifying pseudotumor. (a) Prominent fibrosclerosis and numerous calcifications (H&E, ×0.7). (b) Lymphoid aggregates (H&E, ×5.0). (c) Plump oval spindle cells with intermixing ropey collagen fibers and scattered mononuclear inflammatory cells (H&E, ×20.7). (d) Psammoma body-type laminated calcifications (H&E, ×20).

thickening rather than a localized mass of calcified tissue. Diffuse pleural thickening away from the mass has not been reported in patients with calcifying fibrous pseudotumor. Chronic inflammation is a common finding in pleuritis and dystrophic calcification may occur, but psammomatous calcifications are not seen. In some cases, chronic fibrous pleuritis is associated with fibrous pleural plaques that show dense fibrous tissue with a basket-weave arrangement of slit-like spaces running parallel to the pleural surface a finding not seen in CFPT.

The fibrosis in old hyalinized and calcified granulomas is usually nodular and concentric, unlike the randomly oriented fibrosclerosis with chronic inflammation that CFPT show.

IMTs are usually more cellular, less hyalinized and show greater degrees of chronic inflammatory infiltrates than CFPT, and although calcifications may be present, psammomatous calcifications are usually absent. It has been postulated that CFPTs may be within the spectrum of IMTs; however, the negative or only focal expression of ALK in CFPT argues against this theory (93,96,97).

Nodular amyloid may mimic CFPT given its eosinophilic hypocellular appearance, but they show the characteristic extracellular deposits of eosinophilic waxy-like material that shows apple green.

References

1. Ahmed RA, Marrie TJ, Huang JQ. Thoracic empyema in patients with community-acquired pneumonia. *Am J Med.* 2006;119(10):877–83.

2. Maskell NA, Batt S, Hedley EL, Davies CWH, Gillespie SH, Davies RJO. The bacteriology of pleural infection by genetic and standard methods and its mortality significance. *Am J Respir Crit Care Med.* 2006;174(7):817–23.

3. Foster S, Maskell N. Bacteriology of complicated parapneumonic effusions.

Curr Opin Pulm Med. 2007;13(4):319–23.

4. Nestor J, Huggins T, Kummerfeldt C, DiVietro M, Walters K, Sahn S. Viral diseases affecting the pleura. *J Clin Virol.* 2013;58(2):367–73.

5. Kummerfeldt CE, Huggins JT, Sahn SA. Unusual bacterial infections and the pleura. *Open Respir Med J.* 2012;6:75.

6. Dobbie JW. Serositis: comparative analysis of histological findings and pathogenetic mechanisms in nonbacterial serosal inflammation. *Perit Dial Int.* 1993;13(4):256–69.

7. Esther CR, Barker PM. Pulmonary lymphangiectasia: diagnosis and clinical course. *Pediatr Pulmonol.* 2004;38(4):308–13.

8. Ryu JH, Tomassetti S, Maldonado F. Update on uncommon pleural effusions. *Respirology.* 2011;16(2):238–43.

9. Panchabhai TS, Bandyopadhyay D, Yadav R, Arrossi AV, Mehta AC, Faress JA. A 42-year-old woman with abnormal chest CT scan and chylous ascites. *Chest.* 2016;149(1):e25–28.

10. Lama A, Ferreiro L, Toubes ME, Golpe A, Gude F, Álvarez-Dobaño JM, et al. Characteristics of patients with pseudochylothorax – a systematic review. *J Thorac Dis.* 2016;8(8):2093.

11. Padeh S, Berkun Y. Familial Mediterranean fever. *Curr Opin Rheumatol.* 2016;28(5):523–29.

12. Sarı İ, Birlik M, Kasifoğlu T. Familial Mediterranean fever: an updated review. *Eur J Rheumatol.* 2014;1(1):21–33.

13. Tschopp J-M, Bintcliffe O, Astoul P, Canalis E, Driesen P, Janssen JP, et al. ERS task force statement: diagnosis and treatment of primary spontaneous pneumothorax. *Eur Respir J.* 2015;46(2):321–35.

14. Noppen M. Spontaneous pneumothorax: epidemiology, pathophysiology and cause. *Eur Respir Rev.* 2010;19(117):217–19.

15. Ohata M, Suzuki H. Pathogenesis of spontaneous pneumothorax. With special reference to the ultrastructure of emphysematous bullae. *Chest.* 1980;77(6):771–76.

16. Noppen M, Dekeukeleire T, Hanon S, Stratakos G, Amjadi K, Madsen P, et al. Fluorescein-enhanced autofluorescence thoracoscopy in patients with primary spontaneous pneumothorax and normal subjects. *Am J Respir Crit Care Med.* 2006;174(1):26–30.

17. Lichter I, Gwynne JF. Spontaneous pneumothorax in young subjects. A clinical and pathological study. *Thorax.* 1971;26(4):409–17.

18. Askin FB, McCann BG, Kuhn C. Reactive eosinophilic pleuritis: a lesion to be distinguished from pulmonary eosinophilic granuloma. *Arch Pathol Lab Med.* 1977;101(4):187–91.

19. McDonnell TJ, Crouch EC, Gonzalez JG. Reactive eosinophilic pleuritis. A sequela of pneumothorax in pulmonary eosinophilic granuloma. *Am J Clin Pathol.* 1989;91(1):107–11.

20. Shekhel TA, Ricciotti RW, Blair JE, Colby TV, Sobonya RE, Larsen BT. Surgical pathology of pleural coccidioidomycosis: a clinicopathological study of 36 cases. *Hum Pathol.* 2014;45(5):961–69.

21. Evison M, Holme J, Alaloul M, Doran H, Bishop P, Booton R, et al. Olanzapine-induced eosinophilic pleuritis. *Respir Med Case Rep.* 2015;14:24–26.

22. Sobonya RE, Yanes J, Klotz SA. Cavitary pulmonary coccidioidomycosis: pathologic and clinical correlates of disease. *Hum Pathol.* 2014;45(1):153–59.

23. Cudzilo C, Aragaki A, Guitron J, Benzaquen S. Methotrexate-induced pleuropericarditis and eosinophilic pleural effusion. *J Bronchology Interv Pulmonol.* 2014;21(1):90–92.

24. Middleton KL, Santella R, Couser JI. Eosinophilic pleuritis due to propylthiouracil. *Chest.* 1993;103(3):955–56.

25. Sen N, Ermis H, Karatasli M, Habesoglu MA, Eyuboglu FO. Propylthiouracil-associated eosinophilic pleural effusion: a case report. *Respiration.* 2007;74(6):703–05.

26. Belchis DA, Shekitka K, Gocke CD. A unique, histopathologic lesion in a subset of patients with spontaneous pneumothorax. *Arch Pathol Lab Med.* 2012;136(12):1522–27.

27. Sauter JL, Butnor KJ. Pathological findings in spontaneous pneumothorax specimens: does the incidence of unexpected clinically significant findings justify routine histological examination? *Histopathology.* 2015;66(5):675–84.

28. Butnor KJ, Guinee DG. Pleuropulmonary pathology of Birt–Hogg–Dubé syndrome. *Am J Surg Pathol.* 2006;30(3):395–99.

29. Joseph J, Sahn SA. Thoracic endometriosis syndrome: new observations from an analysis of 110 cases. *Am J Med.* 1996;100(2):164–70.

30. Ghigna M-R, Mercier O, Mussot S, Fabre D, Fadel E, Dorfmuller P, et al. Thoracic endometriosis: clinicopathologic updates and issues about 18 cases from a tertiary referring center. *Ann Diagn Pathol.* 2015;19(5):320–25.

31. Flieder DB, Moran CA, Travis WD, Koss MN, Mark EJ. Pleuro-pulmonary endometriosis and pulmonary ectopic deciduosis: a clinicopathologic and immunohistochemical study of 10 cases with emphasis on diagnostic pitfalls. *Hum Pathol.* 1998;29(12):1495–503.

32. Baker PM, Clement PB, Young RH. Selected topics in peritoneal pathology. *Int J Gynecol Pathol.* 2014;33(4):393–401.

33. Oparka R, McCluggage WG, Herrington CS. Peritoneal mesothelial hyperplasia associated with gynaecological disease: a potential diagnostic pitfall that is commonly associated with endometriosis. *J Clin Pathol.* 2011;64(4):313–18.

34. Cheung AN, Young RH, Scully RE. Pseudocarcinomatous hyperplasia of the fallopian tube associated with salpingitis. A report of 14 cases. *Am J Surg Pathol.* 1994;18(11):1125–30.

35. Clement PB, Young RH. Florid mesothelial hyperplasia associated with ovarian tumors: a potential source of error in tumor diagnosis and staging. *Int J Gynecol Pathol.* 1993;12(1):51–58.

36. Chiosea S, Krasinskas A, Cagle PT, Mitchell KA, Zander DS, Dacic S. Diagnostic importance of 9p21 homozygous deletion in malignant mesotheliomas. *Mod Pathol.* 2008;21(6):742–47.

37. Ito T, Hamasaki M, Matsumoto S, Hiroshima K, Tsujimura T, Kawai T, et al. p16/CDKN2A FISH in differentiation of diffuse malignant peritoneal mesothelioma from mesothelial hyperplasia and epithelial ovarian cancer. *Am J Clin Pathol.* 2015;143(6):830–38.

38. Hwang HC, Pyott S, Rodriguez S, Cindric A, Carr A, Michelsen C, et al.

BAP1 immunohistochemistry and p16 FISH in the diagnosis of sarcomatous and desmoplastic mesotheliomas. *Am J Surg Pathol.* 2016;40(5):714–18.

39. Hida T, Hamasaki M, Matsumoto S, Sato A, Tsujimura T, Kawahara K, et al. BAP1 immunohistochemistry and p16 FISH results in combination provide higher confidence in malignant pleural mesothelioma diagnosis: ROC analysis of the two tests. *Pathol Int.* 2016;66(10):563–70.

40. Takeda M, Kasai T, Enomoto Y, Takano M, Morita K, Kadota E, et al. 9p21 deletion in the diagnosis of malignant mesothelioma, using fluorescence in situ hybridization analysis. *Pathol Int.* 2010;60(5):395–99.

41. Sheffield BS, Hwang HC, Lee AF, Thompson K, Rodriguez S, Tse CH, et al. BAP1 immunohistochemistry and p16 FISH to separate benign from malignant mesothelial proliferations. *Am J Surg Pathol.* 2015;39(7):977–82.

42. Monaco SE, Shuai Y, Bansal M, Krasinskas AM, Dacic S. The diagnostic utility of p16 FISH and GLUT-1 immunohistochemical analysis in mesothelial proliferations. *Am J Clin Pathol.* 2011;135(4):619–27.

43. Walts AE, Hiroshima K, McGregor SM, Wu D, Husain AN, Marchevsky AM. BAP1 immunostain and CDKN2A (p16) FISH analysis: clinical applicability for the diagnosis of malignant mesothelioma in effusions. *Diagn Cytopathol.* 2016;44(7):599–606.

44. Husain AN, Colby T, Ordonez N, Krausz T, Attanoos R, Beasley MB, et al. Guidelines for pathologic diagnosis of malignant mesothelioma: 2012 update of the consensus statement from the International Mesothelioma Interest Group. *Arch Pathol Lab Med.* 2013;137(5):647–67.

45. Churg A, Sheffield BS, Galateau-Sallé F. New markers for separating benign from malignant mesothelial proliferations: are we there yet? *Arch Pathol Lab Med.* 2016;140(4):318–21. PubMed PMID: 26288396

46. Hillerdal G. The pathogenesis of pleural plaques and pulmonary asbestosis: possibilities and impossibilities. *Eur J Respir Dis.* 1980;61(3):129–38.

47. Ren H, Lee DR, Hruban RH, Kuhlman JE, Fishman EK, Wheeler PS, et al. Pleural plaques do not predict asbestosis: high-resolution computed tomography and pathology study. *Mod Pathol.* 1991;4(2):201–09.

48. Clarke CC, Mowat FS, Kelsh MA, Roberts MA. Pleural plaques: a review of diagnostic issues and possible nonasbestos factors. *Arch Environ Occup Health.* 2006;61(4):183–92.

49. Hara A, Kinoshita Y, Hosoi K, Okumura Y, Song M, Min K. Pleural vasculitides of microscopic polyangiitis with asbestos-related plaques. *Respirol Case Rep.* 2015;3(4):148–50.

50. Hillerdal G. Rounded atelectasis. Clinical experience with 74 patients. *Chest.* 1989;95(4):836–41.

51. Dernevik L, Gatzinsky P. Pathogenesis of shrinking pleuritis with atelectasis – "rounded atelectasis." *Eur J Respir Dis.* 1987;71(4):244–49.

52. Dernevik L, Gatzinsky P, Hultman E, Selin K, William-Olsson G, Zettergren L. Shrinking pleuritis with atelectasis. *Thorax.* 1982;37(4):252–58.

53. Sinner WN. Rounded atelectasis or pleuroma? *Chest.* 1985;88(2):312–13.

54. Onishi Y, Nakahara Y, Hirano K, Sasaki S, Kawamura T, Mochiduki Y. IgG4-related disease in asbestos-related pleural disease. *Respirol Case Rep.* 2016;4(1):22–24.

55. Tetikkurt C, Tetikkurt S, Ozdemir I, Bayar N. Round atelectasis in sarcoidosis. *Multidisc Respir Med.* 2011;6(3):180.

56. Scala R, Maccari U, Madioni C, Venezia D, La Magra LC. Amyloidosis involving the respiratory system: 5-year's experience of a multi-disciplinary group's activity. *Ann Thorac Med.* 2015;10(3):212–16.

57. Bontemps F, Tillie-Leblond I, Coppin MC, Frehart P, Wallaert B, Ramon R, et al. Pleural amyloidosis: thoracoscopic aspects. *Eur Respir J.* 1995;8(6):1025–27.

58. Kavuru MS, Adamo JP, Ahmad M, Mehta AC, Gephardt GN. Amyloidosis and pleural disease. *Chest.* 1990;98(1):20–23.

59. Horger M, Vogel M, Brodoefel H, Schimmel H, Claussen C. Omental and peritoneal involvement in systemic amyloidosis: CT with pathologic correlation. *AJR Am J Roentgenol.* 2006;186(4):1193–95.

60. Weinrauch LA, Desautels RE, Christlieb AR, Kaldany A, D'Elia JA. Amyloid deposition in serosal membranes. Its occurrence with cardiac tamponade, bilateral ureteral obstruction, and gastrointestinal bleeding. *Arch Intern Med.* 1984;144(3):630–32.

61. Adams AL, Castro CY, Singh SP, Moran CA. Pleural amyloidosis mimicking mesothelioma: a clinicopathologic study of two cases. *Ann Diagn Pathol.* 2001;5(4):229–32.

62. Coumbaras M, Chopier J, Massiani MA, Antoine M, Boudghène F, Bazot M. Diffuse mesenteric and omental infiltration by amyloidosis with omental calcification mimicking abdominal carcinomatosis. *Clin Radiol.* 2001;56(8):674–76.

63. Akl MN, Kho RM, McCullough AE, Collins JM, Lund JT, Magtibay PM. Mesenteric and omental amyloidosis mimicking intraperitoneal carcinomatosis. *Surgery.* 2008;144(3):473–75.

64. Weiss SW, Tavassoli FA. Multicystic mesothelioma. An analysis of pathologic findings and biologic behavior in 37 cases. *Am J Surg Pathol.* 1988;12(10):737–46.

65. McFadden DE, Clement PB. Peritoneal inclusion cysts with mural mesothelial proliferation. A clinicopathological analysis of six cases. *Am J Surg Pathol.* 1986;10(12):844–54.

66. Figueira PGM, Abrão MS, Krikun G, Taylor HS, Taylor H. Stem cells in endometrium and their role in the pathogenesis of endometriosis. *Ann N Y Acad Sci.* 2011;1221:10–17.

67. Signorile PG, Baldi A. Endometriosis: new concepts in the pathogenesis. *Int J Biochem Cell Biol.* 2010;42(6):778–80.

68. Rahmioglu N, Nyholt DR, Morris AP, Missmer SA, Montgomery GW, Zondervan KT. Genetic variants underlying risk of endometriosis: insights from meta-analysis of eight genome-wide association and replication datasets. *Hum Reprod Update.* 2014;20(5):702–16.

69. Clement PB. The pathology of endometriosis: a survey of the many faces of a common disease emphasizing diagnostic pitfalls and unusual and newly appreciated aspects. *Adv Anat Pathol.* 2007;14(4):241–60.

70. Büttner A, Bässler R, Theele C. Pregnancy-associated ectopic decidua (deciduosis) of the greater omentum. An analysis of 60 biopsies with cases of

fibrosing deciduosis and leiomyomatosis peritonealis disseminata. *Pathol Res Pract.* 1993;189(3):352–59.

71. Pal L, Parkash V, Rutherford TJ. Omental trophoblastic implants and hemoperitoneum after laparoscopic salpingostomy for ectopic pregnancy. A case report. *J Reprod Med.* 2003;48(1):57–59.

72. Fremont RD, Rice TW. Splenosis: a review. *South Med J.* 2007;100(6): 589–93.

73. Liang L, Zhang Y, Malpica A, Ramalingam P, Euscher ED, Fuller GN, et al. Gliomatosis peritonei: a clinicopathologic and immunohistochemical study of 21 cases. *Mod Pathol.* 2015;28(12):1613–20.

74. Ludwig K, Alaggio R, Dall'Igna P, Lazzari E, d'Amore ESG, Chou PM. Omental mesenteric myxoid hamartoma, a subtype of inflammatory myofibroblastic tumor? Considerations based on the histopathological evaluation of four cases. *Virchows Arch.* 2015;467(6):741–47.

75. Coffin CM, Hornick JL, Fletcher CDM. Inflammatory myofibroblastic tumor: comparison of clinicopathologic, histologic, and immunohistochemical features including ALK expression in atypical and aggressive cases. *Am J Surg Pathol.* 2007;31(4):509–20.

76. Coffin CM, Watterson J, Priest JR, Dehner LP. Extrapulmonary inflammatory myofibroblastic tumor (inflammatory pseudotumor). A clinicopathologic and immunohistochemical study of 84 cases. *Am J Surg Pathol.* 1995;19(8):859–72.

77. IARC. *WHO Classification of tumours of soft tissue and bone.* 4th edition. Lyon: World Health Organization; 2013.

78. Gonzalez-Crussi F, deMello DE, Sotelo-Avila C. Omental–mesenteric myxoid hamartomas. Infantile lesions simulating malignant tumors. *Am J Surg Pathol.* 1983;7(6):567–78.

79. Su LD, Atayde-Perez A, Sheldon S, Fletcher JA, Weiss SW. Inflammatory myofibroblastic tumor: cytogenetic evidence supporting clonal origin. *Mod Pathol.* 1998;11(4):364–68.

80. Chun YS, Wang L, Nascimento AG, Moir CR, Rodeberg DA. Pediatric inflammatory myofibroblastic tumor: anaplastic lymphoma kinase (ALK) expression and prognosis. *Pediatr Blood Cancer.* 2005;45(6):796–801.

81. Griffin CA, Hawkins AL, Dvorak C, Henkle C, Ellingham T, Perlman EJ. Recurrent involvement of 2p23 in inflammatory myofibroblastic tumors. *Cancer Res.* 1999;59(12):2776–80.

82. Coffin CM, Patel A, Perkins S, Elenitoba-Johnson KS, Perlman E, Griffin CA. ALK1 and p80 expression and chromosomal rearrangements involving 2p23 in inflammatory myofibroblastic tumor. *Mod Pathol.* 2001;14(6):569–76.

83. Treissman SP, Gillis DA, Lee CL, Giacomantonio M, Resch L. Omental–mesenteric inflammatory pseudotumor. Cytogenetic demonstration of genetic changes and monoclonality in one tumor. *Cancer.* 1994;73(5):1433–37.

84. Ma Z, Hill DA, Collins MH, Morris SW, Sumegi J, Zhou M, et al. Fusion of ALK to the Ran-binding protein 2 (RANBP2) gene in inflammatory myofibroblastic tumor. *Genes Chromosomes Cancer.* 2003;37(1):98–105.

85. Mariño-Enríquez A, Wang W-L, Roy A, Lopez-Terrado D, Lazar AJ, Fletcher CD, et al. Epithelioid inflammatory myofibroblastic sarcoma: an aggressive intra-abdominal variant of inflammatory myofibroblastic tumor with nuclear membrane or perinuclear ALK. *Am J Surg Pathol.* 2011;35(1):135–44.

86. Cook JR, Dehner LP, Collins MH, Ma Z, Morris SW, Coffin CM, et al. Anaplastic lymphoma kinase (ALK) expression in the inflammatory myofibroblastic tumor: a comparative immunohistochemical study. *Am J Surg Pathol.* 2001;25(11):1364–71.

87. Taheri D, Zahavi DJ, Del Carmen Rodriguez M, Meliti A, Rezaee N, Yonescu R, et al. For staining of ALK protein, the novel D5F3 antibody demonstrates superior overall performance in terms of intensity and extent of staining in comparison to the currently used ALK1 antibody. *Virchows Arch.* 2016;469(3):345–50.

88. Meis-Kindblom JM, Kjellström C, Kindblom LG. Inflammatory fibrosarcoma: update, reappraisal, and perspective on its place in the spectrum of inflammatory myofibroblastic tumors. *Semin Diagn Pathol.* 1998;15(2):133–43.

89. Meis JM, Enzinger FM. Inflammatory fibrosarcoma of the mesentery and retroperitoneum. A tumor closely simulating inflammatory pseudotumor. *Am J Surg Pathol.* 1991;15(12):1146–56.

90. Yu L, Liu J, Lao IW, Luo Z, Wang J. Epithelioid inflammatory myofibroblastic sarcoma: a clinicopathological, immunohistochemical and molecular cytogenetic analysis of five additional cases and review of the literature. *Diagn Pathol.* 2016;11(1):67.

91. Jain A, Maheshwari V, Alam K, Jain V. Calcifying fibrous pseudotumor of peritoneum. *J Postgrad Med.* 2007;53(3):189–90.

92. Minerowicz C, Jagpal S, Uppaluri L, Deen M, Langenfeld J. Calcifying fibrous pseudotumor of the pleura. *Am J Respir Crit Care Med.* 2015;192(11): e57–58.

93. Nascimento AF, Ruiz R, Hornick JL, Fletcher CDM. Calcifying fibrous "pseudotumor": clinicopathologic study of 15 cases and analysis of its relationship to inflammatory myofibroblastic tumor. *Int J Surg Pathol.* 2002;10(3):189–96.

94. Pinkard NB, Wilson RW, Lawless N, Dodd LG, McAdams HP, Koss MN, et al. Calcifying fibrous pseudotumor of pleura. A report of three cases of a newly described entity involving the pleura. *Am J Clin Pathol.* 1996;105(2):189–94.

95. Medina AM, Alexis JB. A 27-year-old woman with incidental omental nodules. Calcifying fibrous pseudotumor of the omentum. *Arch Pathol Lab Med.* 2006;130(4):563–64.

96. Sigel JE, Smith TA, Reith JD, Goldblum JR. Immunohistochemical analysis of anaplastic lymphoma kinase expression in deep soft tissue calcifying fibrous pseudotumor: evidence of a late sclerosing stage of inflammatory myofibroblastic tumor? *Ann Diagn Pathol.* 2001;5(1):10–14.

97. Hill KA, Gonzalez-Crussi F, Chou PM. Calcifying fibrous pseudotumor versus inflammatory myofibroblastic tumor: a histological and immunohistochemical comparison. *Mod Pathol.* 2001;14(8):784–90.

Chapter 7

Surgical Pathology of Benign Lesions of Mesothelial Origin

Aliya N. Husain and Marina Ivanovic

Nodular Pleural Plaque

Pleural plaques are flattened or nodular tan, firm, well-circumscribed lesions that develop in the lower two-thirds of the parietal pleura and the outer two-thirds of the diaphragm.

The lesions are often bilateral and symmetric, and are frequently associated with asbestos exposure (1). The frequency of pleural plaques is reported between 5.8 percent and 19.1 percent in the general population, rising to 30–73.6 percent in the population with high environmental/occupational asbestos exposure (2).

Pleural plaques are characterized by accumulation of dense acellular collagen in the submesothelial layer of the pleura (Figure 7.1) with occasional bone formation or calcification, especially in longstanding nodules.

Simple Mesothelial Cyst of the Peritoneum

Simple mesothelial cysts of peritoneum are unilocular cysts that most likely develop as the result of incomplete fusion of the mesothelial-lined surfaces (3) and represent a reactive lesion or inclusion cyst rather than true neoplasms (1).

The cysts vary in size from a few centimeters up to 40 cm and can be found in mesentery and omentum, most often in women. The simple mesothelial cysts are asymptomatic; however, they occasionally present with non-specific symptoms, related to their size and location. Acute abdomen due to rupture or torsion has also been reported.

Simple mesothelial cysts are unilocular thin-walled cysts filled with serous fluid. The cyst wall is composed of fibrous

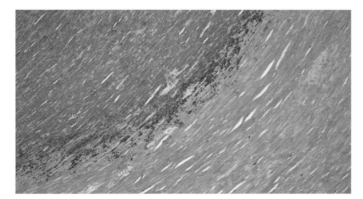

Figure 7.1 Microscopic view of pleural plaque shows characteristic basket-weave pattern of collagen bundles and calcifications (left upper corner).

tissue lined by flat, cuboidal mesothelial cells (Figure 7.2a,b). Diagnosis is confirmed by positive staining of the lining cells for mesothelial markers (calretinin, CK5/6 and/or WT-1).

Complete resection is the treatment of choice with no local recurrence.

Multicystic Mesothelioma of the Peritoneum

Multicystic peritoneal mesothelioma is a rare multilocular cystic lesion involving mostly the peritoneal cavity of women of reproductive age. Cases of multicystic mesothelioma involving pleura and pericardium, or spermatic cord in men, have also been reported (1).

The etiology and pathogenesis are controversial regarding hyperplastic/reactive or neoplastic nature of the lesion. Authors favoring hyperplastic/reactive ethology refer to the lesion as a *multilocular inclusion cyst*. The new term, *benign multicystic mesothelial proliferation*, has been proposed to reflect the benign clinical course of the lesion and to avoid confusion with malignant mesothelioma.

Multicystic peritoneal mesothelioma often presents with abdominal pain, or with abdominal swelling and as a painful abdominal mass (4). Pleural lesions present with chest pain and dyspnea (5).

Multicystic peritoneal mesothelioma consists of multilocular thin-walled cysts filled with serous fluid or gelatinous material, ranging in size from 0.2 to 3.5 cm (Figure 7.3a). The cyst wall is composed of fibrovascular stroma lined by flattened or cuboidal mesothelial cells (Figure 7.3b). Adenomatoid changes or squamous metaplasia are found in approximately 30 percent of the cases (1). The cysts present in clusters as multifocal lesions involving the peritoneal surface of the bladder or retrovesical space.

Differential diagnosis includes lymphangioma and malignant peritoneal mesothelioma. Positive staining of the lining cells for mesothelial markers (Figure 7.3c) and negative staining for D2–40 (podoplanin) and absence of chylous fluid, smooth muscle and lymphoid aggregates in the cyst wall distinguishes it from lymphangioma. Widespread nodular thickening of peritoneum with history of asbestos exposure should raise suspicion for malignant mesothelioma.

Complete surgical resection is the treatment of choice; however, local recurrence occurs in 50 percent of the cases (6,7). The possibility of progression to malignant mesothelioma is controversial.

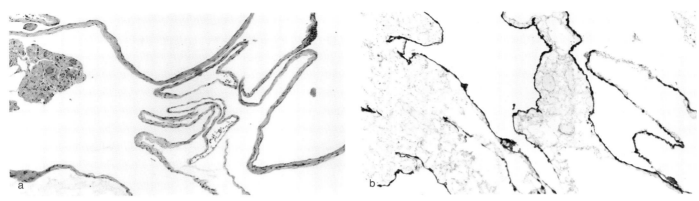

Figure 7.2 Thin fibrotic cyst wall lined by flattened mesothelial cells (a) that stain positive for calretinin (b).

Well-differentiated Papillary Mesothelioma

Well-differentiated papillary mesothelioma is an uncommon subtype of epithelioid mesothelioma with papillary growth pattern involving primarily peritoneal cavity of young women (8). They also can occur in men and involve pleura, pericardium, and tunica vaginalis. These lesions are often asymptomatic and are incidentally found during surgery for other causes, or present with pain, ascites, or pleural effusions.

Earlier literature reported no correlation between well-differentiated papillary mesothelioma and asbestos exposure; however, some more recent publications have shown association with asbestos exposure.

Well-differentiated papillary mesothelioma involves peritoneal surface diffusely, as multiple nodules ranging in size from a few millimeters to a few centimeters or present as a single nodule (1). Histologically these lesions are composed of broad fibrovascular papillae lined by flattened or cuboidal mesothelial cells (Figure 7.4a,b). Occasionally myxoid changes of the papillary cord, psammomatous bodies and central scars are seen. Small numbers of cases show tubulo-glandular structures or solid nests in the cyst wall (9). No or only minimal invasion is present (10). Occasionally, subnuclear vacuoles are seen. No mitosis or necrosis is present.

Differential diagnosis includes mesothelial hyperplasia, malignant mesothelioma, and borderline serous tumor.

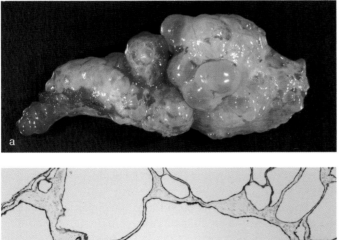

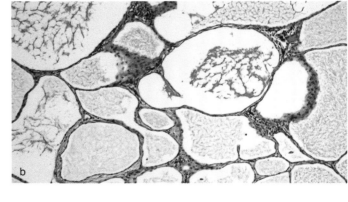

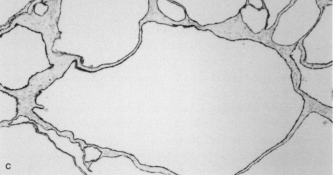

Figure 7.3 Peritoneal mass consisting of multiple thin-walled cysts filled with serous fluid (a). The cyst wall is lined by flattened mesothelial cells (b) that stain positive for calretinin (c).

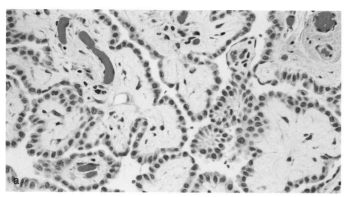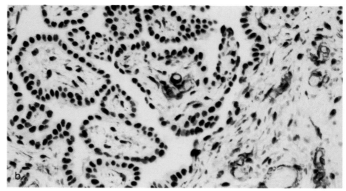

Figure 7.4 Broad papillae with myxoid stroma lined by flattened or cuboidal mesothelial cells (a) that stain positive for WT-1 (b).

Reactive hyperplasia is composed almost exclusively of mesothelial cells and does not show extensive papillary formations. Malignant mesothelioma can have areas resembling well-differentiated papillary mesothelioma and extensive sampling is necessary to confirm invasion. Bulky disease and marked cytologic atypia are additional features seen in malignant mesothelioma that help distinguish it from well-differentiated papillary mesothelioma (11).

Well-differentiated papillary mesothelioma is considered an indolent lesion with favorable outcome after tumor debulking surgery.

Adenomatoid Tumor of Pleura

Adenomatoid tumors of pleura are uncommon, benign neoplasms of mesothelial origin, most commonly occurring in genital tract in men and women; however, they have also have been reported to occur in pleura, mesentery, heart, adrenal gland, and lymph nodes (12,13). Pleural adenomatoid tumors are exceedingly rare.

Adenomatoid tumors are incidentally found during surgery or autopsy as non-encapsulated, relatively circumscribed, firm red–gray to yellow–tan mass measuring 0.5–2.5 cm in greatest dimension.

Pleural adenomatoid tumors are identical to their counterpart in testis/epididymis or uterus and are composed of multiple complex tubules, microcystic and capillary-like spaces anastomosing or embedded in a fibrous stroma. Spaces are lined by plump to flat mesothelial cells, and occasional cuboidal cells, with eccentric, vesicular nuclei and abundant eosinophilic or vacuolated cytoplasm (Figure 7.5a,b).

Sampling the entire tumor is recommended to rule out malignant mesothelioma with a focal or extensive microcystic component. Other entities such as lymphangioma, hemangioma, and metastatic carcinoma should be excluded. Lining cells of lymphangioma/hemangioma are positive for endothelial markers (CD31, CD34, and factor VIII) and are negative for mesothelial markers (calretinin, CK5/6, keratin, and vimentin). Metastatic carcinoma will stain positive for epithelial markers (CEA, claudin-4, EMA, and, if from the lung, TTF-1).

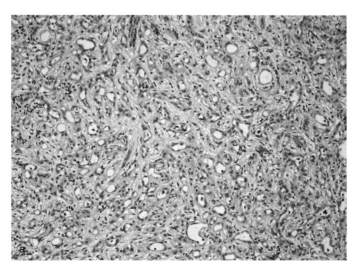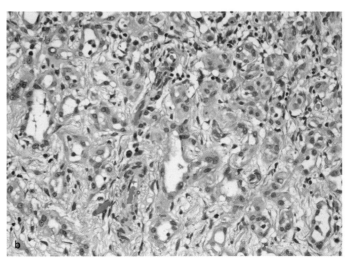

Figure 7.5 Adenomatoid tumor is composed of small tubular structures formed by bland mesothelial cells separated by collagenous stroma (a); the cytoplasm varies from abundant eosinophilic to scant (b).

Calcifying Fibrous Tumor

Calcifying fibrous tumors are benign lesions most commonly occurring in soft tissue of children and young adults. Rarely, they involve pleura and mediastinum either as a solitary mass or multifocal masses. Most patients are asymptomatic or present with symptoms related to the mass effect.

The nodules are firm, gray–white, and well circumscribed (14), ranging in size from 0.6 to 25 cm (15). Microscopically they are composed of hyalinized collagenous bundles with lymphoplasmacytic infiltrate, scattered fibroblasts, and extensive psammomatous/dystrophic calcifications (Figure 7.6). No mitosis or necrosis is present.

Calcified fibrous tumors can be distinguished from solitary fibrous tumors based on the presence of hypercellular and hypocellular areas in solitary fibrous tumors. Solitary fibrous tumors usually lack the calcifications that are the hallmark of calcifying fibrous tumor. Calcifying fibrous tumors occasionally are positive for CD34, a marker expressed in a solitary fibrous tumor.

Complete surgical resection is necessary to prevent recurrence.

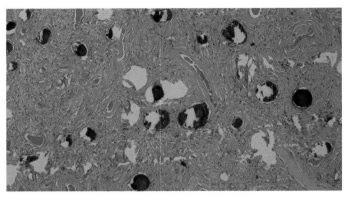

Figure 7.6 Dense hyalinized collagenous stroma with fibroblasts and psammomatous/dystrophic calcifications.

References

1. Churg A, Cagle PT, Roggli VL. Localized benign tumors and tumor-like condition of the serosal membranes. In: *Tumors of the serosal membranes*. Washington, DC: American Registry of Pathology Press; 2006: 107.

2. Mitchev K, Dumortier P, DeVuyst P. "Black spots" and hyaline pleural plaques on the parietal pleura of 150 urban necropsy cases. *Am J Surg Pathol*. 2002;26(9):1198–206.

3. Ousadded A, Elbouhaddouti H, Ibnmajdoub HK, Harmouch T, Mazaz K, Aittaleb K. A giant peritoneal simple mesothelial cyst: a case report. *J Med Case Rep*. 2011;5:361.

4. Dzieniecka M, Kaluzynski A. Benign multicystic peritoneal mesothelioma (BMPM) – case report and review of the literature. *Pol J Pathol*. 2011;2:122–24.

5. Senturk E, Cokpinar S, Sen S, Meteoglu I. Pleural multicystic mesothelial proliferation that presented with hemothorax. *Tuberk Torax*. 2013;61(1):47–49.

6. Wang TB, Dai WG, Liu DW, Shi HP, Dong WG. Diagnosis and treatment of benign multicystic peritoneal mesothelioma. *World J Gastroenterol* 2013;19(39):6689–92.

7. van Ruth S, Bronkhorst MWGA, von Coeverden F, Zoetmulder FAN. Peritoneal cystic mesothelioma: a case report and review of the literature. *Eur J Surg Oncol*. 2002;28(2):192–95.

8. Hoekstra AV, Riben MW, Frumovitz M, Liu J, Ramirez JT. Well-differentiated papillary mesothelioma of the peritoneum: a pathological analysis and review of the literature. *Gynecol Oncol* 2005;98: 161–67.

9. Chen X, Sheng W, Wang J. Well-differentiated papillary mesothelioma: a clinicopathological and immunohistochemical study of 18 cases with additional observation. *Histopathology*. 2013;62:805–13.

10. Ribeiro C, Campelos S, Moura CS, Moura CS, Machado JC, Justino A, et al. Well-differentiated papillary mesothelioma: clustering in a Portuguese family with a germline BAP1 mutation. *Ann Oncol*. 2013; 24:2147–50.

11. Malcipa A, Ambrogio SS, Deavers MT, Silva EG. Well-differentiated papillary mesothelioma of the peritoneum: a clinicopathologic study of 26 cases. *Am J Surg Pathol*. 2012;36(10):117–27.

12. Kaplan M, Tazelaar HD, Tomayoshi H, Schroer KR, Travis WD. Adenomatoid tumors of the pleura. *Am J of Surg Pathol*. 1996;20(10):1219–23.

13. Minato H, Nojima T, Kurose N, Kinoshita E. Adenomatoid tumor of the pleura. *Pathol Int*. 2009;59:567–71.

14. Mito K, Kashima, K, Daa T, Kondoh Y, Miura T, Kawahara K, et al. Multiple calcifying fibrous tumors of the pleura. *Virchows Arch*. 2005; 446:78–81.

15. Nascimento AF, Ruiz R, Hornick JL, Fletcher CDM. Calcifying fibrous 'pseudotumor'. Clinicopathologic study of 15 cases and analysis of its relationship to inflammatory myofibroblastic tumor. *Int J Surg Pathol*. 2002;1(3):189–96.

Chapter 8

Epidemiology, Etiology, and Pathogenesis of Malignant Mesothelioma

Alberto M. Marchevsky

Malignant mesothelioma is one of the human neoplasms where the role of an occupational exposure to a carcinogen, asbestos, has been extensively documented in multiple epidemiologic, experimental pathology, tissue burden analysis, and other studies (1–5). However, the association between asbestos and malignant mesothelioma is complex and the available evidence shows that the type of asbestos fiber, timing and length of exposure, exposure dose, location of the lesion (pleural, peritoneal, other), the type of tumor (diffuse malignant mesothelioma, localized malignant mesothelioma, well-differentiated papillary mesothelioma), and other considerations are important variables in assessing the etiologic role of asbestos exposure in a patient with "mesothelioma." There are extensive data showing significant associations between selected occupations and increased risk of malignant mesothelioma, documenting the induction of these tumors in animals under particular experimental conditions and demonstrating the potential of asbestos fibers to induce cellular transformation in tissue-culture models (1–4, 6–57). However, these data have been interpreted quite variably by different investigators. For example, some authors have postulated that mesotheliomas are almost always caused by asbestos, based on the assumption that mesotheliomas are "signal tumors" that are caused by asbestos (58,59). Based on this interpretation of the literature, the etiology of a malignant mesothelioma in any patient with any well-documented or alleged exposure to asbestos-containing products can be attributed to "asbestos." In contrast, other authors have taken a considerably more skeptical viewpoint and have postulated that pure chrysotile asbestos may not cause malignant mesothelioma altogether, that exposures to low doses of chrysotile asbestos in brake mechanics, drywallers, and other workers do not cause malignant mesothelioma, and that chrysotile asbestos does not cause peritoneal mesothelioma (10,11,32,34,60–65). These variable opinions are particularly difficult to reconcile during the assessment of the etiology of malignant mesotheliomas in patients with an occupational or non-occupational history of contact with multiple products containing variable concentrations of amphibole and/or chrysotile asbestos (4,66).

This chapter will briefly summarize basic concepts about the epidemiology, etiology, and pathogenesis of malignant mesothelioma. This author is not an epidemiologist, has worked as a pathologist medico-legal defense expert, and has a long-standing interest in evidence-based pathology and evaluation of scientific information (67–70).

Incidence and Other Demographic Aspects of Malignant Mesothelioma

According to the most recently available data from the Surveillance, Epidemiology and End Results (SEER) Program data, the incidence of mesothelioma during the 2012–2013 period is 0.9/million in the USA and approximately 2500–3000 new cases develop per year (71). The tumor can occur at all ages, but its incidence increases with age after the fifth decade of life, and has the highest incidence in patients older than 84 years (19.1/million). It is more than three times more frequent in male patients than in women, with a M:F ratio of 1.7:0.5. The incidence of malignant mesothelioma is variable by region of the USA and country, with a higher incidence in regions where asbestos was used more frequently in the past. For example, the incidence of malignant mesothelioma in Western Australia, a region where amphibole asbestos was mined and used in various products, has been reported as high as 47.7/million (72). The incidence of malignant mesothelioma has remained stable or slightly declined in the USA while it has increased in Denmark, Scotland, and other regions (19).

Pleural mesothelioma is considerably more frequent than peritoneal mesothelioma, and the tumor develops in the abdomen in only approximately 10 percent of cases (73). Approximately 250 peritoneal mesotheliomas develop per year in the USA.

Etiologic Agents of Diffuse Malignant Mesothelioma

Since the seminal studies by Wagner et al. in 1960 showing a high incidence of diffuse malignant mesothelioma in South African miners extracting crocidolite and Selikoff et al. in the 1960s of American insulators working with amosite asbestos, amphibole asbestos has been recognized as the most frequent cause of malignant mesothelioma (74,75) (Table 8.1). These initial clinical and epidemiologic studies suggested that all forms of asbestos can cause malignant mesothelioma, but subsequent studies of Canadian miners by McDonald and others have shown that miners working with chrysotile asbestos containing tremolite, a form of amphibole asbestos, had a considerably higher incidence of the disease than those miners exposed to chrysotile asbestos contaminated with smaller concentrations of tremolite, an amphibole, suggesting that tremolite rather than "pure chrysotile" was the cause of the disease (32,34,76).

Table 8.1 Etiologic agents of malignant mesothelioma*

Amphibole asbestos

? Chrysotile asbestos**

Erionite

Therapeutic radiation therapy

? SV40 virus***

* The etiologic agent cannot be identified in a substantial number of malignant mesotheliomas, particularly in women. These tumors have been described in the literature as "idiopathic."

** It is disputed in the epidemiologic literature whether chrysotile asbestos in high exposure doses is an etiologic agent of mesothelioma or whether the carcinogenic effect for this tumor results from contamination by the amphibole tremolite.

*** It is uncertain whether the oncogenic SV40 virus contributes to the causation of malignant mesothelioma. It may have a role as tumor promoter during the development of these tumors.

Table 8.2 Occupations and professions with elevated proportionate mortality ratios for mesothelioma

Plumbers

Pipefitters

Mechanical engineers in selected work sites

Shipyard workers

Electricians

Selected sheet metal workers

Asbestos miners

Asbestos manufacturer workers

Textile workers in industries using asbestos

Railroad workers

Asbestos and Diffuse Malignant Mesothelioma

Asbestos fibers occur naturally in different concentrations in most locations throughout the world, exposing individuals to what has been described as "ambient" or "background" asbestos levels. For example, the Environmental Protection Agency (EPA) estimates average concentrations of asbestos in outdoor US ambient air that range between 1E-05 and 4E-04 fiber/cc (77). Current estimates suggest that approximately 50–80 percent of malignant mesothelioma in men and 20–30 percent in women develop in individuals that have been exposed to significantly higher levels of mineral fiber than "ambient" or "background" asbestos levels (14). It is also generally accepted that the tumors develop many years after exposure, after a latency period of 15 years or longer (14,78,79). Asbestos appears to be a relatively weak carcinogen for malignant mesothelioma, as the tumor is relatively infrequent while millions of individuals have been exposed to occupational levels in the past.

Different asbestos fibers have considerably different carcinogenic potency for mesothelioma. This topic has been the subject of multiple epidemiologic studies that have provided variable and sometimes controversial data. It is beyond the scope of this chapter to discuss this literature in detail, but most studies agree that amphibole fibers are more carcinogenic than chrysotile asbestos for malignant mesothelioma and that crocidolite asbestos is a more potent carcinogen for this tumor than amosite asbestos. Different estimates of relative potency have been proposed. For example, Hodgson et al. have proposed that the relative potencies of crocidolite, amosite, and chrysotile for the development of malignant mesothelioma are 500:100:1 (80). A more recent meta-analysis of the epidemiological literature by Berman et al. suggests that the relative potency of pure chrysotile (uncontaminated by amphibole) relative to amphiboles ranges from 0 to 1/200th in various models (81). There is no consistent epidemiologic evidence supporting the hypothesis than in patients exposed to products containing mixed amphibole and chrysotile asbestos, the presence of

chrysotile increases the risk for the development of malignant mesothelioma over that accounted for the amphibole exposures (80–83).

Non-occupational and para-occupational asbestos exposures resulting from household contact with "asbestos workers" that brought dirty clothes to be laundered at home, bystander exposure to other workers, and/or exposure to amphibole asbestos as a building occupant or because of living or working near facilities that release asbestos fibers into the ambient air have also been described (84,85).

There is no epidemiologic evidence showing a significant association between asbestos exposure and increased risk for the development of unusual mesothelial neoplasms, such as localized mesothelioma or well-differentiated papillary mesothelioma (see Chapter 11).

Occupations at High Risk for the Development of Diffuse Malignant Mesothelioma Because of Past Exposure to Asbestos

An association between amphibole asbestos exposure and high risk for pleural malignant mesothelioma was initially described in asbestos miners, shipyard workers, and insulators, but several other occupations have been shown to expose workers to an increased risk of developing this tumor, as shown in Table 8.2 (86,87). An association between amphibole asbestos and peritoneal mesothelioma has been shown only in patients exposed to very high exposure doses (5). There is no significant evidence to support the hypothesis that chrysotile asbestos with or without tremolite contamination causes peritoneal mesothelioma (73).

Other Etiologic Agents for Diffuse Malignant Mesothelioma

Erionite and ionizing radiation are the other two known causes of malignant mesothelioma (Table 8.1) (79,88). Erionite is a non-asbestiform mineral fiber that has been widely used in the Cappadocia region of Turkey and is also present in other regions, such as North Dakota in the USA (16,21,88–92). It has a carcinogenic activity for mesothelioma like that of crocidolite asbestos. Malignant mesothelioma has also been associated with a history of prior radiation therapy to treat previous malignancies (93,94).

Several studies have suggested that the simian virus SV40 may play a role as a promoter in the pathogenesis of malignant mesothelioma (95,96). SV40 is a DNA virus of the family papovaviridae that is known to be oncogenic in rodents and able to transform human and animal cells *in vitro* (95). It has contaminated early polio vaccines and SV40 DNA sequences have been detected in up to 40–50 percent of human malignant mesotheliomas in the USA (79). However, there is no epidemiologic evidence showing an increased risk for mesothelioma in individuals exposed to the virus, and it remains controversial whether the virus can initiate mesothelial tumors in humans (97).

The terminology "idiopathic mesothelioma" has been applied to tumors of unknown etiology (4,78,79).

Genetic Risk for Malignant Mesothelioma

Germline mutations of *BAP1* gene have been described in a recently identified cancer syndrome that has been described in over 50 families worldwide, characterized by a markedly increased incidence of skin and uveal malignant melanoma, clear cell renal cell carcinoma, cholangiocarcinoma, and other tumors (78). Familial cases of malignant melanoma have also been described and the possible role of *BAP1* and other mutations in these individuals is under investigation (3,21,98–100). Ascoli et al. described losses at 1p, 6q, 13q, and 14q in patients with familial mesothelioma using comparative genomic hybridization, but similar findings have been seen in sporadic mesotheliomas, and it is unknown whether these genetic alterations increase the risk for malignant mesothelioma development or develop during the tumor evolution (101). Other studies have shown a history of asbestos exposure in familial clusters of malignant mesothelioma, so it is unclear whether these cases developed as a result of genetic susceptibility or household exposure to asbestos fibers (100).

Pathogenesis of Malignant Mesotheliomas Caused By Asbestos Exposure

It is beyond the scope of this chapter to review in detail the extensive available literature regarding the pathogenesis of malignant mesothelioma in asbestos-exposed individuals (14,24,38,51,97,102–104).

A relatively small proportion of inhaled asbestos fibers are deposited in the lungs, and many fibers are trapped in the airways and expelled through the muco-ciliary apparatus of the respiratory epithelium. The asbestos fibers that reach the lungs tend to deposit in peribronchiolar areas. Amphibole fibers are more efficient than chrysotile fibers to reach the lungs, due to their shape, rigidity, size, and other physicochemical characteristics. Intrapulmonary fibers are ingested by macrophages, broken into smaller mineral fragments and are eventually removed from the lungs by macrophages and lymphatics. Amphibole fibers tend to remain in lung tissues for many years while chrysotile fibers are considerably more biodegradable and are removed from the lung tissues in weeks or months (48,49). Asbestos fibers that are split or decomposed within the lungs by macrophages undergo chemical transformation and probably lose their carcinogenic potential.

The macrophage response triggered by the presence of asbestos fibers in tissues induces a local inflammatory reaction with release of high mobility group box 1 (HMGB1), various growth factors, reactive oxygen species, and other cytokines that promote sustained cell injury, DNA damage and cell growth resulting in carcinogenesis. Lung tissues undergo chronic inflammation, fibrosis and occasionally develop lung neoplasms in smokers and individuals exposed to high asbestos doses.

As asbestos fibers are mostly deposited in the lung parenchyma rather than pleural linings, it remains somewhat uncertain how they can initiate and promote carcinogenesis in mesothelial cells. Boutin et al. have shown the presence of amphibole fibers in thoracoscopic biopsies of parietal pleural from "black spots," in much higher concentrations than other pleural biopsies (105). This finding has suggested the hypothesis that amphibole asbestos fibers are deposited in a heterogeneous distribution following lymphatics in the parietal pleura reaching their highest concentrations in the pleural black spots visible by thoracoscopy. Microscopically, these areas show fibrosis and the deposition of environmental pigment and asbestos fibers that have been removed from the lungs by macrophages and lymphatics. Studies by Suzuki et al. have shown the presence of numerous chrysotile fibers shorter than 5 μm in length within pleural tissues from patients with malignant mesothelioma, and have proposed the hypothesis that short chrysotile asbestos fibers are the main cause of pleural mesothelioma (106). However, epidemiologic data do not show a significant association between short chrysotile fiber exposure and increased risk of developing malignant mesothelioma, and experimental pathology experiments have shown that short chrysotile fibers do not cause the tumor or other significant disease in animals due to their short biopersistence in lung tissues and other physicochemical characteristics (48,49,107). In addition, workers in occupations that have been exposed mostly to chrysotile fibers shorter than 5 μm in length, such as brake mechanics, have not been shown in a majority of epidemiological studies to be at an increased risk of developing malignant mesothelioma (61–63,66).

Mesothelial cell transformation is probably enhanced by epigenetic mechanisms, such as deletion of the key regulator gene *INK4a/ARF* by methylation, autophosphorylation of the epithelial growth factor EGF, activation of the *MET* gene, activation of mitogen-activated protein (MAP) kinases, increase in tumor necrosis alpha (TNF-α), and other mechanisms that are still poorly understood (14,79,96,108).

References

1. Beebe-Dimmer JL, Fryzek JP, Yee CL, Dalvi TB, Garabrant DH, Schwartz AG, et al. Mesothelioma in the United States: a Surveillance, Epidemiology, and End Results (SEER)–Medicare investigation of treatment patterns and overall survival. *Clin Epidemiol.* 2016;8:743–50.

2. Magnani C, Bianchi C, Chellini E, Consonni D, Fubini B, Gennaro V, et al. III Italian Consensus Conference on Malignant Mesothelioma of the Pleura. Epidemiology, Public Health and Occupational Medicine related issues. *Med Lav.* 2015;106:325–32.

3. Marinaccio A, Binazzi A, Bonafede M, Corfiati M, Di Marzio D, Scarselli A, et al. Malignant mesothelioma due to non-occupational asbestos exposure from the Italian national surveillance system (ReNaM): epidemiology and public health issues. *Occup Environ Med.* 2015;72:648–55.

4. Craighead JE. Epidemiology of mesothelioma and historical background. *Recent Results Cancer Res.* 2011;189:13–25.

5. Roggli VL, Sharma A, Butnor KJ, Sporn T, Vollmer RT. Malignant mesothelioma and occupational exposure to asbestos: a clinicopathological correlation of 1445 cases. *Ultrastruct Pathol.* 2002;26: 55–65.

6. Geltner C, Errhalt P, Baumgartner B, Ambrosch G, Machan B, Eckmayr J, et al. Management of malignant pleural mesothelioma – part 1: epidemiology, diagnosis, and staging: Consensus of the Austrian Mesothelioma Interest Group (AMIG). *Wien Klin Wochenschr.* 2016;128:611–17.

7. Taioli E, Wolf AS, Camacho-Rivera M, Kaufman A, Lee DS, Nicastri D, et al. Determinants of survival in malignant pleural mesothelioma: a Surveillance, Epidemiology, and End Results (SEER) study of 14,228 patients. *PLoS ONE.* 2015;10:e0145039.

8. Meyerhoff RR, Yang CF, Speicher PJ, Gulack BC, Hartwig MG, D'Amico TA, et al. Impact of mesothelioma histologic subtype on outcomes in the Surveillance, Epidemiology, and End Results database. *J Surg Res.* 2015;196:23–32.

9. Budroni M, Cossu A, Paliogiannis P, Palmieri G, Attene F, Cesaraccio R, et al. Epidemiology of malignant pleural mesothelioma in the province of Sassari (Sardinia, Italy). A population-based report. *Ann Ital Chir.* 2014;85:244–48.

10. Akl Y, Kaddah S, Abdelhafeez A, Salah R, Lotayef M. Epidemiology of mesothelioma in Egypt. A ten-year (1998–2007) multicentre study. *Arch Med Sci.* 2010;6:926–31.

11. McDonald JC. Epidemiology of malignant mesothelioma–an outline. *Ann Occup Hyg.* 2010;54:851–57.

12. Flores RM, Riedel E, Donington JS, Alago W, Ihekweazu U, Krug L, et al. Frequency of use and predictors of cancer-directed surgery in the management of malignant pleural mesothelioma in a community-based (Surveillance, Epidemiology, and End Results [SEER]) population. *J Thorac Oncol.* 2010;5:1649–54.

13. Ugolini D, Neri M, Canessa PA, Casilli C, Catrambone G, Ivaldi GP, et al. The CREST biorepository: a tool for molecular epidemiology and translational studies on malignant mesothelioma, lung cancer, and other respiratory tract diseases. *Cancer Epidemiol Biomarkers Prev.* 2008;17:3013–19.

14. Yang H, Testa JR, Carbone M. Mesothelioma epidemiology, carcinogenesis, and pathogenesis. *Curr Treat Options Oncol.* 2008;9:147–57.

15. Chapman A, Mulrennan S, Ladd B, Muers MF. Population based epidemiology and prognosis of mesothelioma in Leeds, UK. *Thorax.* 2008;63;435–39.

16. Metintas M, Metintas S, Ak G, Erginel S, Alatas F, Kurt E, et al. Epidemiology of pleural mesothelioma in a population with non-occupational asbestos exposure. *Respirology.* 2008;13:117–21.

17. Mak V, Davies E, Putcha V, Choodari-Oskooei B, Moller H. The epidemiology and treatment of mesothelioma in South East England 1985–2002. *Thorax.* 2008;63:160–66.

18. Larson T, Melnikova N, Davis SI, Jamison P. Incidence and descriptive epidemiology of mesothelioma in the United States, 1999–2002. *Int J Occup Environ Health.* 2007;13:398–403.

19. Boffetta P. Epidemiology of peritoneal mesothelioma: a review. *Ann Oncol.* 2007;18:985–90.

20. Yarborough CM. Chrysotile as a cause of mesothelioma: an assessment based on epidemiology. *Crit Rev Toxicol.* 2006;36:165–87.

21. Bertazzi PA. Descriptive epidemiology of malignant mesothelioma. *Med Lav.* 2005;96:287–303.

22. Bolognesi C, Martini F, Tognon M, Filiberti R, Neri M, Perrone E, et al. A molecular epidemiology case control study on pleural malignant mesothelioma. *Cancer Epidemiol Biomarkers Prev.* 2005;14:1741–46.

23. Abratt RP, White NW, Vorobiof DA. Epidemiology of mesothelioma – a South African perspective. *Lung Cancer.* 2005;49(Suppl 1):S13–15.

24. Zellos L, Christiani DC. Epidemiology, biologic behavior, and natural history of mesothelioma. *Thorac Surg Clin.* 2004;14:469–77, viii.

25. Lange JH. Re: "Mesothelioma trends in the United States: an update based on surveillance, epidemiology, and end results program data for 1973 through 2003". *Am J Epidemiol.* 2004;160:823.

26. Filiberti R, Montanaro F. Epidemiology of pleural mesothelioma in Italy. *Lung Cancer.* 2004;45(Suppl 1):S25–27.

27. Musk AW, de Klerk NH. Epidemiology of malignant mesothelioma in Australia. *Lung Cancer.* 2004;45(Suppl 1):S21–23.

28. Price B, Ware A. Mesothelioma trends in the United States: an update based on Surveillance, Epidemiology, and End Results Program data for 1973 through 2003. *Am J Epidemiol.* 2004;159:107–12.

29. Puntoni R. Molecular epidemiology of mesothelioma. *Pathologica.* 2003;95: 291–97.

30. Puntoni R, Filiberti R, Cerrano PG, Neri M, Andreatta R, Bonassi S. Implementation of a molecular epidemiology approach to human pleural malignant mesothelioma. *Mutat Res.* 2003;544:385–96.

31. Britton M. The epidemiology of mesothelioma. *Semin Oncol.* 2002;29;18–25.

32. McDonald AD, Case BW, Churg A, Dufresne A, Gibbs GW, Sebastien P, et al. Mesothelioma in Quebec

chrysotile miners and millers: epidemiology and aetiology. *Ann Occup Hyg.* 1997;41:707–19.

33. McLean AN, Patel KR. Clinical features and epidemiology of malignant pleural mesothelioma in west Glasgow 1987–1992. *Scott Med J.* 1997;42:37–39.

34. McDonald JC, McDonald AD. The epidemiology of mesothelioma in historical context. *Eur Respir J.* 1996;9:1932–42.

35. Ross D, McDonald JC. Occupational and geographical factors in the epidemiology of malignant mesothelioma. *Monaldi Arch Chest Dis.* 1995;50:459–63.

36. Antman KH. Natural history and epidemiology of malignant mesothelioma. *Chest.* 1993;103: 373S–76S.

37. Walz R, Koch HK. Malignant pleural mesothelioma: some aspects of epidemiology, differential diagnosis and prognosis. Histological and immunohistochemical evaluation and follow-up of mesotheliomas diagnosed from 1964 to January 1985. *Pathol Res Pract.* 1990;186:124–34.

38. Craighead JE. The epidemiology and pathogenesis of malignant mesothelioma. *Chest.* 1989;96:92S–93S.

39. Huncharek M. The epidemiology of pleural mesothelioma: current concepts and controversies. *Cancer Invest.* 1989;7:93–99.

40. Demopoulos RI, Kahn MA, Feiner HD. Epidemiology of cystic mesothelioma. *Int J Gynecol Pathol.* 1986;5:379–81.

41. Armstrong BK, Musk AW, Baker JE, Hunt JM, Newall CC, Henzell HR, et al. Epidemiology of malignant mesothelioma in Western Australia. *Med J Aust.* 1984;141:86–88.

42. Browne K. The epidemiology of mesothelioma. *J Soc Occup Med.* 1983;33:190–94.

43. McDonald JC, McDonald AD. Epidemiology of mesothelioma from estimated incidence. *Prev Med.* 1977;6:426–42.

44. Lemesch C, Steinitz R, Wassermann M. Epidemiology of mesothelioma in Israel. *Environ Res.* 1976;12:255–61.

45. Rubino GF, Scansetti G, Donna A, Palestro G. Epidemiology of pleural mesothelioma in North-western Italy (Piedmont). *Br J Ind Med.* 1972;29:436–42.

46. Stumphius J. Epidemiology of mesothelioma on Walcheren Island. *Br J Ind Med.* 1971;28:59–66.

47. Stanton MF, Wrench C. Mechanisms of mesothelioma induction with asbestos and fibrous glass. *J Natl Cancer Inst.* 1972;48:797–821.

48. Bernstein DM, Chevalier J, Smith P. Comparison of Calidria chrysotile asbestos to pure tremolite: final results of the inhalation biopersistence and histopathology examination following short-term exposure. *Inhal Toxicol.* 2005;17:427–49.

49. Bernstein DM, Chevalier J, Smith P. Comparison of Calidria chrysotile asbestos to pure tremolite: inhalation biopersistence and histopathology following short-term exposure. *Inhal Toxicol.* 2003;15:1387–419.

50. Berry G. Models for mesothelioma incidence following exposure to fibers in terms of timing and duration of exposure and the biopersistence of the fibers. *Inhal Toxicol.* 1999;11:111–30.

51. Kane AB. Animal models of malignant mesothelioma. *Inhal Toxicol.* 2006;18:1001–04.

52. Miller BG, Searl A, Davis JM, Donaldson K, Cullen RT, Bolton RE, et al. Influence of fibre length, dissolution and biopersistence on the production of mesothelioma in the rat peritoneal cavity. *Ann Occup Hyg.* 1999;43:155–66.

53. Whitaker D, Shilkin KB, Walters MN. Cytologic and tissue culture characteristics of asbestos-induced mesothelioma in rats. *Acta Cytol.* 1984;28:185–89.

54. Minami D, Takigawa N, Kato Y, Kudo K, Isozaki H, Hashida S, et al. Downregulation of *TBXAS1* in an iron-induced malignant mesothelioma model. *Cancer Sci.* 2015;106:1296–302.

55. Cunniff B, Newick K, Nelson KJ, Wozniak AN, Beuschel S, Leavitt B, et al. Disabling mitochondrial peroxide metabolism via combinatorial targeting of peroxiredoxin 3 as an effective therapeutic approach for malignant mesothelioma. *PLoS ONE.* 2015;10:e0127310.

56. Blackshear PE, Pandiri AR, Nagai H, Bhusari S, Hong HH, Ton TV, et al. Gene expression of mesothelioma in vinylidene chloride-exposed F344/N rats reveal immune dysfunction, tissue

damage, and inflammation pathways. *Toxicol Pathol.* 2015;43:171–85.

57. Zhong J, Lardinois D, Szilard J, Tamm M, Roth M. Rat mesothelioma cell proliferation requires p38delta mitogen activated protein kinase and C/EBP-alpha. *Lung Cancer.* 2011;73:166–70.

58. Mark EJ, Kradin RL. Pathological recognition of diffuse malignant mesothelioma of the pleura: the significance of the historical perspective as regards this signal tumor. *Semin Diagn Pathol.* 2006;23:25–34.

59. Smith AH, Wright CC. Chrysotile asbestos is the main cause of pleural mesothelioma. *Am J Ind Med.* 1996;30:252–66.

60. Teschke K. Thinking about occupation–response and exposure–response relationships: vehicle mechanics, chrysotile, and mesothelioma. *Ann Occup Hyg.* 2016;60:528–30.

61. Garabrant DH, Alexander DD, Miller PE, Fryzek JP, Boffetta P, Teta MJ, et al. Mesothelioma among motor vehicle mechanics: an updated review and meta-analysis. *Ann Occup Hyg.* 2016;60:8–26.

62. Hessel PA, Teta MJ, Goodman M, Lau E. Mesothelioma among brake mechanics: an expanded analysis of a case-control study. *Risk Anal.* 2004;24:547–52.

63. Goodman M, Teta MJ, Hessel PA, Garabrant DH, Craven VA, Scrafford CG, et al. Mesothelioma and lung cancer among motor vehicle mechanics: a meta-analysis. *Ann Occup Hyg.* 2004;48:309–26.

64. Robinson CF, Petersen M, Sieber WK, Palu S, Halperin WE. Mortality of Carpenters' Union members employed in the US construction or wood products industries, 1987–1990. *Am J Ind Med.* 1996;30:674–94.

65. Case BW, Abraham JL, Meeker G, Pooley FD, Pinkerton KE. Applying definitions of "asbestos" to environmental and "low-dose" exposure levels and health effects, particularly malignant mesothelioma. *J Toxicol Environ Health B Crit Rev.* 2011;14:3–39.

66. Welch LS. Asbestos exposure causes mesothelioma, but not this asbestos exposure: an amicus brief to the

Michigan Supreme Court. *Int J Occup Environ Health*. 2007;13:318–27.

67. Marchevsky AM, Walts AE, Wick MR. Evidence-based pathology in its second decade: toward probabilistic cognitive computing. *Hum Pathol*. 2017;61:1–8.

68. Marchevsky AM, Wick MR. Evidence-based guidelines for the utilization of immunostains in diagnostic pathology: pulmonary adenocarcinoma versus mesothelioma. *Appl Immunohistochem Mol Morphol*. 2007;15:140–44.

69. Marchevsky AM. Evidence-based medicine in pathology: an introduction. *Semin Diagn Pathol*. 2005;22:105–15.

70. Marchevsky AM, Wick MR. Current controversies regarding the role of asbestos exposure in the causation of malignant mesothelioma: the need for an evidence-based approach to develop medicolegal guidelines. *Ann Diagn Pathol*. 2003;7:321–32.

71. Malignant mesothelioma mortality. United States, 1999–2015. www.cdc.gov .mmwr/volumes/66/wr/mm608a3.htm.

72. Leigh J, Driscoll T. Malignant mesothelioma in Australia, 1945–2002. *Int J Occup Environ Health*. 2003;9:206–17.

73. Hassan R, Alexander R, Antman K, Boffetta P, Churg A, Coit D, et al. Current treatment options and biology of peritoneal mesothelioma: meeting summary of the first NIH peritoneal mesothelioma conference. *Ann Oncol*. 2006;17:1615–19.

74. Wagner JC, Sleggs CA, Marchand P. Diffuse pleural mesothelioma and asbestos exposure in the North Western Cape Province. *Br J Ind Med*. 1960;17:260–71.

75. Selikoff IJ, Churg J, Hammond EC. Relation between exposure to asbestos and mesothelioma. *N Engl J Med*. 1965;272:560–65.

76. Roggli VL, Vollmer RT, Butnor KJ, Sporn TA. Tremolite and mesothelioma. *Ann Occup Hyg*. 2002;46:447–53.

77. EPA summary of published measurements of asbestos levels in ambient air. www.epa.gov/sites/ production/files/2013-08/documents/ libbyasbestos_ambientairlitsearch5- 20-2013.pdf.

78. Carbone M, Kanodia S, Chao A, Miller A, Wali A, Weissman D, et al.

Consensus Report of the 2015 Weinman International Conference on Mesothelioma. *J Thorac Oncol*. 2016;11:1246–62.

79. Carbone M, Ly BH, Dodson RF, Pagano I, Morris PT, Dogan UA, et al. Malignant mesothelioma: facts, myths, and hypotheses. *J Cell Physiol*. 2012;227:44–58.

80. Hodgson JT, Darnton A. The quantitative risks of mesothelioma and lung cancer in relation to asbestos exposure. *Ann Occup Hyg*. 2000;44:565–601.

81. Berman DW, Crump KS. A meta-analysis of asbestos-related cancer risk that addresses fiber size and mineral type. *Crit Rev Toxicol*. 2008;38(Suppl 1):49–73.

82. Berman DW, Crump KS. Update of potency factors for asbestos-related lung cancer and mesothelioma. *Crit Rev Toxicol*. 2008;38(Suppl 1):1–47.

83. Hodgson JT, Darnton A. Mesothelioma risk from chrysotile. *Occup Environ Med*. 2010;67:432.

84. Ferrante D, Mirabelli D, Tunesi S, Terracini B, Magnani C. Pleural mesothelioma and occupational and non-occupational asbestos exposure: a case-control study with quantitative risk assessment. *Occup Environ Med*. 2016;73:147–53.

85. Marchevsky AM, Harber P, Crawford L, Wick MR. Mesothelioma in patients with nonoccupational asbestos exposure. An evidence-based approach to causation assessment. *Ann Diagn Pathol*. 2006;10:241–50.

86. Bang KM, Pinheiro GA, Wood JM, Syamlal G. Malignant mesothelioma mortality in the United States, 1999–2001. *Int J Occup Environ Health*. 2006;12:9–15.

87. Goldberg M, Imbernon E, Rolland P, Gilg Soit Ilg A, Saves M, de Quillacq A, et al. The French National Mesothelioma Surveillance Program. *Occup Environ Med*. 2006;63:390–95.

88. Carbone M, Baris YI, Bertino P, Brass B, Comertpay S, Dogan AU, et al. Erionite exposure in North Dakota and Turkish villages with mesothelioma. *Proc Natl Acad Sci U S A*. 2011;108:13618–23.

89. Tanrikulu AC, Senyigit A, Dagli CE, Babayigit C, Abakay A. Environmental malignant pleural mesothelioma in

Southeast Turkey. *Saudi Med J*. 2006;27:1605–07.

90. Senyigit A, Dalgic A, Kavak O, Tanrikulu AC. Determination of environmental exposure to asbestos (tremolite) and mesothelioma risks in the southeastern region of Turkey. *Arch Environ Health*. 2004;59:658–62.

91. Lilis R. Fibrous zeolites and endemic mesothelioma in Cappadocia, Turkey. *J Occup Med*. 1981;23:548–50.

92. Baris YI, Artvinli M, Sahin AA. Environmental mesothelioma in Turkey. *Ann N Y Acad Sci*. 1979;330:423–32.

93. Teta MJ, Lau E, Sceurman BK, Wagner ME. Therapeutic radiation for lymphoma: risk of malignant mesothelioma. *Cancer*. 2007;109:1432–38.

94. Witherby SM, Butnor KJ, Grunberg SM. Malignant mesothelioma following thoracic radiotherapy for lung cancer. *Lung Cancer*. 2007;57:410–13.

95. Cerrano PG, Jasani B, Filiberti R, Neri M, Merlo F, De Flora S, et al. Simian virus 40 and malignant mesothelioma (Review). *Int J Oncol*. 2003;22:187–94.

96. Carbone M, Pass HI, Rizzo P, Marinetti M, Di Muzio M, Mew DJ, et al. Simian virus 40-like DNA sequences in human pleural mesothelioma. *Oncogene*. 1994;9:1781–90.

97. Henzi T, Blum WV, Pfefferli M, Kawecki TJ, Salicio V, Schwaller B. SV40-induced expression of calretinin protects mesothelial cells from asbestos cytotoxicity and may be a key factor contributing to mesothelioma pathogenesis. *Am J Pathol*. 2009;174:2324–36.

98. Bianchi C, Brollo A, Ramani L, Bianchi T, Giarelli L. Familial mesothelioma of the pleura–a report of 40 cases. *Ind Health*. 2004;42:235–39.

99. Musti M, Cavone D, Aalto Y, Scattone A, Serio G, Knuutila S. A cluster of familial malignant mesothelioma with del(9p) as the sole chromosomal anomaly. *Cancer Genet Cytogenet*. 2002;138:73–76.

100. Ascoli V, Mecucci C, Knuutila S. Genetic susceptibility and familial malignant mesothelioma. *Lancet*. 2001;357:1804.

101. Ascoli V, Aalto Y, Carnovale-Scalzo C, Nardi F, Falzetti D, Mecucci C, et al. DNA copy number changes in familial

malignant mesothelioma. *Cancer Genet Cytogenet.* 2001;127:80–82.

102. Kubo T, Toyooka S, Tsukuda K, Sakaguchi M, Fukazawa T, Soh J, et al. Epigenetic silencing of microRNA-34b/c plays an important role in the pathogenesis of malignant pleural mesothelioma. *Clin Cancer Res.* 2011;17:4965–74.

103. Weiner SJ, Neragi-Miandoab S. Pathogenesis of malignant pleural mesothelioma and the role of environmental and genetic factors. *J Cancer Res Clin Oncol.* 2009;135:15–27.

104. Carbone M, Albelda SM, Broaddus VC, Flores RM, Hillerdal G, Jaurand MC, et al. Eighth international mesothelioma interest group. *Oncogene.* 2007;26:6959–67.

105. Boutin C, Dumortier P, Rey F, Viallat JR, De Vuyst P. Black spots concentrate oncogenic asbestos fibers in the parietal pleura. Thoracoscopic and mineralogic study. *Am J Respir Crit Care Med.* 1996;153:444–49.

106. Suzuki Y, Yuen SR, Ashley R. Short, thin asbestos fibers contribute to the development of human malignant mesothelioma: pathological evidence. *Int J Hyg Environ Health.* 2005;208:201–10.

107. Iigren E. The fiber length of Coaling chrysotile: Enhanced clearance due to its short nature in aqueous solution with a brief critique on "short fiber toxicity". *Indoor Built Environ.* 2008;17:5–26.

108. Carbone M, Gaudino G, Yang H. Recent insights emerging from malignant mesothelioma genome sequencing. *J Thorac Oncol.* 2015;10:409–11.

Chapter 9

Pathologic "Markers" of Above Background Asbestos Exposure

Allen Gibbs

The lung can exhibit a wide range of pathological responses to particle exposure depending on the physiochemical characteristics and dosage of the inhaled material, whether it is inhaled singly or in combination with other materials, on the immunological makeup of the individual exposed, and on whether the individual is suffering from any other disease which interferes with the normal lung defense mechanisms. The response may range from a mild fibrosis reaction around a collection of dust-laden macrophages, e.g., tin or titanium; to gross fibrosis, e.g., free silica, and neoplasia, e.g., asbestos.

The determination of whether asbestos exposure took place in a subject is important in cases of malignant mesothelioma, lung cancer, and pulmonary fibrosis. The identification of markers of exposure by histopathological means is important in a considerable proportion of cases, particularly where the occupational history is rather nebulous and ill-defined. It should be recognized that not all mesotheliomas are related to asbestos exposure and assessment of whether a lung cancer or pulmonary fibrosis is due to asbestos exposure can be extremely difficult unless strict criteria are utilized. It should be recognized that there is a continuum from background exposure to industrially derived exposures to asbestos and there is no sharp boundary between them. This can give rise to problems in determining the background ranges of asbestos for various populations (1). The latent period for asbestos-related diseases is generally measured in decades and therefore recall of exposures to asbestos may be inaccurate (2).

Indicators of above background exposure to asbestos which a pathologist may utilize to determine above background exposures include (a) pleural plaques (Figure 9.1), (b) identification of asbestos bodies on hematoxylin and eosin (Figure 9.2a), or iron-stained (Figure 9.2b) slides by light microscopy, and (c) quantification of asbestos fibers and bodies on lung tissue digests (3). Asbestosis results from relatively high exposures to asbestos and therefore a good history of exposure to asbestos should be obtained easily. Diffuse pleural fibrosis, which can result from exposure to asbestos, is relatively non-specific and its diagnosis relies on finding pleural plaques or an elevated level of asbestos bodies or fibers. It can result from other conditions such as tuberculosis, collagen vascular diseases, drugs, and idiopathic forms.

Mineralogy

Asbestos is a generic term for a family of naturally occurring fibrous crystalline hydrous silicate minerals. To qualify as a fiber the length to breadth (aspect) ratio has to be at least three to one – generally, the asbestos minerals have a high aspect ratio often ranging from 20:1 to 100:1 or higher and the fibers exceed 5 μm in length. The fibers are thin and usually < 0.5 μm in width. This mineral family is widespread in nature and due to its high tensile strength, pliability, and heat resistance, it had been increasingly used in industry from the beginning of the twentieth century. Production of asbestos rose from approximately a few hundred thousand tons in 1920 to more than five million tons in 1974 (4). However, since the 1980s, use of asbestos in developed countries has dropped and in the European Union its use has been banned.

Based on their physical configuration the various types of asbestos fibers can be divided into two major subfamilies – the serpentines and the amphiboles. They have distinctly different physical characteristics and geologic origins and as a consequence have different health implications. Chrysotile, which is the only serpentine form, has a wavy, coiled configuration (Figure 9.3), whereas the amphiboles, which include all the others, are long and straight and consist of double chains of silicate tetrahedral (Figure 9.4). The biopersistence of chrysotile and amphibole fibers differ significantly; chrysotile is substantially less durable in the lung, its half-life being measured in weeks or months, whereas the half-lives of the various amphibole fibers are measured in decades (5–7). The physical dimensions and configuration have implications for their pathogenicity.

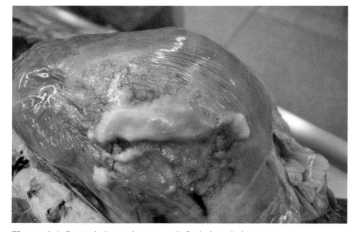

Figure 9.1 Parietal pleura showing calcified pleural plaque.

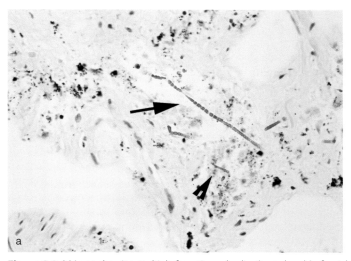

Figure 9.2 (a) Lung showing multiple ferruginous bodies (arrowheads) of variable length. Please note their "beaded" appearance with multiple yellow deposits arranged around a transparent core (H&E, ×100). (b) Ferruginous body with characteristic morphology (Perl's iron stain, ×1000).

Chrysotile accounted for between 90 percent and 95 percent of the world's production of asbestos, whereas crocidolite accounted for 3 percent and amosite 2–3 percent of the world's production. Crocidolite and amosite asbestos are known as the commercial forms of amphibole asbestos fibers. The other non-commercial amphibole forms – tremolite, actinolite and anthophyllite – were rarely used commercially, but they have occurred as minor contaminants of asbestos products.

Asbestos Bodies

In 1927 a publication by Cooke described asbestos bodies in the lungs of asbestos workers, and in 1932 Gloyne demonstrated the fiber forming the core of the body (8,9). They are golden brown, beaded structures often with clubbed ends producing a dumb-bell appearance (Figure 9.2a). They measure between 2

and 5 μm in width and from 30 to 300 μm in length. On careful inspection, a transparent, needle-shaped core may be observed. This distinguishes them from other types of ferruginous body which can form on carbon and sheet silicates (10). The brown coat is composed of haemosiderin and glycoprotein, so a Prussian blue stain may be useful in their demonstration (Figure 9.2b).

Asbestos body formation is influenced by a number of factors (Table 9.1). It has been found that, in the general population, 98 percent of ferruginous bodies have an amphibole core and 2 percent serpentine, i.e., chrysotile, core (11,12). Asbestos bodies show a greater propensity to form on longer fibers (10,13). Generally they are 20–50 μm in length with diameters of 2–5 μm. Bodies smaller than 10 μm in length are rarely encountered, while for fibers longer than 80 μm the probability of coating is close to 100 percent (14,15). The ratio of asbestos

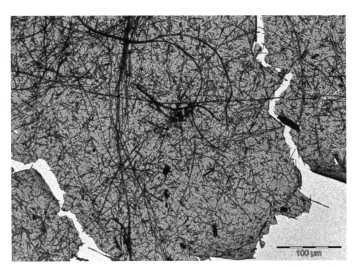

Figure 9.3 Electron microscopy grid showing multiple chrysotile fibers with characteristic curly appearance.

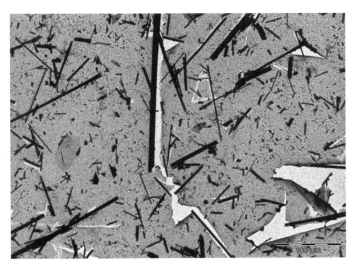

Figure 9.4 Electron microscopy grid showing multiple amosite fibers. The fibers are thicker and have a straight appearance, in contrast to those seen in Figure 9.3.

Table 9.1 Factors influencing the formation of asbestos bodies

Fiber type

Fiber length

Fiber diameter

Total amphibole fiber burden

Host biological factors

fibers to bodies is variably ranging: (a) between 5 and 100 to 1 in high-level amphibole exposure; (b) 10,000 to 1 in the general autopsy population; and (c) 100 to 1 in patients with pleural plaques in the absence of asbestosis. Counts of asbestos bodies do not show a consistent relationship to numbers of fibers and therefore one cannot easily extrapolate from a count of asbestos bodies to numbers of uncoated fibers (16). The proportion of

asbestos bodies formed is higher with amosite than crocidolite. This probably relates to fiber width, as bodies appear to more readily form on fibers of greater diameter. When there is a large amount of iron deposition in the lung, for example in association with welding or long-standing chronic passive venous congestion, a greater proportion of asbestos fibers become coated to form bodies. It is likely that the coating of asbestos fibers is part of the lung's defense mechanisms.

In order for a pathologist to see even one asbestos body in a tissue section, a fairly high asbestos exposure is required (11). It has been estimated that the finding of two asbestos bodies in a 2×2 cm by $5\ \mu m$ thick iron-stained tissue section is equivalent to 200 asbestos bodies per gram of wet-fixed lung tissue (17). Clusters of three or more asbestos bodies in the microscopic field usually indicate high exposure (Figure 9.3) (18).

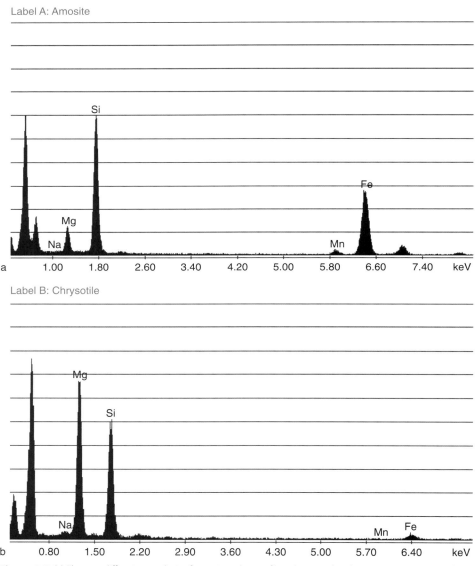

Figure 9.5 (a) Electron diffraction analysis of amosite asbestos fiber showing the characteristic presence of magnesium, silica, and iron minerals. (b) Electron diffraction analysis of chrysotile asbestos fiber showing the presence of magnesium and silica.

Table 9.2 Asbestos fiber concentrations in control subjects

Location	Method	Median fiber/g dry × 10⁶	Reference
UK	PCM	0.007 (ND – 0.521)	Whitwell et al. 1977 (58)
USA	SEM	0.031	Roggli 2004 (59)
France	TEM	11.2	Gaudichet et al. 1988 (60)
USA	TEM	1.29 (0.26–7.55)	Churg & Warnock 1980 (12)
Canada	TEM	0.62	Case & Sebastien 1987 (61)

Nearly all of the general population has experienced some background exposure to asbestos and this has been reflected in the finding of asbestos bodies in the digested lung tissue of control subjects. Therefore, it is important that laboratories performing such analyses should establish ranges for background controls because there is interlaboratory variation resulting from different protocols and counting rules (1).

Asbestos Fibers

These cannot be identified accurately in tissue sections by light microscopy because they are beyond the resolution of the light microscope and analytical equipment (EDXA) is needed for their identification (Figure 9.5a, b). There are a number of different methods for mineral fiber analysis which differ in sensitivity, specificity, complexity, and cost. In general, the tissue has to be digested and the digested material filtered and prepared for examination by phase-contrast microscopy (PCM) or the scanning (SEM) or transmission (TEM) electron microscope.

PCM analysis is a relatively easy, inexpensive method, but it does not provide accurate identification of mineral fiber type and lacks sensitivity. SEM can be used to quantify the number and dimensions of fibers, but it does not resolve the finest fibers, and the analytical capabilities are more limited than with TEM. Therefore, results from one laboratory cannot be directly compared with the results from another laboratory because the counting rules may be different and TEM is more sensitive than SEM. Asbestos fibers have been fairly ubiquitous in the air and so present in the lungs of the general population. A laboratory performing these analyses should determine the range for the background population in order to determine the significance of a result from a specific case. Table 9.2 lists the background control concentrations of asbestos fibers from a number of studies, and Table 9.3 the asbestos fiber concentrations by fiber type.

Pleural Plaques

Pleural plaques are located mainly in the parietal pleura but occasionally affect the visceral pleura (Figure 9.1) (19). They are shiny, waxy, gray–white raised nodular lesions located in the posterolateral, basal, and diaphragmatic zones of the parietal pleura (Figure 9.6). They do not involve apices or costophrenic angles and are either elongated in the vertical axis or follow the contours of the ribs. They are often calcified. Calcification of pleural plaques usually takes place two to three decades after the initial exposure (20).

Table 9.3 Asbestos fibers by type in control subjects

Location	Method	Median fiber/g dry × 10⁶	Reference
UK	TEM	Chrysotile 1.4 (ND – 11.7)*	Gibbs et al. 1991 (62)
		Amphibole 0.02 (ND – 1.7)*	
UK	TEM	Chrysotile 0.4	Howel et al. 1999 (63)
		Amphibole < 0.1	
UK	TEM	Chrysotile 9.3#	Wagner et al. 1988 (64)
		Amphibole 1.93#	
Canada	TEM	Chrysotile 0.2* (ND – 1.3)	Churg 1986 (65)
		Tremolite 0.2* (ND – 1.2)	
USA	SEM	Chrysotile 0.09 (ND – 4.2)	Dodson et al. 1988 (66)
		Amphibole 0.26 (0.05–5.2)	
Finland	SEM	Amphibole 0.16 (ND – 2.9)	Karjalainen et al. 1994 (67)
Germany (male)	TEM	Chrysotile ND!	Rodelsperger et al. 1999 (68)
		Amphibole 0.03!	
Germany (female)	TEM	Chrysotile 0.02!	Rodelsperger et al. 1999 (68)
		Amphibole 0.04!	

* Geometric mean.
# Arithmetic mean.
! Fibers > 5 μm in length counted only.

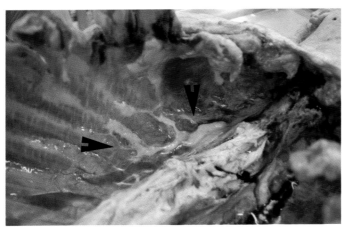

Figure 9.6 Pleural plaques located on the parietal pleura (arrowheads).

Histologically, the collagenous hyalinized plaque shows a basket-weave pattern with underlying small collections of lymphocytes and plasma cells (Figure 9.7). The mesothelial layer over the surface of the plaque is not always preserved. The center of the plaque is often calcified.

Pleural plaques are non-neoplastic and a great majority of individuals with plaques alone have no symptoms or changes detectable by lung function studies. Radiographic surveys of general populations have shown a 1–2 percent prevalence in males. In contrast, autopsy surveys have shown an increased prevalence of 4–39 percent (21,22). Computerized tomography (CT) scan studies are more specific and sensitive than ordinary chest x-ray studies for the detection of pleural plaques and calcifications. The majority of studies have shown no symptoms relative to pleural plaques nor impairment of lung function (23–26). In contrast, some studies of lung function have shown minor ventilatory defects (27,28).

The development of pleural plaques is highly correlated with increasing age and years since first exposure to asbestos and exposure duration. The greater the interval after first exposure to asbestos, the more likely is radiological detection because cal-

cification increases with age of the plaque – in one series, more than 50 percent of individuals showed radiological evidence of plaques 30–40 years after exposure (29). In a radiological survey of dockyard workers by Shears and Templeton the prevalence of pleural plaques increased with intensity of exposure (30). Similar findings were found in an autopsy series by Mollo et al. (31). However, Jones et al. found that the occurrence of plaques was more directly related to time from first exposure to asbestos than to cumulative exposure (32). Pleural plaques can result from brief, intermittent, and low-level exposures to asbestos (20,22).

Electron-microscopic investigations of lung tissue digests in subjects with parietal pleural plaques have shown that it is primarily amphibole asbestos fibers that are seen in increased amounts (18,22,33,34). Churg studied autopsy subjects of the general public and compared those with pleural plaques and those without plaques and no exposure to asbestos and found that plaques were associated with increased levels of commercial amphibole asbestos (amosite and crocidolite), but there was no association with numbers of chrysotile and noncommercial amphiboles (tremolite and anthophyllite) (33). However, approximately half of the pleural plaque cases did not appear to be related to increases in asbestos fibers. Similar findings have been found in other studies (6,34,35). Epidemiological studies have also shown that pleural plaques correlate with amphibole exposure rather than chrysotile asbestos exposure. For example, in Canadian chrysotile miners and millers the pleural plaques correlated with the presence of tremolite, which was associated with chrysotile in certain mines (36,37). In general, autopsy series investigating plaques have described cases that have occurred without an identifiable asbestos exposure (38). Therefore, in the individual case a degree of circumspection should be exercised before leaping to the conclusion that a pleural plaque automatically signifies an above-background exposure to asbestos.

Endemic pleural plaques have also been associated with environmental exposures to soils containing non-commercial amphibole fibers (tremolite and anthophyllite), for example, in Bulgaria, Greece, Turkey, Austria, and north-east Corsica (39–43).

Associations of plaques with factors other than exposure to asbestos include trauma, tuberculosis, exposures to titanium (44), mica, talc, and zeolites (45). Tobacco consumption appears to potentiate plaque development (34,36).

The question has arisen as to whether the presence of parietal pleural plaques increases the risk of lung cancer in individuals. Not surprisingly, general surveys have shown an increased risk of mesothelioma and lung cancer in subjects with pleural plaques compared to those without (46–49). However, when one controls for asbestos exposure in various industrial cohorts, the presence of pleural plaques does not result in an increased risk of lung cancer or mesothelioma compared to workers in the same industrial cohort without pleural plaques. This has been shown in Quebec chrysotile miners (36), dockyard employees (50), and other surveys (51–53).

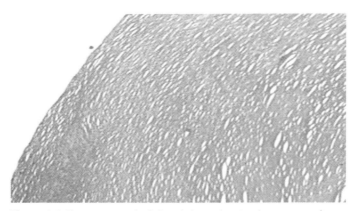

Figure 9.7 Photomicrograph of pleural plaque showing the presence of hyalinized, fibrotic tissue with characteristic basket-weave appearance (H&E, ×40).

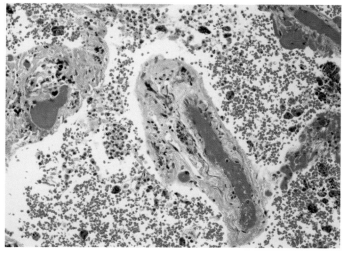

Figure 9.8 Early asbestosis, showing the presence of mild peribronchiolar fibrosis and elastosis and ferruginous bodies (H&E, ×40).

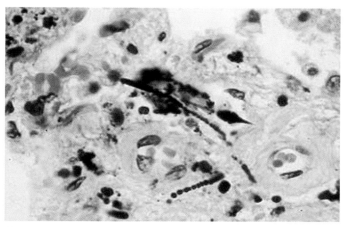

Figure 9.9 More advanced asbestosis with interstitial fibrosis and numerous ferruginous bodies (H&E, ×200).

Asbestosis

In 1924, Cooke introduced this term for pulmonary fibrosis consequent upon asbestos exposure (54). The earliest lesions of fibrosis are seen around the respiratory bronchioles (Figure 9.8) (55) and, if sufficiently numerous, they may lead to the obstruction of small airways, as evidenced by lung function tests (56). The fibrosis later extends to link up the respiratory bronchioles via adjacent alveolar walls and ducts (Figure 9.9). Progression of the lesion results in varying degrees of distortion of the pulmonary architecture with combinations of more solid fibrosis and honeycombing (5). The earliest macroscopical lesions are usually found in the subpleural zones of the posterior basal segments. They can progress to involve most of the lung so that it becomes contracted and exhibits honeycombing of the fine character, most severe at the bases. In the early stages, the patient is frequently asymptomatic, but by the time a third or so of the lung tissue has been involved, breathlessness is manifest. Radiological examination underestimates the degree of fibrosis, as it does not become detectable until the disease is relatively advanced. Severe asbestosis with clinical symptoms is a consequence of a high level of exposure to asbestos and is now rare in developed countries. It results from direct, heavy, and prolonged exposure to asbestos.

There is an increasing clinical problem with differentiating the fibrosis resulting from asbestos exposure to that occurring idiopathically. The average age of people living in developed countries has increased significantly and with it an increasing number of idiopathic pulmonary fibrosis cases has occurred. The light-microscopic findings of asbestosis are now well established and defined by the recent 2010 College of Pathologists – Pulmonary Pathology Society (CAP-PPS) Asbestosis Guidelines committee (57). First there is a requirement to confirm the presence of diffuse interstitial fibrosis *of an appropriate pattern* described as "always acellular and collagenous rather than fibroblastic and inflammatory." The second component is the presence of a necessary minimum number of either asbestos bodies or fibers (see below). Their assessment is made in Perls stained routine thickness (5 μm) sections (Figure 9.2b), and the average (arithmetic mean) number is calculated by counting all present within the available lung section area. For bonafide asbestosis, an average rate of > 2 asbestos bodies/cm² section area is necessary (in the presence of diffuse interstitial fibrosis). Most persons with bona fide asbestosis meet these morphological criteria set by the 2010 CAP-PPS Asbestosis committee. In most persons there is a correlation between inhaled and retained amphibole asbestos fibers and asbestos body counts.

References

1. Gibbs AR, Pooley F. Mineral fiber analysis and asbestos-related diseases. In: Craighead JE, Gibbs AR, editors. *Asbestos and its diseases*. New York, NY: Oxford University Press; 2008: 299–316.

2. Lanphear BP, Buncher CR. Latent period for malignant mesothelioma of occupational origin. *J Occup Med*. 1992;34:718–21.

3. Gibbs AR, Pooley F. Analysis and interpretation of inorganic mineral particles in "lung" tissues. *Thorax*. 1996;51:327–34.

4. Becklake MR. Asbestos related disease of the lung and other organs. Their epidemiology and implications for clinical practise. *Am Rev Respir Dis*. 1976;114:187–227.

5. Berry G, Pooley FD, Gibbs AR, Harris J, McDonald JC. Lung fibre burden in the Nottingham gas mask cohort. *Inhal Toxicol*. 2009;21:168–72.

6. Churg A, Vedal S. Fibre burden and patterns of asbestos related disease in workers with heavy mixed amosite and chrysotile exposure. *Am J Respir Critic Care Med*. 1994;150:663–69.

7. Bernstein D, Dunnigan J, Hesternerg T, Brown R, Legaspi Velasco JA, Barrera R, et al. Health risk of chrysotile revisited. *Crit Rev Toxicol*. 2013;43:154–83.

8. Cooke WE. Pulmonay asbestosis. *Br Med J*. 1927;2:1024–25.

9. Gloyne SR. The asbestos body. *Lancet*. 1932;1:1351–55.

10. Churg A, Warnock ML. Asbestos and other ferruginous bodies. Their formation and clinical significance. *Am J Pathol*. 1981;102:447–56.

11. Churg A, Golden J. Current problems in the pathology of asbestos related disease. In: Sommers SC, Rosen PP, editors. *Pathology annual*, Part 2. Norwalk, NJ: Appleton-Century-Crofts; 1982: 33–66.

12. Churg A, Warnock ML. Asbestos fibres in the general population. *Am Rev Respir Dis*. 1980;122:669–77.

13. Pooley FD. Asbestos bodies, their formation, composition and character. *Environ Res*. 1972;5:363–79.

14. Morgan A. Effect of length on the clearance of fibres from the lung and on body formation. In: Wagner JC, editor. *Biological effects of mineral fibres*. Lyon: IARC Scientific Publications; 1980: 329–35.

15. Morgan A, Holmes A. The enigmatic asbestos body. *Environ Res*. 1985;38: 283–92.

16. Pooley FD, Ranson DL. Comparison of the results of asbestos fibre dust counts in lung tissue obtained by analytical electron microscopy and light microscopy. *J Clin Pathol*. 1986;39:313–17.

17. Roggli VL, Pratt PC. Number of asbestos bodies on iron stained tissue sections in relation to asbestos body counts in lung tissue digestates. *Hum Pathol*. 1983;14:355–61.

18. Warnock ML, Prescott BT, Kuwahara TJ. Correlation of asbestos bodies and fibres in lungs of subjects with and without asbestosis. *Scan Electron Microsc*. 1982;2:845–57.

19. Solomon A, Sluis-Kremer GK, Goldstein B. Visceral pleural plaque formation in asbestosis. *Environ Res*. 1979;19:258–64.

20. Hillerdal G. Nonmalignant pleural disease related to asbestos exposure. *Clin Chest Med*. 1985;6:141–52.

21. Hourihane D, Lessof L, Richardson PC. Hyaline and calcified pleural plaques as an index of exposure to asbestos. A study of radiological and pathological features of one hundred cases with consideration of epidemiology. *Br Med J*. 1966;1:1069–74.

22. Wain SL, Roggli VL, Foster WL. Parietal pleural plaques, asbestos bodies, and neoplasia. *Chest*. 1984;86:707–13.

23. Leathart GL. Pulmonary function tests in asbestos workers. *Trans Soc Occup Med*. 1968;18:49–55.

24. Jarvolm B, Sanden A. Pleural plaques and respiratory function. *Am J Ind Med*. 1986;10:419–26.

25. Clin B, Paris C, Ameille J, Brochard P, Conso F, Gislard A, et al. Do asbestos related pleural plaques on HRCT scans cause restrictive impairment in the absence of pulmonary fibrosis? *Thorax*. 2011;66:985–91.

26. Kerper LE, Lynch HN, Zu K, Tao G, Utell MJ, Goodman JE. Systematic review of pleural plaques and lung function. *Inhal Toxicol*. 2015;27:15–44.

27. Schwartz DA, Fuortes LJ, Galvin JR, Burmeister LF, Schmidt LE, Lestikow BN, et al. Asbestos-induced pleural fibrosis and impaired lung function. *Am Rev Respir Dis*. 1990;141:321–26.

28. Shih JF, Wilson JS, Broderick A, Watt JL, Galvin JR, Merchant JA, et al. Asbestos-induced pleural fibrosis and impaired exercise physiology. *Chest*. 1994;105:1370–76.

29. Harries PG, Mackenzie FAF, Sheer G, Kemp JH, Oliver TP, Wright DS. Radiological survey of men exposed to asbestos in naval dockyards. *Br J Indust Med*. 1972;29:274–79.

30. Sheers G, Templeton AR. Effects of asbestos in dockyard workers. *Br Med J*. 1968;3;574–79.

31. Mollo F, Andrion A, Pira E, Barocelli MP. Indicators of asbestos exposure in autopsy routine. *Med Lav*. 1983;74: 137–42.

32. Jones RN, Diem JE, Glindemeyer H, Weill H, Gilson JC. Progression of asbestos radiographic abnormalities. In: Wagner JC, editor. *Biological effects of mineral fibres*. Lyon: IARC Scientific Publication; 1980: 537–44.

33. Churg A. Asbestos fibres and pleural plaques in a general autopsy population. *Am J Pathol*. 1982;109:88–96.

34. Karjalainen A, Karhunen PJ, Lalu K, Pentillä A, Vanhala E, Kyyrönen P, et al. Pleural plaques and exposure to mineral fibres in a male urban necropsy population. *Occup Environ Med*. 1994;51:456–60.

35. Gibbs AR, Pooley FD, Griffiths DM. Lung fibrous content of subjects with pleural plaques. *Eur Respir J*. 1994;7(Suppl 18):425.

36. Gibbs GW. Aetiology of pleural calcification. *Archs Environ Health*. 1979;2:76–83.

37. Churg A, dePaoli L. Environmental pleural plaques in residents of a Quebec mining town. *Chest*. 1988;94:58–60.

38. Andrion A, Pira E, Mollo F. Pleural plaques at autopsy, smoking habits and asbestos exposure. *Eur J Respir Dis*. 1984;65:125–30.

39. Burilkov T, Michailova L. Asbestos content of the soil and endemic pleural asbestosis. *Environ Res*. 1970;3:443.

40. Langer AM, Nolan RP, Constantopoulos SA, Moutsopoulos M. Association of Metsovo lung and pleural mesothelioma with exposure to tremolite containing whitewash. *Lancet*. 1987;1:965.

41. Yazicioglu S, Ibcayto R, Balci K, Sayli BS, Yorulmaz B, et al. Pleural calcification, pleural mesotheliomas and bronchial cancers caused by tremolite dust. *Thorax*. 1980;35: 564–69.

42. Boutin C, Viallat J, Steinbauer J, Gaudichet A, Dufour G. Pleural plaques and environmental asbestosis in North Corsica. In: Bignon J, Peto J, Saracci R, editors. *Non-occupational exposure to mineral fibres*. Lyon: IARC Scientific Publication; 1989; vol. 90: 406–10.

43. McConnochie K, Simonato L, Mevrides P, Cristofides P, Mitha R, Wagner JC. In: Bignon J, Peto J, Saracci R, editors. *Non-occupational exposure to mineral fibres*. Lyon: IARC Scientific Publication; 1989; vol. 90: 411–19.

44. Garabrant DH, Fine LJ, Oliver C, Bernstein L, Peters J. Abnormalities of pulmonary function and pleural disease among titanium metal production workers. *Scand J Environ Health*. 1987;13:47–51.

45. Artvinli M, Baris YI. Environmental fibre-induced pleuro-pulmonary disease in an Anatolian village: an epidemiologic study. *Arch Environ Health*. 1982;37:177–81.

46. Fletcher DE. A mortality study of shipyard workers with pleural plaques. *Br J Ind Med*. 1972;29:142–45.

47. Edge JR. Incidence of bronchial carcinoma in shipyard workers with

pleural plaques. *Ann N Y Acad Sci.* 1979;330:289–94.

48. Hillerdal G. Pleural plaques and risk for cancer in the County of Uppsala. *Eur J Respir Dis.* 1980;Suppl 107:111–17.

49. Pairon JC, Laurent F, Rinaldo M, Clin B, Andujar P, Ameille J, et al. Pleural plaques and the risk of pleural mesothelioma. *J Nat Cancer Inst.* 2013;105:293–301.

50. Sheers G. Asbestos associated disease in employees of Devenport dockyard. *Ann N Y Acad Sci.* 1979;330:281–87.

51. Weiss W. Asbestos-related pleural plaques and lung cancer. *Chest.* 1993;103:1854–59.

52. Kiviluto R, Meurman LO, Hakama M. Pleural plaques and neoplasia in Finland. *Ann N Y Acad Sci.* 1979;330:31–33.

53. Ameille JA, Brochard P, Letourneux M, Paris C, Pairon JC. Asbestos-related cancer risk in patients with asbestosis or pleural plaques. *Rev Mal Respir.* 2011;6:e11–e17.

54. Cooke WE. Fibrosis of the lungs due to inhalation of asbestos dust. *Br Med J.* 1924;2:147.

55. Wagner JC. The pneumoconioses due to mineral dusts. *J Geol Soc.* 1980;137:537–45.

56. Jodoin G, Gibbs GW, Macklem PT, McDonald JC, Becklake M. Early effects of asbestos exposure on lung function. *Am Rev Respir Dis.* 1971;104:525–34.

57. Roggli VL, Gibbs AR, Attanoos RL, Churg A, Popper H, Cagle P, et al. Pathology of asbestosis – an update of the diagnostic criteria. Report of the Asbestosis Committee of the College of American Pathologists and Pulmonary Pathology Society. *Arch Pathol Lab Med.* 2010;134:462–80.

58. Whitwell F, Scott J, Grimshaw M. Relationship between occupations and asbestos-fibre content of the lungs in patients with pleural mesothelioma, lung cancer and other diseases. *Thorax.* 1977;32:377–86.

59. Roggli VL. Asbestos bodies and non-asbestos ferruginous bodies. In: Roggli VL, Oury TD, Sporn TA, editors. *Pathology of asbestos-associated diseases.* 2nd edition. New York, NY: Springer; 2004: 34–70.

60. Gaudichet A, Janson X, Monchaux G, Dufour G, Sebastien P, De Lajartre AY, et al. Assessment by analytical microscopy of the total lung fibre burden in mesothelioma patients matched with four other pathological series. *Ann Occup Hyg.* 1988;32(Suppl 1):213–23.

61. Case BW, Sebastien P. Environmental and occupational exposures to chrysotile asbestos: a comparative microanalytic study. *Arch Environ Health.* 1987;42:185–91.

62. Gibbs AR, Stephens M, Griffiths DM, Blight BJ, Pooley FD. Fibre distribution in the lung and pleura of subjects with asbestos-related diffuse pleural fibrosis. *Br J Ind Med.* 1991;48:762–70.

63. Howel D, Gibbs AR, Arblaster L, Swinburne L, Schweiger M, Hatton P, et al. Mineral fibre analysis and routes of exposure to asbestos in the development of mesothelioma in an English region. *Occup Environ Med.* 1999;56:51–58.

64. Wagner JC, Newhouse ML, Corrin B, Rossiter CE, Griffiths DM. Correlation between fibre content of the lung and disease in East London asbestos factory workers. *Br J Ind Med.* 1988;45:305–08.

65. Churg A. Lung asbestos content in long-term residents of a chrysotile mining town. *Am Rev Respir Dis.* 1986;134:125–27.

66. Dodson RF, Williams Jr MG, Corn CJ, Rankin TL. A comparison of asbestos burden in nonurban patients with and without lung cancer. *Cytobios.* 1988;56:7–15.

67. Karjalainen A, Vanhala E, Karhunen PJ, Lalu K, Penttilä A, Tossavainen A. Asbestos exposure and pulmonary fibre concentrations of 300 Finnish urban men. *Scand J Work Environ Health.* 1994;20:34–41.

68. Rodelsperger K, Woitowitz HJ, Brukel B, Arhelger R, Pohlaben H, Jöckel KH. Dose–response relationship between amphibole fibre lung burden and mesothelioma. *Cancer Detect Prev.* 1999;23:183–93.

Chapter 10

Molecular Aspects of Malignant Mesothelioma and Other Tumors of the Pleura and Peritoneum

Sanja Dacic

Introduction

The evolution of molecular platforms that permit rapid identification of genetic alterations has played a significant role in the detection of major genomic events in the development of carcinomas, mesotheliomas, and other neoplasms. Molecular approaches have evolved from a single gene test approach, so-called first-generation of molecular diagnostics (Sanger sequencing and FISH), to second-generation polymerase chain reaction (PCR) amplicon multiplex gene panel testing-based platforms (i.e., Sequenom, SNaPShot, PCR-based massively parallel next-generation sequencing) for detection of an ever-expanding number of genes of interest. The single-gene approach used in the earlier studies was rather disappointing in the detection of oncogenic events responsible for the development and progression of mesotheliomas. Furthermore, a single gene test approach did not lead to the discovery of potentially targetable oncogenic alterations. Therefore, the third generation of molecular diagnostics, hybrid capture-based massively parallel NGS, represents a major breakthrough in the detection of the full spectrum of genomic alterations (mutations, insertions, deletions, copy number alterations, gene fusions) in a single assay. The NGS is highly dependent on sophisticated bioinformatics analysis programs and faces significant data management and interpretation challenges. The sequencing instruments generate millions of short sequence reads, which are strings of data representing the order of the DNA nucleotides in each fragment. Complex computational algorithms are used to process the large amounts of data and to reliably detect genomic alterations. The sequence reads are aligned to specific positions in the human genome reference sequence with the use of appropriate computer algorithm.

The output file is computationally filtered according to the research/clinical objective and provides information regarding the number of sequence reads generated (depth of coverage) and the accuracy of the genotype at each position. Data output is implemented in constantly updated databases that allow distinction of polymorphisms and germline mutations from somatic events.

This chapter summarizes the results of studies that used all of the above-mentioned approaches in the analysis of mesothelioma and to a lesser extent other neoplasms occurring in the pleura.

Malignant Mesothelioma

Gene Mutations and Copy Number Changes

Various methods including traditional cytogenetic karyotypic studies, comparative genomic hybridization (CGH), array CGH, and single nucleotide polymorphism (SNP) arrays have demonstrated many structural and numeric chromosomal alterations in malignant mesotheliomas (MM). Chromosomal losses are more common than gains in MM. Regardless of the MM histological subtype, the most common losses are on chromosomal arms 1p, 3p, 4q, 6q, 9p, 13q, 14q, and 22q. The most common gains are on chromosomal arms 1q, 5p, 7p, 8q, and 17q (1–3). Most genomic changes overlap between different histological subtypes of MM, although losses at chromosomal regions 3p14–21p, 8p12-pter and 17p12-pter and gains at 7q are more common in epithelioid mesotheliomas (1). Deletions in 6q, 14q, 17p and 22q, and gain of 17q were seen in asbestos-associated but not radiation-related cases (4). Overall, regions of copy number gain are more common in peritoneal MM, whereas losses are more common in pleural MM, with regions of loss containing known tumor suppressor genes and regions of gain encompassing genes encoding receptor tyrosine kinase pathway members (4).

Major somatic mutations occur in tumor suppressor genes including *CDKN2A* ($p16^{INK4a}$), *NF2*, and *BAP1* (Table 10.1) (5–14). Recent whole-exome analysis revealed other mutations not previously reported in MM, such as mutations in *SETD2* (8 percent), *DDX3X* (4 percent), *ULK2, RYR2* (4 percent), *CFAP45* (3 percent), *SETDB1* (3 percent), *SF3B1* (2 percent), *TRAF7* (2 percent), and *DDX51* (1 percent) (13,15). *TRAF7* mutations seem to be mutually exclusive with *NF2* alterations. Oncogene point mutations are uncommon in MM and rare cases with *PTEN, RB1, FBXW7, APC, KRAS,* and *NRAS* mutations have been reported (13,16,17).

CDKN2A (***p16***^{INK4a}). Deletions of the 9p21 are the most common genetic abnormality in MM resulting in loss of *CDKN2A* ($p16^{INK4a}$), *CDKN2B* ($p15^{INK4b}$), *p53* regulator *CDKN2A/p14*^{ARF}, and *MTAP*. The loss of *p14*^{ARF} leads to destabilization and functional loss of p53, which is very rarely mutated in MM. Loss of *p16/CDKN2A* in MM is a result of deletion, promoter hypermethylation, or point mutation, with homozygous deletion being the most common (5,6,18).

Table 10.1 Summary of major somatic alterations in tumor suppressor genes in malignant mesothelioma

Gene	Associated histology	Prognosis	Methods of detection	Treatment response
P16/CDKN2A	Sarcomatoid	Poor	FISH	None
NF2	None	None	FISH	mTOR inhibitors CRL inhibitors FAK inhibitors
BAP1	Epithelioid	None*	IHC DNA sequencing	Presumable PARP-inhibitor DNA-PK inhibitor EZH2 inhibitor HDAC inhibitor

CRL, Cullin-RING ligase; FAK, focal adhesion kinase; PARP, poly ADP ribose polymerase; DNA-PK, DNA-dependent protein kinase; HDAC, histone deacetylase.
* BAP1 germline mutations are associated with favorable prognosis.

Frequency of *p16/CDKN2A* deletion depends on the histological subtype of MM (100 percent sarcomatoid, 60–70 percent epithelioid, and biphasic pleural MM). In contrast to pleural MM, *p16* deletions occur less frequently in peritoneal MM (up to 35 percent) (19). Numerous studies demonstrated the diagnostic usefulness of *p16* deletion in separating benign from malignant mesothelial proliferations in the body cavity effusion specimens and formalin-fixed paraffin embedded surgical specimens (6,20–25) (Figure 10.1a–c). Genetic alterations of 9p are one of the most frequent events in other tumor types

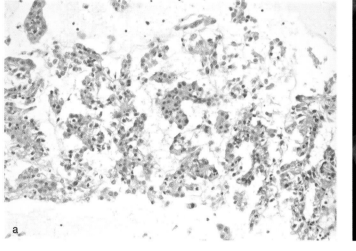
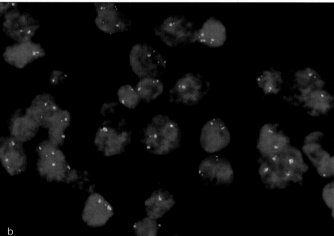
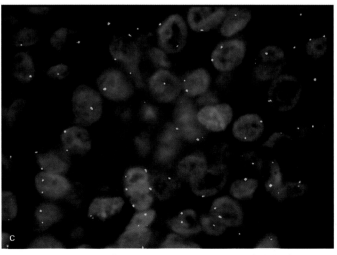

Figure 10.1 (a) Pleural effusion with highly atypical mesothelial cells in a patient with diffuse pleural thickening and pleural nodules (H&E, ×10). (b) Example of a normal p16 FISH assay. Normal cells demonstrate two green (9 centromere CEP9) and two red signals (p16). (c) Positive FISH assay demonstrating only two green signals (9 centromere) and the lack of red (p16) signals in the atypical nuclei.

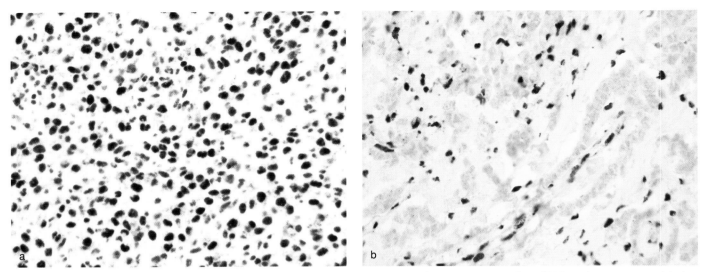

Figure 10.2 (a) Example of intact *BAP1* showing nuclear immunoreactivity in all cells (IHC, ×40). (b) Positive *BAP1* test: loss of *BAP1* nuclear immunoreactivity in mesothelioma cells. In contrast, the benign stromal cells show *BAP1* nuclear immunoreactivity, a finding that can be used as an internal positive control for the immunostain (IHC, ×40).

including non-small cell lung carcinomas and sarcomas, and, therefore, deletion cannot be used to differentiate these neoplasms from MM (26). Deletions of *CDKN2A* ($p16^{INK4a}$) are associated with poor prognosis in all histological subtypes of pleural and peritoneal MM (19,27).

NF2. The neurofibromin 2 (*NF2*) located on 22q12.1 was one of the first neurofibromatosis-related genes shown to be inactivated in MM (8,10). The *NF2* gene is inactivated by deletions, nonsense and missense mutations in about 60 percent of MM, while mutations occur in about 20 percent of MM. Recently, comprehensive genomic analysis of MM identified recurrent fusions in *NF2* that were mutually exclusive with *NF2* mutations (13). *NF2* inactivation has not been associated with histological subtype of MM or prognosis in pleural MM. In contrast, hemizygous loss of *NF2* in peritoneal MM has been associated with poor prognosis (28). The neurofibromin 2 protein (merlin) is a membrane cytoskeleton-associated protein downstream of integrin-like kinase (8). Merlin is thought to be one of the key molecules in the signaling cascades that determine invasion, cell growth, and survival of malignant mesothelial cells (8–10). *NF2* inactivation results in increased mTOR signaling and Hippo pathway activation (9,29,30). Targeting Hippo and mTOR pathways has been recently suggested as possible treatment strategies (31–35). A phase I study of the dual PI3K/mTOR inhibitor GDC-0980 (Apitolisib) showed a 15 percent partial response rate in MM (36).

BAP1. BRCA-associated protein 1 (*BAP1*) somatic alterations occur in about 20 percent of sporadic MM in Western patients and in 60 percent of Japanese patients (37). Somatic alterations are the result of large deletions, point mutations, fusions, and insertions (11–14). Germline *BAP1* mutations have been identified in patients with *BAP1* tumor predisposing syndrome, which is inherited in an autosomal dominant manner

and is characterized by uveal melanoma, mesothelioma, cutaneous melanocytic lesions, renal cell carcinoma, basal cell carcinoma, and possibly intrahepatic cholangiocarcinoma (12,38–43). Less than 5 percent of sporadic MM harbor *BAP1* germline mutations. Patients with *BAP1* somatic mutations are more frequently tobacco smokers, and no other distinct clinical feature has been reported (44). *BAP1* alterations appear to be more common in epithelioid-type MM (44,45). Prognostic significance of *BAP1* is controversial, but it appears that outcomes are more favorable in MM with germline mutations (46,47). Recent studies suggested that loss of *BAP1* as determined by immunohistochemistry can be used to support the diagnosis of MM in small biopsy and cytology samples (Figure 10.2a,b) (48–52). *BAP1* mutations might be a potential therapeutic target. *BAP1* loss results in increased expression of *EZH2* and preclinical studies showed that mesothelioma cells that lack *BAP1* are sensitive to *EZH2* pharmacologic inhibition, suggesting a novel therapeutic approach for *BAP1*-mutant malignancies. *EZH2* inhibitors have recently entered clinical trials (NCT01897571, NCT01395601, NCT01082977) (53).

LATS2. The *LATS2* (large tumor suppressor homolog 2) gene located at chromosome 13q12 encodes a serine/threonine kinase, a component of the Hippo signaling pathway. Inactivation of *LATS2* results in activation of Hippo signaling through YAP. Recurrent inactivating mutations in *LATS2* have been reported in approximately 5–15 percent of MM and 35 percent in cell lines (29,54). It is uncertain if *LATS2* inactivation is associated with the MM histology or prognosis.

TP53. Mutations of *p53* are frequent in different cancer types, but occur only in about 8 percent of MM (13). Mutations in *TP53* are associated with shorter overall survival in patients with MM (55). *TP53* was reported to be absent from the epithelioid subtype (13). *TP53* polymorphisms in intron 7 were more

Table 10.2 Summary of predicted gene fusions in malignant mesothelioma

Gene	Fusion partners
NF2	EWSR1
	D2HGDH
	CABP7
	GSTT1
	RHOT1
	THRB
	IFT140
	CABP7
	PIEZO2
	OSBP2
	PI4KA
	RHOT1
	NFATC1
BAP1	WDR6
	ALDH3B1
	TNNC1
	PBRM1
	CCDC66
SETD2	NBEAL2
	PHF7
	SPATA12
	CCDC12
PBRM1	CYB561D2
	NISCH
	WDR82
	ALAS1
	DNAH1
PTEN	SH3RF1
	PAPSS2
Other	STK11–NOSIP
	LIFR–C20orf24
	CLTC–BDNF
	RRBP1–DTD1

* Modified with permission from reference 13.

frequently identified in MM associated with asbestos exposure than in MM occurring in asbestos-unexposed patients (56).

Gene Fusions

Analysis of RNA-seq data for presence of gene fusions identified many recurrent fusions involving tumor suppressor genes such as *NF2*, *BAP1*, *SETD2*, *PBRM1*, and *PTEN* (Table 10.2) (13). It has been shown that fusions are mutually exclusive with other alterations occurring in the same genes such as mutations. A gene fusion between *GSTT1* and *NF2* does not lead to a copy number change, and it may be undetected in the absence of fusion data.

DNA Methylation

Numerous genes have been shown to be downregulated by DNA methylation in MM, most notably the genes in the Wnt pathway. MM epigenetic profiles differ from normal mesothelial cells and from other tumor types (57). The DNA methylation profile of MM depends on the patient's age, ethnic background, histologic subtype, and asbestos exposure. The DNA methylation of

TRAIL receptor genes and of tumor suppressor gene *RSSF1* is more frequent in epithelioid than in sarcomatoid MM (58,59). Methylation of several genes have been described to be useful in the diagnosis of MM (57,60,61).

A significant association between asbestos fiber burden and methylation status of *CDKN2A*, *CDKN2B*, *RASSF1*, and *MT1A* has been demonstrated (62). MM with a low frequency of DNA methylation are associated with longer survival (61).

Gene Expression Profiles

Expression profiling using microarray has been used to identify new diagnostic and prognostic markers of MM (18,63–67). Studies also tried to link the gene expression profiles to fibers/asbestos exposure. The main limitation of the published studies is the very limited overlap in gene expression results. Gene expression profiles can differentiate between epithelioid and non-epithelioid MM, but they do not enhance the classification beyond traditional histological approach. Furthermore, the predictive value of published studies is only around 65 percent, which is below the level of clinical usefulness. Nevertheless, one study identified gene *Aurora Kinase B* to be overexpressed in both sarcomatoid and epithelioid pleural MM (18). Aurora kinases A and B (and their binding partners survivin and TPX2, respectively) belong to a small family of serine/threonine kinase that function in various stages of mitosis and its overexpression is known to contribute to oncogenesis. The interest in Aurora kinase relates to its potential as a therapeutic target (68).

Bueno et al. recently defined four major molecular clusters of MM using RNA-seq-derived expression data (13). The clusters included sarcomatoid, epithelioid, biphasic–epithelioid and biphasic–sarcomatoid. Although molecular clusters mostly concurred with the histological classification, there were some differences, particularly in the biphasic type. The biphasic–sarcomatoid cluster was a group of biphasic MM with a high proportion of sarcomatoid component. The biphasic–epithelioid cluster was histologically more heterogeneous and included pure epithelioid and biphasic MM with mostly epithelioid component. Interestingly, molecular clustering was a better predictor of prognosis than histology alone. Histologically classified epithelioid mesothelioma that were molecularly classified as biphasic–epithelioid, biphasic–sarcomatoid, or sarcomatoid showed shorter overall survival. The epithelioid cluster showed the longest survival. Similar to earlier studies, the differential expression analysis of sarcomatoid and epithelioid clusters demonstrated differences in upregulated and downregulated genes. The most significantly upregulated gene in the epithelioid group was *CLDN15*, a gene that is downregulated in cells undergoing epithelial-to-mesenchymal transition. The most significantly upregulated genes in the sarcomatoid group were *LOXL2* and *VIM*, both of which are upregulated during epithelial-to-mesenchymal transition.

miRNA

miRNA is a group of endogenous, small, non-coding RNA that can modulate protein expression by regulating translational efficiency or cleavage of target. They regulate the expression of known tumor suppressor genes and oncogenes. miRNA genes are frequently located at fragile sites, regions of loss of heterozygosity, minimal regions of amplifications or common chromosomal breakpoint regions. They are expressed in a tissue-specific manner, and the pattern of expression accurately defines the specific cancer types. Microarray profiling, confirmed by qRT-PCR, revealed a differential expression of miRNAs between benign and malignant mesothelial cells. The expression of several miRNAs (miR-17–5p, miR-21, miR-29a, miR-30c, miR-30e-5p, miR-106a, and miR-143) was significantly associated with the histological subtypes of malignant pleural mesothelioma (MPM) (69). miRNA downregulation (miR-141, MiR-200a, MiR-200b, miR-200c, miR-203, miR-205, and miR-429) can differentiate between MM and adenocarcinoma (70). Upregulation of miR-29c in epithelioid mesothelioma was associated with better prognosis, while upregulation of miR-31 was a negative prognostic indicator in the sarcomatoid subtype (69,71). The predicted target genes for upregulated and downregulated miRNAs included tumor suppressor genes and oncogenes well known to play a role in MPM. The most common targets included *CDKN2A*, *NF2*, *HGF*, *PDGF*, *EGF*, and *JUN*.

Tyrosine Kinase Receptors

Many studies have confirmed the significance of tyrosine kinase receptors in malignant mesothelioma, including the epidermal growth factor (EGF), platelet-derived growth factor (PDGF), hepatocyte growth factor, and insulin-like growth factor (IGF) pathways and their downstream signaling molecules, such as the mitogen-activating protein kinase (MAPK) and phosphatidylinositol 3-kinase (PI3-K)/Akt kinase, respectively (72). There is *in vitro* evidence of efficacy of EGFR TKIs in MPM (73). Somatic mutations of the tyrosine kinase domain of the EGFR receptor were reported in peritoneal mesothelioma including EGFR TKI-sensitizing mutations (74,75). In contrast, unknown polymorphisms in the EGFR gene were identified in pleural mesothelioma, but no EGFR TKI-sensitizing mutations (76–78). Targeted therapies are under investigation in clinical trials (79).

Pathway Analysis of Mesothelioma

Table 10.3 summarizes significantly altered pathways identified by MuSiC pathway analysis (13). Integrated analysis of the genomics data identified Hippo, mTOR, histone methylation, RNA helicases, and p53 signaling pathways to be altered in MM (Figure 10.3) (13).

Immune Biomarkers in Mesothelioma

Tumor-infiltrating lymphocytes and macrophages have been proposed as prognostic markers in MPM patients. Recent studies demonstrated PD-L1 expression in up to 40 per cent of pleural mesothelioma, predominantly in the sarcomatoid subtype (13,80,81). Expression of PD-L1 was associated with poor survival (13,80,81). The expression of PD-L1 may have important therapeutic implications (82,83).

Table 10.3 Summary of significantly altered pathways in malignant mesothelioma*

Significant pathways in malignant mesothelioma*
Signaling by Hippo
RHO GTPases activate PAKs
Transcriptional activation of cell cycle inhibitor p21
Transcriptional activation of p53-responsive genes
Activation of PUMA and translocation to mitochondria
Activation of NOXA and translocation to mitochondria
Formation of Senescence-Associated Heterochromatin Foci (SAHF)
Activation of BH3-only proteins
Intrinsic pathway for apoptosis
Oncogene-induced senescence
DNA damage/telomere stress-induced senescence
TP53 regulates metabolic genes
Transcriptional regulation by TP53
Pre-NOTCH expression and processing
Pre-NOTCH transcription and translation
Termination of *O*-glycan biosynthesis
Stabilization of *p53*
Autodegradation of the E3 ubiquitin ligase COP1
Olfactory signaling pathway
G1/S DNA damage checkpoints
Oxidative stress-induced senescence
PKMTs methylate histone lysines
O-linked glycosylation of mucins
O-linked glycosylation
Cellular senescence
Factors involved in megakaryocyte development and platelet production

* Modified with permission from reference 13.

Table 10.4 Summary of gene fusion in mesenchymal tumors of the pleura and peritoneum

Tumor type	Gene fusions
Synovial sarcoma	*SS18–SSx4* *SS18L1–SSX1*
Epithelioid hemangioendothelioma	*WWTR1–CAMTA1* *YAP1–TFE3*
Angiosarcoma	*CIC–LEUTX* *NUP160–SLC43A3* *EWSR1–ATF1* *CEP85L–ROS1*
Solitary fibrous tumor	*NAB2–STAT6*
Desmoplastic small round cell tumor	*EWSR1–WT1*

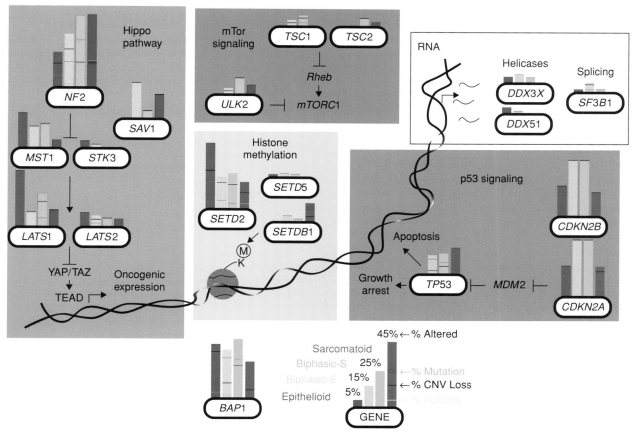

Figure 10.3 Integrated analysis of pathway alterations observed in MPM. Reproduced with permission from (13).

Molecular Alterations of Other Tumors of the Pleura and Peritoneum

The molecular alterations of mesenchymal tumors and carcinomas of the pleura and peritoneum are identical to those of their counterparts occurring at other anatomic sites. Table 10.4 summarizes gene fusions occurring in mesenchymal tumors, some of which are of diagnostic importance.

References

1. Krismann M, Muller KM, Jaworska M, Johnen G. Molecular cytogenetic differences between histological subtypes of malignant mesotheliomas: DNA cytometry and comparative genomic hybridization of 90 cases. *J Pathol.* 2002;197(3):363–71.

2. Lindholm PM, Salmenkivi K, Vauhkonen H, Nicholson AG, Anttila S, Kinnula VL, et al. Gene copy number analysis in malignant pleural mesothelioma using oligonucleotide array CGH. *Cytogenet Genome Res.* 2007;119(1–2):46–52.

3. Musti M, Kettunen E, Dragonieri S, Lindholm P, Cavone D, Serio G, et al. Cytogenetic and molecular genetic changes in malignant mesothelioma. *Cancer Genet Cytogenet.* 2006;170(1):9–15.

4. Borczuk AC, Pei J, Taub RN, Levy B, Nahum O, Chen J, et al. Genome-wide analysis of abdominal and pleural malignant mesothelioma with DNA arrays reveals both common and distinct regions of copy number alteration. *Cancer Biol Ther.* 2016;17(3):328–35.

5. Hirao T, Bueno R, Chen CJ, Gordon GJ, Heilig E, Kelsey KT. Alterations of the p16(INK4) locus in human malignant mesothelial tumors.

Carcinogenesis. 2002;23(7): 1127–30.

6. Illei PB, Rusch VW, Zakowski MF, Ladanyi M. Homozygous deletion of CDKN2A and codeletion of the methylthioadenosine phosphorylase gene in the majority of pleural mesotheliomas. *Clin Cancer Res.* 2003;9(6):2108–13.

7. Xio S, Li D, Vijg J, Sugarbaker DJ, Corson JM, Fletcher JA. Codeletion of p15 and p16 in primary malignant mesothelioma. *Oncogene.* 1995;11(3):511–15.

8. Bianchi AB, Mitsunaga SI, Cheng JQ, Klein WM, Jhanwar SC, Seizinger B,

et al. High frequency of inactivating mutations in the neurofibromatosis type 2 gene (*NF2*) in primary malignant mesotheliomas. *Proc Natl Acad Sci U S A*. 1995;92(24):10854–58.

9. Hamaratoglu F, Willecke M, Kango-Singh M, Nolo R, Hyun E, Tao C, et al. The tumour-suppressor genes NF2/Merlin and Expanded act through Hippo signalling to regulate cell proliferation and apoptosis. *Nat Cell Biol*. 2006;8(1):27–36.

10. Sekido Y, Pass HI, Bader S, Mew DJ, Christman MF, Gazdar AF, et al. Neurofibromatosis type 2 (*NF2*) gene is somatically mutated in mesothelioma but not in lung cancer. *Cancer Res*. 1995;55(6):1227–31.

11. Bott M, Brevet M, Taylor BS, Shimizu S, Ito T, Wang L, et al. The nuclear deubiquitinase BAP1 is commonly inactivated by somatic mutations and 3p21.1 losses in malignant pleural mesothelioma. *Nat Genet*. 2011;43(7): 668–72.

12. Testa JR, Cheung M, Pei J, Below JE, Tan Y, Sementino E, et al. Germline *BAP1* mutations predispose to malignant mesothelioma. *Nat Genet*. 2011;43(10):1022–25.

13. Bueno R, Stawiski EW, Goldstein LD, Durinck S, De Rienzo A, Modrusan Z, et al. Comprehensive genomic analysis of malignant pleural mesothelioma identifies recurrent mutations, gene fusions and splicing alterations. *Nat Genet*. 2016;48(4):407–16.

14. Nasu M, Emi M, Pastorino S, Tanji M, Powers A, Luk H, et al. High incidence of somatic *BAP1* alterations in sporadic malignant mesothelioma. *J Thorac Oncol*. 2015;10(4):565–76.

15. Guo G, Chmielecki J, Goparaju C, Heguy A, Dolgalev I, Carbone M, et al. Whole-exome sequencing reveals frequent genetic alterations in *BAP1*, *NF2*, *CDKN2A*, and *CUL1* in malignant pleural mesothelioma. *Cancer Res*. 2015;75(2):264–69.

16. Lo Iacono M, Monica V, Righi L, Grosso F, Libener R, Vatrano S, et al. Targeted next-generation sequencing of cancer genes in advanced stage malignant pleural mesothelioma: a retrospective study. *J Thorac Oncol*. 2015;10(3):492–99.

17. Shukuya T, Serizawa M, Watanabe M, Akamatsu H, Abe M, Imai H, et al. Identification of actionable mutations in malignant pleural mesothelioma. *Lung Cancer*. 2014;86(1):35–40.

18. Lopez-Rios F, Chuai S, Flores R, Shimizu S, Ohno T, Wakahara K, et al. Global gene expression profiling of pleural mesotheliomas: overexpression of aurora kinases and *P16/CDKN2A* deletion as prognostic factors and critical evaluation of microarray-based prognostic prediction. *Cancer Res*. 2006;66(6):2970–79.

19. Krasinskas AM, Bartlett DL, Cieply K, Dacic S. *CDKN2A* and *MTAP* deletions in peritoneal mesotheliomas are correlated with loss of p16 protein expression and poor survival. *Mod Pathol*. 2010;23(4):531–38.

20. Chiosea S, Krasinskas A, Cagle PT, Mitchell KA, Zander DS, Dacic S. Diagnostic importance of 9p21 homozygous deletion in malignant mesotheliomas. *Mod Pathol*. 2008;21(6):742–47.

21. Monaco SE, Shuai Y, Bansal M, Krasinskas AM, Dacic S. The diagnostic utility of p16 FISH and GLUT-1 immunohistochemical analysis in mesothelial proliferations. *Am J Clin Pathol*. 2011;135(4):619–27.

22. Hida T, Matsumoto S, Hamasaki M, Kawahara K, Tsujimura T, Hiroshima K, et al. Deletion status of p16 in effusion smear preparation correlates with that of underlying malignant pleural mesothelioma tissue. *Cancer Sci*. 2015;106(11):1635–41.

23. Churg A, Sheffield BS, Galateau-Sallé F. New Markers for Separating Benign From Malignant Mesothelial Proliferations: Are We There Yet? *Arch Pathol Lab Med*. 2016;140(4):318–21.

24. Wu D, Hiroshima K, Matsumoto S, Nabeshima K, Yusa T, Ozaki D, et al. Diagnostic usefulness of p16/CDKN2A FISH in distinguishing between sarcomatoid mesothelioma and fibrous pleuritis. *Am J Clin Pathol*. 2013;139(1):39–46.

25. Savic S, Franco N, Grilli B, Barascud Ade V, Herzog M, Bode B, et al. Fluorescence *in situ* hybridization in the definitive diagnosis of malignant mesothelioma in effusion cytology. *Chest*. 2010;138(1):137–44.

26. Tochigi N, Attanoos R, Chirieac LR, Allen TC, Cagle PT, Dacic S. p16 Deletion in sarcomatoid tumors of the lung and pleura. *Arch Pathol Lab Med*. 2013;137(5):632–36.

27. Dacic S, Kothmaier H, Land S, Shuai Y, Halbwedl I, Morbini P, et al. Prognostic significance of p16/cdkn2a loss in pleural malignant mesotheliomas. *Virchows Arch*. 2008;453(6):627–35.

28. Singhi AD, Krasinskas AM, Choudry HA, Bartlett DL, Pingpank JF, Zeh HJ, et al. The prognostic significance of *BAP1*, *NF2*, and *CDKN2A* in malignant peritoneal mesothelioma. *Mod Pathol*. 2016;29(1):14–24.

29. Mizuno T, Murakami H, Fujii M, Ishiguro F, Tanaka I, Kondo Y, et al. *YAP* induces malignant mesothelioma cell proliferation by upregulating transcription of cell cycle-promoting genes. *Oncogene*. 2012;31(49):5117–22.

30. Thurneysen C, Opitz I, Kurtz S, Weder W, Stahel RA, Felley-Bosco E. Functional inactivation of *NF2*/merlin in human mesothelioma. *Lung Cancer*. 2009;64(2):140–47.

31. Hassan R, Schweizer C, Lu KF, Schuler B, Remaley AT, Weil SC, et al. Inhibition of mesothelin–CA-125 interaction in patients with mesothelioma by the anti-mesothelin monoclonal antibody MORAb-009: implications for cancer therapy. *Lung Cancer*. 2010;68(3):455–59.

32. Hassan R, Cohen SJ, Phillips M, Pastan I, Sharon E, Kelly RJ, et al. Phase I clinical trial of the chimeric anti-mesothelin monoclonal antibody MORAb-009 in patients with mesothelin-expressing cancers. *Clin Cancer Res*. 2010;16(24):6132–38.

33. Kelly RJ, Sharon E, Pastan I, Hassan R. Mesothelin-targeted agents in clinical trials and in preclinical development. *Mol Cancer Ther*. 2012;11(3):517–25.

34. Hassan R, Miller AC, Sharon E, Thomas A, Reynolds JC, Ling A, et al. Major cancer regressions in mesothelioma after treatment with an anti-mesothelin immunotoxin and immune suppression. *Sci Transl Med*. 2013;5(208):208ra147.

35. Ou SH, Moon J, Garland LL, Mack PC, Testa JR, Tsao AS, et al. SWOG S0722: phase II study of mTOR inhibitor everolimus (RAD001) in advanced malignant pleural mesothelioma (MPM). *J Thorac Oncol*. 2015;10(2): 387–91.

36. Dolly SO, Wagner AJ, Bendell JC, Kindler HL, Krug LM, Seiwert TY, et al.

Phase I study of Apitolisib (GDC-0980), dual phosphatidylinositol-3-kinase and mammalian target of rapamycin kinase inhibitor, in patients with advanced solid tumors. *Clin Cancer Res.* 2016;22(12):2874–84.

37. Emi M, Yoshikawa Y, Sato C, Sato A, Sato H, Kato T, et al. Frequent genomic rearrangements of *BRCA1* associated protein-1 (*BAP1*) gene in Japanese malignant mesothelioma-characterization of deletions at exon level. *J Hum Genet.* 2015;60(10): 647–49.

38. Wiesner T, Obenauf AC, Murali R, Fried I, Griewank KG, Ulz P, et al. Germline mutations in *BAP1* predispose to melanocytic tumors. *Nat Genet.* 2011;43(10):1018–21.

39. Harbour JW, Onken MD, Roberson ED, Duan S, Cao L, Worley LA, et al. Frequent mutation of *BAP1* in metastasizing uveal melanomas. *Science.* 2010;330(6009):1410–13.

40. Carbone M, Ferris LK, Baumann F, Napolitano A, Lum CA, Flores EG, et al. *BAP1* cancer syndrome: malignant mesothelioma, uveal and cutaneous melanoma, and MBAITs. *J Transl Med.* 2012;10:179.

41. Pena-Llopis S, Vega-Rubin-de-Celis S, Liao A, Leng N, Pavia-Jimenez A, Wang S, et al. *BAP1* loss defines a new class of renal cell carcinoma. *Nat Genet.* 2012;44(7):751–59.

42. Abdel-Rahman MH, Pilarski R, Cebulla CM, Massengill JB, Christopher BN, Boru G, et al. Germline *BAP1* mutation predisposes to uveal melanoma, lung adenocarcinoma, meningioma, and other cancers. *J Med Genet.* 2011;48(12):856–59.

43. Wadt KA, Aoude LG, Johansson P, Solinas A, Pritchard A, Crainic O, et al. A recurrent germline *BAP1* mutation and extension of the *BAP1* tumor predisposition spectrum to include basal cell carcinoma. *Clin Genet.* 2015;88(3):267–72.

44. Zauderer MG, Bott M, McMillan R, Sima CS, Rusch V, Krug LM, et al. Clinical characteristics of patients with malignant pleural mesothelioma harboring somatic *BAP1* mutations. *J Thorac Oncol.* 2013;8(11):1430–33.

45. Yoshikawa Y, Sato A, Tsujimura T, Emi M, Morinaga T, Fukuoka K, et al. Frequent inactivation of the *BAP1* gene in epithelioid-type malignant mesothelioma. *Cancer Sci.* 2012;103(5):868–74.

46. Baumann F, Flores E, Napolitano A, Kanodia S, Taioli E, Pass H, et al. Mesothelioma patients with germline *BAP1* mutations have 7-fold improved long-term survival. *Carcinogenesis.* 2015;36(1):76–81.

47. Farzin M, Toon CW, Clarkson A, Sioson L, Watson N, Andrici J, et al. Loss of expression of *BAP1* predicts longer survival in mesothelioma. *Pathology.* 2015;47(4):302–07.

48. Hwang HC, Sheffield BS, Rodriguez S, Thompson K, Tse CH, Gown AM, et al. Utility of *BAP1* immunohistochemistry and p16 (CDKN2A) FISH in the diagnosis of malignant mesothelioma in effusion cytology specimens. *Am J Surg Pathol.* 2016;40(1):120–26.

49. McGregor SM, Dunning R, Hyjek E, Vigneswaran W, Husain AN, Krausz T. *BAP1* facilitates diagnostic objectivity, classification, and prognostication in malignant pleural mesothelioma. *Hum Pathol.* 2015;46(11):1670–78.

50. Andrici J, Sheen A, Sioson L, Wardell K, Clarkson A, Watson N, et al. Loss of expression of *BAP1* is a useful adjunct, which strongly supports the diagnosis of mesothelioma in effusion cytology. *Mod Pathol.* 2015;28(10):1360–68.

51. Cigognetti M, Lonardi S, Fisogni S, Balzarini P, Pellegrini V, Tironi A, et al. *BAP1* (*BRCA1*-associated protein 1) is a highly specific marker for differentiating mesothelioma from reactive mesothelial proliferations. *Mod Pathol.* 2015;28(8):1043–57.

52. Walts AE, Hiroshima K, McGregor SM, Wu D, Husain AN, Marchevsky AM. BAP1 immunostain and CDKN2A (p16) FISH analysis: clinical applicability for the diagnosis of malignant mesothelioma in effusions. *Diagn Cytopathol.* 2016;44(7):599–606.

53. LaFave LM, Beguelin W, Koche R, Teater M, Spitzer B, Chramiec A, et al. Loss of *BAP1* function leads to EZH2-dependent transformation. *Nat Med.* 2015;21(11):1344–49.

54. Murakami H, Mizuno T, Taniguchi T, Fujii M, Ishiguro F, Fukui T, et al. *LATS2* is a tumor suppressor gene of malignant mesothelioma. *Cancer Res.* 2011;71(3):873–83.

55. Carbone M, Gaudino G, Yang H. Recent insights emerging from malignant mesothelioma genome sequencing. *J Thorac Oncol.* 2015;10(3):409–11.

56. Andujar P, Pairon JC, Renier A, Descatha A, Hysi I, Abd-Alsamad I, et al. Differential mutation profiles and similar intronic TP53 polymorphisms in asbestos-related lung cancer and pleural mesothelioma. *Mutagenesis.* 2013;28(3):323–31.

57. Christensen BC, Marsit CJ, Houseman EA, Godleski JJ, Longacker JL, Zheng S, et al. Differentiation of lung adenocarcinoma, pleural mesothelioma, and nonmalignant pulmonary tissues using DNA methylation profiles. *Cancer Res.* 2009;69(15):6315–21.

58. Toyooka S, Pass HI, Shivapurkar N, Fukuyama Y, Maruyama R, Toyooka KO, et al. Aberrant methylation and simian virus 40 tag sequences in malignant mesothelioma. *Cancer Res.* 2001;61(15):5727–30.

59. Shivapurkar N, Toyooka S, Toyooka KO, Reddy J, Miyajima K, Suzuki M, et al. Aberrant methylation of trail decoy receptor genes is frequent in multiple tumor types. *Int J Cancer.* 2004;109(5):786–92.

60. Fujii M, Fujimoto N, Hiraki A, Gemba K, Aoe K, Umemura S, et al. Aberrant DNA methylation profile in pleural fluid for differential diagnosis of malignant pleural mesothelioma. *Cancer Sci.* 2012;103(3):510–14.

61. Goto Y, Shinjo K, Kondo Y, Shen L, Toyota M, Suzuki H, et al. Epigenetic profiles distinguish malignant pleural mesothelioma from lung adenocarcinoma. *Cancer Res.* 2009;69(23):9073–82.

62. Christensen BC, Houseman EA, Godleski JJ, Marsit CJ, Longacker JL, Roelofs CR, et al. Epigenetic profiles distinguish pleural mesothelioma from normal pleura and predict lung asbestos burden and clinical outcome. *Cancer Res.* 2009;69(1):227–34.

63. Romagnoli S, Fasoli E, Vaira V, Falleni M, Pellegrini C, Catania A, et al. Identification of potential therapeutic targets in malignant mesothelioma using cell-cycle gene expression analysis. *Am J Pathol.* 2009;174(3):762–70.

64. Gordon GJ, Rockwell GN, Jensen RV, Rheinwald JG, Glickman JN, Aronson JP, et al. Identification of novel

candidate oncogenes and tumor suppressors in malignant pleural mesothelioma using large-scale transcriptional profiling. *Am J Pathol.* 2005;166(6):1827–40.

65. Gordon GJ, Jensen RV, Hsiao LL, Gullans SR, Blumenstock JE, Ramaswamy S, et al. Translation of microarray data into clinically relevant cancer diagnostic tests using gene expression ratios in lung cancer and mesothelioma. *Cancer Res.* 2002;62(17):4963–67.

66. Gordon GJ, Jensen RV, Hsiao LL, Gullans SR, Blumenstock JE, Richards WG, et al. Using gene expression ratios to predict outcome among patients with mesothelioma. *J Natl Cancer Inst.* 2003;95(8):598–605.

67. Pass HI, Liu Z, Wali A, Bueno R, Land S, Lott D, et al. Gene expression profiles predict survival and progression of pleural mesothelioma. *Clin Cancer Res.* 2004;10(3):849–59.

68. Crispi S, Fagliarone C, Biroccio A, D'Angelo C, Galati R, Sacchi A, et al. Antiproliferative effect of Aurora kinase targeting in mesothelioma. *Lung Cancer.* 2010;70(3):271–79.

69. Busacca S, Germano S, De Cecco L, Rinaldi M, Comoglio F, Favero F, et al. MicroRNA signature of malignant mesothelioma with potential diagnostic and prognostic implications. *Am J Respir Cell Mol Biol.* 2010;42(3):312–19.

70. Gee GV, Koestler DC, Christensen BC, Sugarbaker DJ, Ugolini D, Ivaldi GP, et al. Downregulated microRNAs in the differential diagnosis of malignant pleural mesothelioma. *Int J Cancer.* 2010;127(12):2859–69.

71. Matsumoto S, Nabeshima K, Hamasaki M, Shibuta T, Umemura T. Upregulation of microRNA-31 associates with a poor prognosis of malignant pleural mesothelioma with sarcomatoid component. *Med Oncol.* 2014;31(12):303.

72. Jean D, Daubriac J, Le Pimpec-Barthes F, Galateau-Sallé F, Jaurand MC. Molecular changes in mesothelioma with an impact on prognosis and treatment. *Arch Pathol Lab Med.* 2012;136(3):277–93.

73. Brevet M, Shimizu S, Bott MJ, Shukla N, Zhou Q, Olshen AB, et al. Coactivation of receptor tyrosine kinases in malignant mesothelioma as a rationale for combination targeted therapy. *J Thorac Oncol.* 2011;6(5):864–74.

74. Kalra N, Ashai A, Xi L, Zhang J, Avital I, Raffeld M, et al. Patients with peritoneal mesothelioma lack epidermal growth factor receptor tyrosine kinase mutations that would make them sensitive to tyrosine kinase inhibitors. *Oncol Rep.* 2012;27(6):1794–800.

75. Foster JM, Radhakrishna U, Govindarajan V, Carreau JH, Gatalica Z, Sharma P, et al. Clinical implications of novel activating *EGFR* mutations in malignant peritoneal mesothelioma. *World J Surg Oncol.* 2010;8:88.

76. Schildgen V, Pabst O, Tillmann RL, Lusebrink J, Schildgen O, Ludwig C, et al. Low frequency of *EGFR* mutations in pleural mesothelioma patients, Cologne, Germany. *Appl Immunohistochem Molec Morphol.* 2015;23(2):118–25.

77. Velcheti V, Kasai Y, Viswanathan AK, Ritter J, Govindan R. Absence of mutations in the epidermal growth factor receptor (*EGFR*) kinase domain in patients with mesothelioma. *J Thorac Oncol.* 2009;4(4):559.

78. Cortese JF, Gowda AL, Wali A, Eliason JF, Pass HI, Everson RB. Common *EGFR* mutations conferring sensitivity to gefitinib in lung adenocarcinoma are not prevalent in human malignant mesothelioma. *Int J Cancer.* 2006;118(2):521–22.

79. Astoul P, Roca E, Galateau-Sallé F, Scherpereel A. Malignant pleural mesothelioma: from the bench to the bedside. *Respiration.* 2012;83(6):481–93.

80. Mansfield AS, Roden AC, Peikert T, Sheinin YM, Harrington SM, Krco CJ, et al. B7-H1 expression in malignant pleural mesothelioma is associated with sarcomatoid histology and poor prognosis. *J Thorac Oncol.* 2014;9(7):1036–40.

81. Combaz-Lair C, Galateau-Sallé F, McLeer-Florin A, Le Stang N, David-Boudet L, Duruisseaux M, et al. Immune biomarkers PD-1/PD-L1 and TLR3 in malignant pleural mesotheliomas. *Hum Pathol.* 2016;52:9–18.

82. Currie AJ, Prosser A, McDonnell A, Cleaver AL, Robinson BW, Freeman GJ, et al. Dual control of antitumor CD8 T cells through the programmed death-1/programmed death-ligand 1 pathway and immunosuppressive CD4 T cells: regulation and counterregulation. *J Immunol.* 2009;183(12):7898–908.

83. Marcq E, Pauwels P, van Meerbeeck JP, Smits EL. Targeting immune checkpoints: new opportunity for mesothelioma treatment? *Cancer Treat Rev.* 2015;41(10):914–24.

Pathology of Malignant Mesothelioma

Alberto M. Marchevsky, Françoise Galateau-Sallé, Lucian Chirieac, and Aliya N. Husain

The mesothelial cells lining the serosal membranes can develop a variety of benign and malignant neoplasms listed in Chapter 2 (1–4) (Table 11.1). Malignant neoplasms originating from mesothelial cells are usually highly malignant tumors that have been historically designated in the literature as malignant mesotheliomas (MMs), a terminology that is somewhat redundant, as there are no "benign mesotheliomas." Indeed, benign neoplasms of mesothelial origin have been classified as adenomatoid tumors or benign multicystic mesotheliomas rather than as benign mesotheliomas (5–19). Well-differentiated papillary mesothelioma (WDPM) has been more recently described as a low-grade neoplasm of mesothelial origin that can recur locally but not metastasize (20). Rare cases of composite mesothelial tumors composed of MM associated with adenomatoid tumor or WDPM associated with adenomatoid tumor have been described, reflecting a common cell of origin for these rare neoplasms (7,8,21,22).

MM are unusual neoplasms, with an incidence of 2000–3000 cases per year in the USA (23–33). The incidence in other countries such as the UK and Australia is somewhat higher. MM can involve patients of all ages and both genders but are more frequent in men (M:F ratio of 3:1) older than 60 years of age (33,34).

Approximately 90 percent of MM arise on the pleural surfaces, and slightly less than 10 percent of MM arise on the peritoneum. MM arising from the pericardium and the tunica albuginea/testis/paratesticular area are rare neoplasms (9,17,34–46).

Diffuse Malignant Mesothelioma

Etiology and Epidemiology

The epidemiology and etiology of MM are discussed in detail in Chapter 8. Approximately 80 percent of MM in men and 50 percent of MM in women have been caused by above-background exposures to commercial amphibole asbestos such as amosite and crocidolite (32,33,47–59). The tumors develop after a longer than 15 years latency period and are often clinically evident 30–40 years after initial asbestos exposure (60–63). Epidemiological studies have suggested that the risk of developing MM after exposure to amphibole asbestos is a linear function of amphibole dose and a power function of time since initial exposure (64,65). The role of chrysotile mesothelioma in the causation of MM has been controversial because most but not all chrysotile asbestos mined in North America, Italy, and other locations has been contaminated with variable concentrations of tremolite, a form of amphibole asbestos (53,66–70). However, epidemiological studies have shown that a small number of MM, such as those developing in Canadian miners or textile factory workers, can be attributed to exposure to high doses of chrysotile asbestos; whether the cause was "pure chrysotile" or tremolite remains uncertain (53,71–76). The marked difference in the incidences of MM developing after exposure to either amphibole or chrysotile asbestos exposure support the concept that amosite and crocidolite asbestos are in 2–3 orders of magnitude more carcinogenic for the development of this neoplasm than chrysotile asbestos (65).

Other causes of MM include exposure to non-asbestiform minerals with similar dimensions to commercial amphibole asbestos and exposure to therapeutic radiation therapy (77). Minerals with similar dimensions to commercial amphiboles include winchite, found in vermiculite mines in Libby, Montana and other locations, and erionite, a mineral extracted in the Cappadocia region of Turkey, North Dakota, and Mexico (55,78–83). Vermiculite has been used in blow-in insulation products (83). Erionite has been used as "white wash" during construction in Turkey and in road surfacing materials used in the USA and Mexico (79,84–87). MM can also develop at the site of previous therapeutic radiation therapy in patients treated for lung cancer, lymphomas, breast cancer, and germ cell neoplasms (88–93). These radiation-induced neoplasms usually appear after a 10-year latency period, although some patients have been described with shorter latency period (88–90).

It has been controversial whether exposure to simian virus SV40 plays a role in the causation of MM (94–98). In the past, the virus contaminated some polio vaccines and it has been found with molecular methods in cases of MM, but there are no epidemiological data showing that patients with exposure to this virus were at an increased risk of developing the neoplasm.

Rarely, MM can develop in children or as a familial disease (99–123). A rare familial cancer syndrome characterized by germline *BAP1* mutations has been described in patients that develop MM, clear cell carcinoma of the kidney, uveal melanoma, cholangiocarcinoma, atypical melanocytic lesions, and/or other neoplasms (120,122–124). It is uncertain whether the mutations alone cause MM or are one of the risk factors for the development of the tumor. Recent studies have suggested that germline or sporadic *BAP1* mutations may

Table 11.1 Classification of mesothelial neoplasms

Benign
　Adenomatoid tumor
　Multicystic mesothelioma

Uncertain malignant potential
　Well-differentiated papillary mesothelioma (WDPM)

Diffuse malignant mesothelioma
　Epithelioid
　Sarcomatoid
　Biphasic

Localized malignant mesothelioma
　Epithelioid
　Sarcomatoid

Combined mesothelial tumors
　Adenomatoid tumor and multicystic mesothelioma
　WDPM and adenomatoid tumor

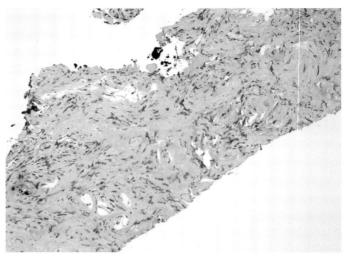

Figure 11.1 Transthoracic needle biopsy of pleural lesion showing an atypical spindle cell proliferation. Needle biopsies often lack the presence of adipose tissue and can be difficult to diagnose definitively as malignant mesothelioma or reactive pleuritis, such as in this example (H&E, ×100). The patient was subsequently diagnosed with desmoplastic mesothelioma with thoracoscopic biopsies.

predispose patients to develop mesothelioma after asbestos exposure (120,123,125).

The etiology of approximately 20 percent of MM in men and 50 percent in women remains unknown; these neoplasms have been characterized in the literature as "background MM" or "idiopathic MM" (32,57,64,126).

Clinical Findings

Patients with diffuse pleural MM usually present with dyspnea, fatigue, weight loss, and/or dull, non-pleuritic chest wall pain that is usually unilateral (127–131). They may also present with fever, cough, and other findings suggestive of an upper respiratory infection and, less often, with cervical lymphadenopathy, hemoptysis, paraneoplastic syndromes, or symptoms secondary to bone or other metastases. Physical examination of the chest usually shows decreased air sounds in the affected hemithorax. Chest x-rays often show pleural effusion that is often recurrent and/or loculated and sometimes results in complete opacification of a hemithorax (132–134). The presence of pleural calcifications and history of asbestos exposure can be helpful to suspect the possibility of MM in a patient with pleural effusion (135,136).

Chest computerized tomograms (CT) can vary in MM patients from cases showing only pleural effusion to the more characteristic findings of diffuse pleural thickening forming a rind with areas of nodularity (137). In advanced cases of MM the chest CT also shows the presence of pleural-based masses of varying size that infiltrate into the chest wall. In addition to clinical diagnosis, chest CT and magnetic resonance (MRI) scans are also helpful to evaluate for the presence of mediastinal adenopathy and invasion of the pericardium, diaphragm or other intrathoracic structures for the staging of the disease (see below) (132,138,139). Larsen et al. described five patients with an unusual presentation of MM as a diffuse intrapulmonary lesion simulating interstitial lung disease on imaging studies (140). These patients lacked findings of pleural disease on chest CT and other imaging studies and were found to have pleural involvement in only four instances on lung biopsies.

Patients with diffuse peritoneal mesothelioma usually present with abdominal pain and distention due to the development of ascites (141,142). CT of the abdomen and pelvis demonstrate the presence of ascites and omental or other intraabdominal masses that need to be distinguished from intraperitoneal carcinomatosis.

The clinical and imaging findings and treatment of patients with diffuse MM are discussed in more detail in Chapters 3 and 8 of this volume.

Pathologic Diagnosis

A history of asbestos exposure has no diagnostic value for diffuse MM as various benign conditions and other malignancies can develop in patients with such exposure history. Diffuse MM can be suspected based on clinical presentation and imaging findings, but there are no pathognomonic clinical or imaging findings that are diagnostic for this neoplasm. Indeed, the diagnosis of MM can only be established by histopathological examination of adequate ultrasound- or CT-guided needle-core biopsies or video-assisted thoracoscopic biopsies (VATS) stained with H&E (Figure 11.1) and appropriate immunostains (3). Mucicarmine stain can also be helpful in selected cases, but it can be positive in both adenocarcinomas and MM. The biopsies need to provide enough tissue to examine the growth features and cytological features of a putative neoplasm, to perform several immunostains, and to evaluate for possible invasion. Evaluation of stromal invasion often requires availability of subpleural adipose tissue and/or lung tissue, materials that usually can only be obtained with surgical biopsies. The diagnostic features of the different subtypes and variants of MM will be discussed further on in this chapter, but it is important to emphasize that reliance on routine histopathology and

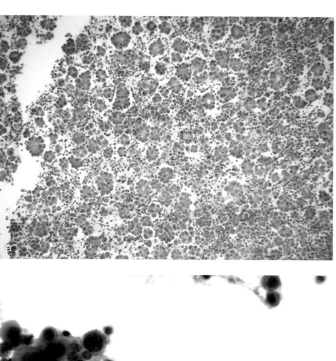
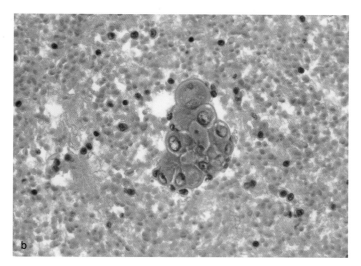
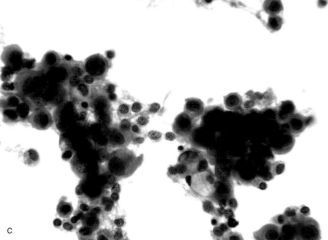

Figure 11.2 (a–c) Cytology from a patient with epithelioid malignant mesothelioma of the pleura. The cell block shows high cellularity (a, H&E, ×100) with numerous clusters of epithelioid cells showing relatively low anisocytosis. Note the presence of intercellular spaces ("windows") between the tumor cells. They show round nuclei with small nucleoli and amphophilic cytoplasm (b, H&E, ×400). Cytospin preparation from the same sample shows papillary clusters of mesothelial cells (c, Pap stain, ×400).

immunohistochemistry showing reactivity for a single epitope such as calretinin can result in diagnostic errors, as none of the so-called mesothelial markers are 100 percent specific for MM (143).

The Role of Cytopathology in the Initial Diagnosis of Malignant Mesothelioma

Patients with MM frequently present with recurrent pleural effusions or ascites and the fluids are often sent for cytologic examination. Direct smears, cytospin, and thin-layer preparations and cell block can be obtained from effusion fluids and used to evaluate for the presence of metastatic lesions, reactive mesothelial hyperplasia, and malignant mesothelioma (144–147). The sensitivity of the cytological diagnosis of MM ranges from 32 percent to 76 percent, depending on various sampling methods and perhaps the degree of experience of individual cytopathologists with this diagnosis.

Cytological techniques have implicit shortcomings for the diagnosis of MM, as they cannot demonstrate the presence of tissue invasion, an important histopathologic feature for diagnosis on biopsies. In addition, sarcomatoid mesotheliomas do not generally shed a significant number of diagnostic malignant cells into effusions. As cytologic examination of effusion samples is therefore insensitive for the diagnosis of sarcomatoid mesothelioma, and it does not reliably provide diagnostic information regarding the presence of biphasic MM. The presence of sarcomatoid or biphasic morphology in a diffuse MM is used by at least some thoracic surgeons to exclude patients from extrapleural pneumonectomy (EPP) (137,148–156).

Cytologic features that can be helpful for the diagnosis of MM include the presence of cell balls composed of > 50 cells with scalloped edges (Figure 11.2a), intercellular

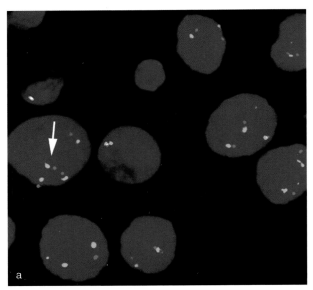 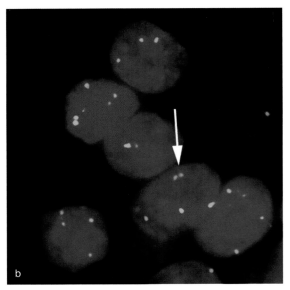

Figure 11.3 (a,b) p16/PDKN2A showing the presence of homozygous deletion in malignant mesothelioma cells. (a) Normal mesothelial cells showing red and blue signals in each nucleus (arrow). (b) The red signals are missing (arrow), indicating a deletion. The finding of p16/PDKN2A deletions in atypical mesothelial cells is 100 percent specific for the diagnosis of malignant mesothelioma.

windows (Figure 11.2b), presence of cells with macronucleoli (Figure 11.2c), submembranous cytoplasmic condensation, and low nuclear/cytoplasmic (N:C) ratios. These findings are not entirely specific for MM and can also be seen, perhaps with lower incidence, in benign effusions from patients with reactive mesothelial hyperplasia. Paradoxically, the presence in effusion cytology specimens of the usual cytologic features of malignancy such as moderate to severe nuclear atypia, marked anisocytosis, hyperchromasia, irregular nuclear membranes, and high N:C ratios are usually absent in MM and their presence in cytologic samples should raise doubts about the diagnosis of MM.

US-guided to CT-guided fine-needle aspiration biopsies (FNA) of MM that show nodular areas on imaging findings can be used for the diagnosis of mesothelial neoplasms. The cytologic features need to be interpreted with caution and correlated with the imaging findings.

It remains controversial whether the initial diagnosis of epithelioid MM can be rendered based solely on effusion cytology (3,144). Most experts probably agree that effusion cytology is not a good method for the initial diagnosis of sarcomatoid MM, as this neoplasm tends not to shed neoplastic cells into the effusion fluids. Recent studies with fluorescence *in-situ* hybridization (FISH) have demonstrated that homozygous deletion of p16/PDKN2A can be helpful to distinguish MM from reactive mesothelial proliferations (Figure 11.3a,b) (157–165). For example, Wu et al. reported a homozygous deletion pattern in 55.6 percent and 100 percent of epithelioid and sarcomatoid MM, respectively (160). However, this finding is not specific for MM and can be seen in other malignancies. The topic is discussed in more detail in Chapter 14.

A recent study by Cigognetti et al. evaluated the presence of *BRCA*-associated protein (BAP-1) immunoreactivity in 212 MM, 12 benign mesothelial tumors, and 42 reactive mesothelial proliferations and reported its loss only in MM (Figure 11.4a,b) with a sensitivity of 69 percent in biopsies and 64 percent in cytological samples (166). None of the cases with reactive mesothelial proliferation exhibited loss of BAP-1 immunoreactivity, suggesting a specificity of 100 percent for the differential diagnosis between benign and malignant mesothelial proliferations. Walts et al. recently demonstrated that BAP-1 immunostains and p16 FISH tests were also helpful for the diagnosis of MM in effusion cytology specimens with 95% specificity (167).

A more detailed description of the cytological features of MM in various cytological samples is provided in Chapter 5.

Pathology of Pleural Diffuse Malignant Mesothelioma

Location

Approximately 90 percent and 10 percent of MM are located in the pleural and peritoneal cavities, respectively (2,3,168–170). MM can also less frequently develop in the pericardium and rarely in the serosal membranes surrounding the testes, albuginea, and paratesticular tissues (17,38–43,171).

Gross Pathology

Pleural MM usually present grossly as small, firm, white–gray nodules distributed along the pleural surfaces (Figure 11.5) (172). They arise more often in the parietal pleura than in the visceral pleura and are more common in the right hemithorax than in the left chest, with a right:left ratio of 3:2 (2). The tumor nodules grow in size and progressively coalesce to form a thick, white–gray, firm tumor rind that progressively encases

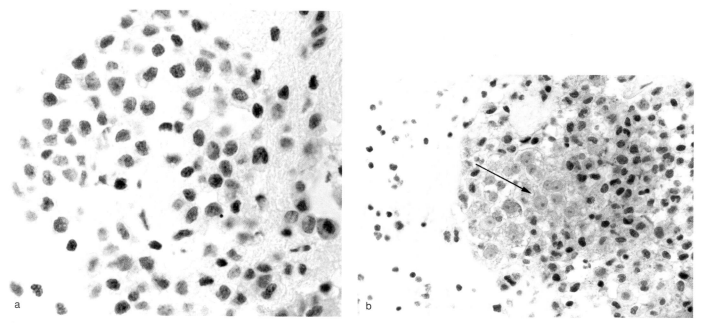

Figure 11.4 (a) Reactive mesothelial cells with normal nuclear immunoreactivity for BAP-1 (Pap stain, ×200). (b) The large, atypical mesothelial cells seen in the center of the photomicrograph (arrow) lack BAP-1 nuclear immunoreactivity, while adjacent lymphoid cells show immunoreactivity (Pap stain, ×200). This finding in atypical mesothelial cells supports a diagnosis of malignancy with a specificity of 95–100 percent.

the lung (Figure 11.6). Over time, pleural MM infiltrate diffusely into the soft tissues of the chest wall, surrounding the ribs (Figure 11.7), but usually without bone invasion except in advanced cases. MMs involving the visceral pleura infiltrate through the lung fissures and eventually into the underlying pulmonary parenchyma. As the MM progresses, the tumor nodules grow in size to form a thick pleural rind that can measure several centimeters in thickness and multiple, large,

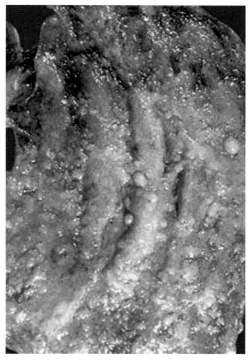

Figure 11.5 Thoracoscopy shows the presence of multiple small, white nodules on the parietal pleural surface of a patient with malignant mesothelioma.

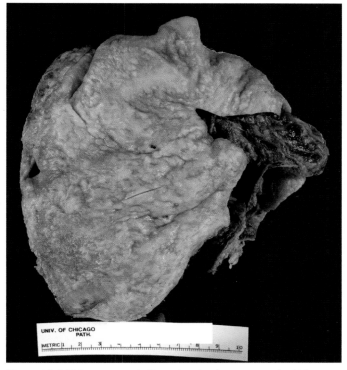

Figure 11.6 Malignant mesothelioma showing the presence of a thick, yellow–gray rind surrounding the majority of the lung surfaces.

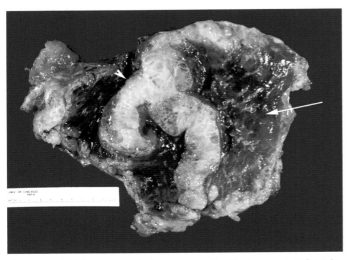

Figure 11.7 Malignant mesothelioma surrounding the lung, seen in the right portion of the gross photograph (arrow) and extending to the chest wall shown on the left portion of the image (arrowhead). The tumor, seen in the center of the lesion shows a diffuse, gray, firm surface.

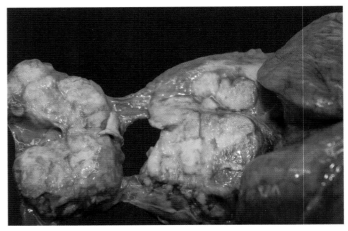

Figure 11.9 Malignant mesothelioma showing a variegated, yellow–gray, mucoid, soft, solid and cystic mass attached to lung tissue shown in the right portion of the image. Multiple areas of yellow necrosis are present.

white–gray masses with variable areas of necrosis, hemorrhage, and/or myxoid change (Figure 11.8). MM are usually solid lesions but can exhibit cystic areas containing myxoid, sticky, yellow–gray mucoid material (Figure 11.9).

Pleural MM spreads through direct invasion to the pericardium and other mediastinal structures and metastasizes to mediastinal lymph nodes that become partially or completely replaced by ill-defined, white–gray tumor.

Microscopic Features: Malignant Mesothelioma Subtypes

MMs have historically been classified based on their microscopic features into three subtypes: epithelioid, sarcomatoid, and biphasic (mixed) (Table 11.1), but multiple growth patterns can be present in each of the subtypes (169). Most neoplasms exhibit more than one growth pattern, and there are no consensus or evidence-based criteria to determine what minimal proportion of a particular growth pattern is needed to subclassify an MM as a specific variant of a subtype, so that terminology remains somewhat variable. For example, some authors have used the terminology "subtype" to described growth patterns within an MM subtype (e.g., papillary, pleomorphic, other "subtypes" of epithelioid MM) (173). The International Mesothelioma Interest Group has recently suggested that, as

Table 11.2 Growth patterns in epithelioid malignant mesothelioma

Common growth patterns
Tubular
Papillary
Tubulo-papillary
Trabecular
Solid

Less common growth patterns
Micropapillary
Adenomatoid (microglandular)
Clear cell
Transitional
Deciduoid
Small cell
Adenoid cystic
Signet ring cell
Rhabdoid
Myxoid
Pleomorphic

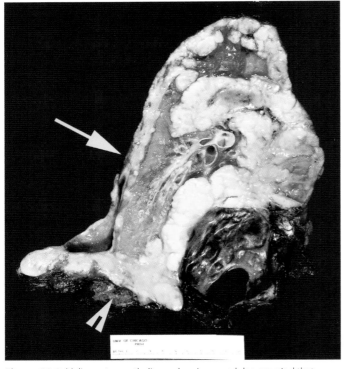

Figure 11.8 Malignant mesothelioma showing a nodular, gray rind that completely encases the lung (arrow) and extends into the diaphragm and pericardium (arrowhead).

Table 11.3 Sarcomatoid malignant mesothelioma: growth patterns

Conventional, spindle cell

Desmoplastic

Heterologous differentiation (osteosarcomatous, chondrosarcomatous, other)

Lymphohistiocytoid*

* It is controversial whether a malignant mesothelioma with lymphohistiocytoid growth pattern should be classified as epithelioid or sarcomatoid.

most mesotheliomas have several growth patterns that may not all be present on a biopsy, it is advisable to describe the patterns in the microscopic description or comment sections of a pathology report rather than attempt to diagnose specific variants of MM subtypes (3).

MMs exhibit epithelioid histopathological features in approximately 90 percent of cases (2,3). The remainder exhibit sarcomatoid or biphasic (mixed) morphology (1). The recent World Health Organization (WHO) classification of pleural neoplasms suggests to use an arbitrary 10 percent threshold of a second component to classify an MM as biphasic (mixed) (169).

Both epithelioid and sarcomatoid MM can exhibit a variety of growth patterns and cytologic features listed in Tables 11.2 and 11.3.

Epithelioid Malignant Mesothelioma

Common Growth Patterns

The majority of epithelioid MMs can be tentatively diagnosed without much difficulty on routine hematoxylin and eosin (H&E) stained slides as they are composed of cytologically bland epithelioid cells that usually exhibit less prominent cytologic atypia than carcinomas. They are typically composed of

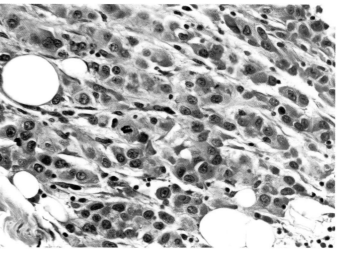

Figure 11.11 Epithelioid mesothelioma cells at higher power showing minimal anisocytosis, low nuclear cytoplasmic ratio, and round nuclei with small nucleoli. This tumor has a slightly higher tumor grade than the neoplasm shown in Figure 11.10 (H&E, ×200).

neoplastic cells that exhibit round nuclei, variable size nucleoli (Figure 11.10), slightly eosinophilic or amphophilic cytoplasm, and relatively low nucleo:cytoplasmic ratio (Figure 11.11). In general, the tumor cells exhibit minimal anisocytosis (Figure 11.12), although higher-grade tumors do exhibit considerable nuclear atypia, small numbers of mitoses (Figure 11.13), usually rare atypical mitoses (Figure 11.14), and variable areas of necrosis (Figure 11.15).

The neoplastic cells of epithelioid MM are arranged in the various growth patterns shown in Table 11.2 in the majority of cases. The tubular growth pattern is characterized by the presence of acinar structures composed of a small central lumen surrounded by uniform epithelioid cells (Figure 11.16). The papillary growth pattern is characterized by the presence of

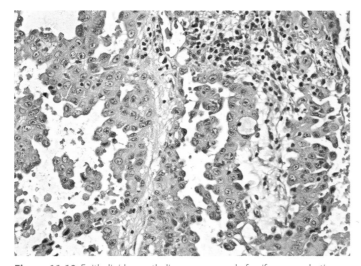

Figure 11.10 Epithelioid mesothelioma composed of uniform neoplastic cells showing round nuclei, amphophilic cytoplasm and inconspicuous nucleoli (H&E, ×100).

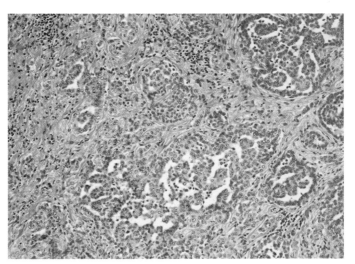

Figure 11.12 Low-grade mesothelioma composed of uniform cells showing tubulo-papillary growth features, minimal anisocytosis, and low mitotic activity (H&E, ×200).

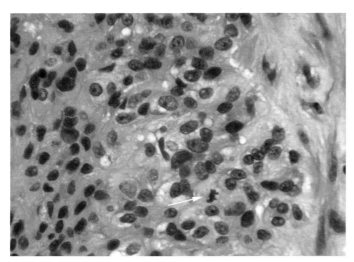

Figure 11.13 The cells of a higher-grade epithelioid mesothelioma show greater anisocytosis than seen in the previous examples, and somewhat irregular-shaped nuclei with some hyperchromasia and focal nucleoli. Nucleo:cytoplasmic ratios are higher than in low-grade neoplasm and mitoses (arrow) are more frequent (H&E, ×400).

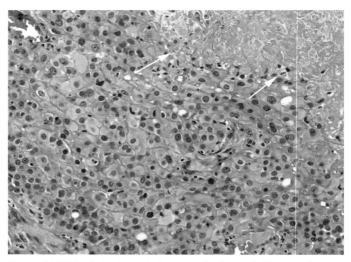

Figure 11.15 Epithelioid mesothelioma usually show variable areas of necrosis (arrows) (H&E, ×100).

presence of somewhat discohesive, amorphous sheets of tumor cells.

Less Common Growth Patterns

Epithelioid MM can also exhibit one or more of the other less frequent growth patterns listed in Table 11.3. Micropapillary growth pattern is characterized by the presence of finger-like papillary structures that lack fibrovascular cores (Figure 11.21) (174,175). This growth pattern has been shown to correlate with a higher incidence of lymphatic invasion (174).

In the adenomatoid (microglandular) growth pattern the neoplastic cells form multiple, confluent, small acinar structures that can be difficult to distinguish on biopsies from benign adenomatoid tumors or metastatic signet-ring cell carcinomas (Figure 11.22) (42,176). The small acinar structures of

finger-like structures composed of a central connective tissue core covered by epithelioid cells that are often multilayered (Figure 11.17a). The papillary and tubular features are often seen combined as a tubulo-papillary growth pattern (Figure 11.17b). The papillary structures can be accompanied by laminated calcifications identical in morphology to the psammoma bodies (Figure 11.18) seen in serous papillary carcinomas of the gynecologic genital tract, and papillary carcinomas of thyroid, lung, and other origin. Indeed, the finding of psammoma bodies in a serosal tumor cannot be used to diagnose either an MM or a metastatic carcinoma. The trabecular growth pattern is characterized by the presence of thin or thick cords of neoplastic cells infiltrating into a fibrotic stroma (Figure 11.19), while the solid growth pattern (Figure 11.20) is characterized by the

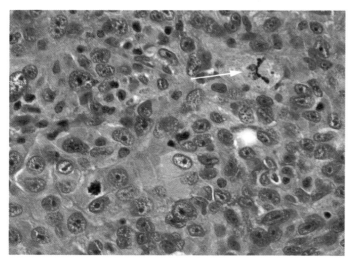

Figure 11.14 High-grade pleomorphic epithelioid mesothelioma showing atypical mitosis (arrow) (H&E, ×400).

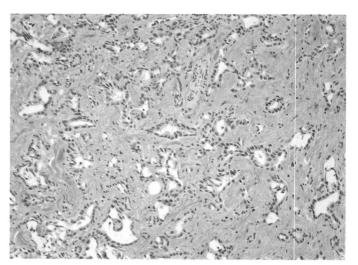

Figure 11.16 Epithelioid mesothelioma with tubular growth features. The tumor exhibits multiple tubules lined by epithelioid cells showing minimal pleomorphism, admixed with a fibrotic stroma (H&E, ×100).

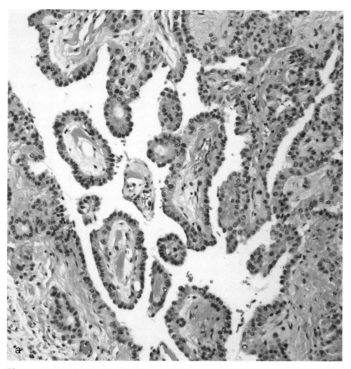

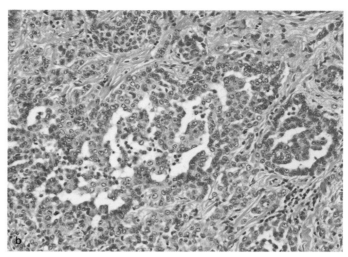

Figure 11.17 (a,b) Epithelioid mesothelioma showing papilla composed of a vascularized fibrous tissue core covered by atypical epithelioid cells (a). A different tumor shows tubulo-papillary growth features with papillary structures closely admixed with tubular formations (b) (H&E, ×200).

adenomatoid tumors and MM are lined by bland flat or cuboidal epithelioid cells that usually lack cytologic atypia. The acinar spaces contain basophilic, amorphous, or myxoid material. MM with adenomatoid growth pattern present as diffuse rather than localized processes involving the pleura, peritoneum, or tunica albuginea and microscopically show invasive features and cytologic atypia, features that allow for distinction from adenomatoid tumors (Figure 11.23a,b) (176). They can exhibit the

presence of signet-ring cells that can be distinguished from metastatic carcinomas with the aid of mucicarmine stain and immunostains, as described later on in this chapter.

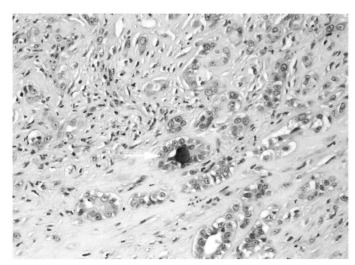

Figure 11.18 Presence of focal psammoma body in epithelioid mesothelioma (arrow). This feature should not be interpreted as evidence for an adenocarcinoma (H&E, ×200).

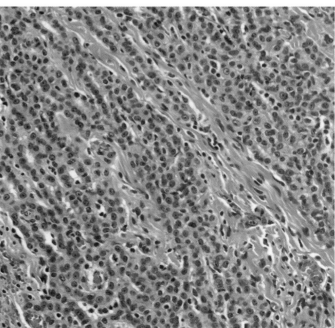

Figure 11.19 Epithelioid mesothelioma showing trabecular features with thick cords of neoplastic cells infiltrating into a fibrotic stroma. Focal acinar spaces are also present (H&E, ×100).

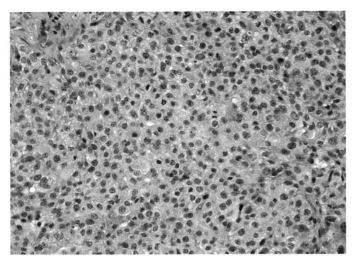

Figure 11.20 Epithelioid mesothelioma with solid growth features (H&E, ×100).

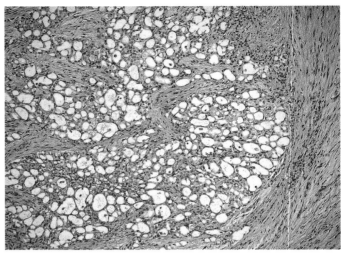

Figure 11.22 Epithelioid mesothelioma with adenomatoid growth feature. The tumor cells form numerous confluent microglandular spaces (H&E, ×100).

Clear cell growth pattern is characterized by the presence of solid sheets of large cells with round nuclei, often prominent nucleoli and abundant clear cytoplasm (Figure 11.24); these neoplasms can closely simulate metastatic renal cell carcinoma (177–179). The cells can contain abundant intracytoplasmic glycogen.

Transitional growth pattern is characterized by the presence of solid sheets of cohesive epithelioid cells that range in shape from polygonal to spindle (Figure 11.25) (2). Some of the spindle cells of tumors with this growth pattern exhibit elongated shapes that are similar to those of sarcomatoid MM (Figure 11.26), and these lesions can be difficult to distinguish from biphasic MM. However, the neoplastic cells are considerably

more discohesive in sarcomatoid MM than in lesions with a transitional growth pattern.

The deciduoid growth pattern is characterized by the presence of solid sheets of large polygonal or ovoid epithelioid cells with single or multiple nuclei, usually prominent nucleoli and abundant eosinophilic cytoplasm that closely resemble the placental decidua (Figure 11.27) (99,180–188). They can exhibit considerable anisocytosis, marked nuclear atypia, and variable mitotic activity that in some lesions is > 5 mitoses/10 HPF, an unusual finding in most epithelioid MM (Figure 11.28). Deciduoid mesothelioma was initially described as a rare, clinically aggressive variant of peritoneal MM in young women that lacked a history of asbestos exposure (182,183,186,187,189–197). However, subsequent reports have shown that some patients with pleural deciduoid MM had a history of asbestos exposure (182,186,187,189–194). In addition, not all patients with deciduoid MM have had a particularly aggressive clinical course. Ordonez has suggested that patients with deciduoid MM that exhibit high-grade histologic findings with marked cytologic atypia and > 5 mitoses/10 HPF have a highly aggressive clinical behavior with a mean survival of 7 months, while those with tumors that are less pleomorphic and exhibit lower mitotic activity had a better prognosis with a mean survival of 23 months (188). However, it must be noted that prognostic assessments based on evaluation of small case series without adequate controls can be biased by various co-morbidities, treatment or other variables.

Small cell is an extremely rare growth pattern of epithelioid MM characterized by the proliferation of irregular, solid sheets of small tumor cells with round or oval shaped nuclei, hyperchromatic cytoplasm and scanty cytoplasm (Figure 11.29a–c) (198). These tumors can be difficult to distinguish from metastatic small cell carcinomas growing in a pseudomesotheliomatous distribution with diffuse pleural thickening (199,200). However, MM with small cell growth pattern usually

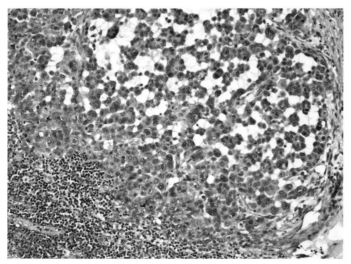

Figure 11.21 Epithelioid mesothelioma showing micropapillary growth features. The tumor cells show multiple finger-like projections that in contrast to the papillary structures seen in Figure 11.11a lack fibrovascular cores (H&E, ×100).

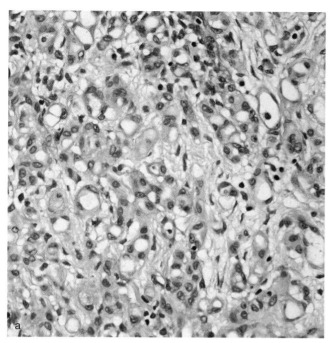
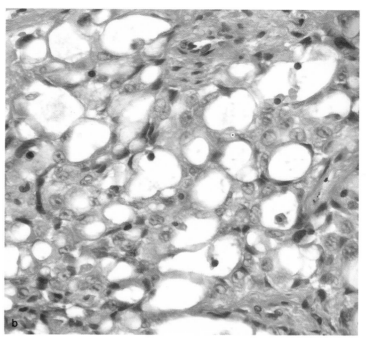

Figure 11.23 (a) Benign adenomatoid tumor composed of multiple small tubules lined by mesothelial cells that exhibit small nuclei without significant anisocytosis or other features of cytologic atypia. (b) Epithelioid mesothelioma with adenomatoid features show similar growth pattern but the neoplastic cells are slightly larger and more atypical than those seen in benign lesions. The distinction between these two entities can be difficult in practice, particularly on small biopsy specimens. The histopathologic features need to be correlated with the gross appearance of the lesion, as adenomatoid tumors present as localized nodules, while malignant mesotheliomas are diffuse or multifocal lesions in most patients (H&E, ×100).

lack features of neuroendocrine differentiation such as nesting and pseudorosettes, occasionally seen in small cell carcinomas, and generally lack the karyorrhexis and basophilic staining of blood vessels (the so-called Azzopardi effect) characteristic of small cell carcinomas. The tumor cells exhibit immunoreactivity for mesothelial markers and lack immunoreactivity for neuroendocrine markers such as chromogranin, synaptophysin,

and CD56. The recent WHO classification of pleural neoplasms discourages the use of the term "small cell mesothelioma" to avoid confusion with the epithelial lesion (169).

Epithelioid MM can rarely exhibit an adenoid cystic growth pattern characterized by the presence of cribriform and tubular structures admixed with variable fibrous stroma (Figure 11.30) (3,201). They can be distinguished from metastatic

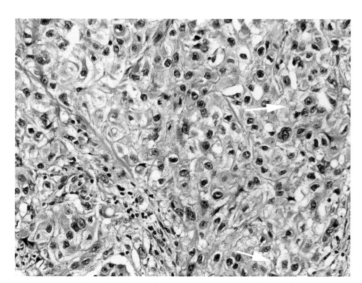

Figure 11.24 Epithelioid mesotheliomas can have variable numbers of cells with clear cytoplasm (arrows) (H&E, ×200).

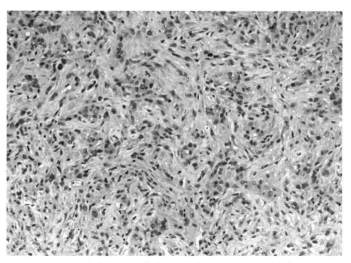

Figure 11.25 Epithelioid mesothelioma with transitional growth features. The lesion is composed of cells with intermediate shape between epithelioid and spindle cells and is difficult to classify as an epithelioid or sarcomatoid lesion (H&E, ×200).

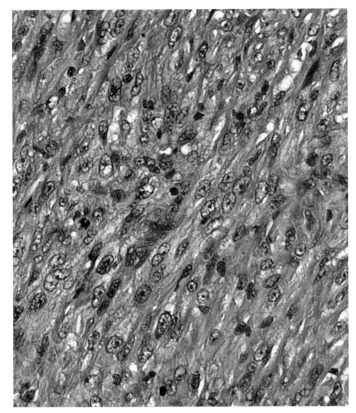

Figure 11.26 Sarcomatoid mesothelioma. In contrast to the tumor seen in Figure 11.25 the lesion is composed of tumor cells with spindle-shaped nuclei (H&E, ×200).

adenoid cystic carcinoma to a serosal surface with the aid of immunostains.

Epithelioid MM with signet-ring cells (lipid-rich) pattern exhibit solid nests, tubules, or solid cords with round cells that exhibit a clear cytoplasm containing large intracytoplasmic vacuoles and peripheral nuclei (Figure 11.31a) (202–205). The intracytoplasmic vacuoles contain lipids and/or glycogen. The nuclei of MM with signet-ring cells are usually displaced by the intracytoplasmic vacuole without indentation, while the latter cytological feature is commonly seen in signet-ring carcinomas (Figure 11.31a,b). Epithelioid MM with this growth pattern can be distinguished from metastatic adenocarcinomas with the aid of immunostains. Use of mucicarmine and diastase periodic acid–Schiff (D-PAS) stains can be misleading in this differential diagnosis, as peritoneal MM composed of signet-ring cells with abundant mucicarmine and D-PAS-positive intracytoplasmic materials have been described (202).

The rhabdoid growth pattern is very rare in MM and has been described in a few patients with epithelioid, sarcomatoid, and biphasic subtypes. These tumors are composed of large cells with round nuclei, prominent nucleoli, and abundant eosinophilic cytoplasm that does not exhibit cross-striations as seen in rhabdomyosarcoma (Figure 11.32) (186,206,207). The tumor cells exhibit immunohistochemical features of mesothelial differentiation and lack the presence of muscle-specific actin

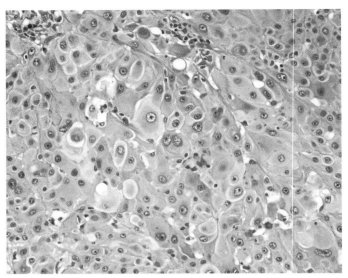

Figure 11.27 Epithelioid mesothelioma with deciduoid features. The tumor cells have round nuclei and abundant amphophilic to eosinophilic cytoplasm resulting in low nucleo:cytoplasmic ratios (H&E, ×400).

and ultrastructural evidence of rhabdomyoblastic differentiation. This growth pattern may be associated with a poor prognosis, as five of six patients with survival information available in the small series of 10 patients reported by Ordonez had a 3.8 months mean survival (207).

The pleomorphic growth pattern is also rare in MM and is characterized by the presence of solid sheets of discohesive large neoplastic cells exhibiting marked anisocytosis (Figure 11.33), multinucleation, prominent nucleoli, eosinophilic cytoplasm, high mitotic activity, atypical mitoses, and patchy areas of necrosis (Figure 11.34), features characteristic of a high-grade neoplasm (208). Patients with pleomorphic growth pattern appear to have a particularly poor prognosis. For example,

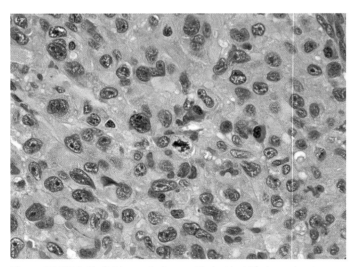

Figure 11.28 Epithelioid mesothelioma with deciduoid features showing neoplastic cells with more prominent cytologic atypia than seen in the previous example (H&E, ×400).

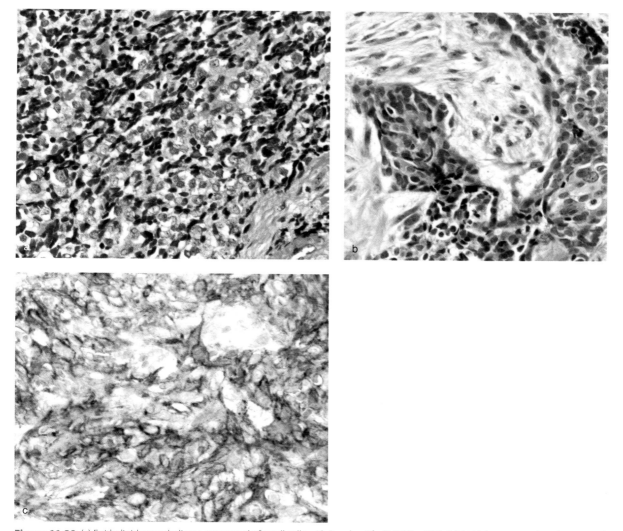

Figure 11.29 (a) Epithelioid mesothelioma composed of small cells with "crush artifact" (H&E, ×100). (b) At higher power they show round to oval hyperchromatic nuclei, scanty cytoplasm and high N:C ratio. They closely resemble the histopathological features of a small cell carcinoma (H&E, 400). (c) However, they lack immunoreactivity for neuroendocrine markers and exhibit immunoreactivity for mesothelial markers such as calretinin (Pap, Calretinin, ×200).

seven patients with MM showing pleomorphic growth pattern treated with extrapleural pneumonectomy at MD Anderson Cancer Center had a median survival of only 8.2 months (208). It has been controversial whether to classify lesions with pleomorphic growth pattern as epithelioid or sarcomatoid MM (2,208,209). The recent WHO classification of pleural tumors groups pleomorphic MM as epithelioid lesions, as these lesions show similar histopathologic features to those of pleomorphic carcinomas of the lung and other organs (169).

Evaluation of Stromal Invasion

An important histopathologic feature for the diagnosis of epithelioid and other subtypes of MM is the presence of stromal invasion, characterized by extension of the tumor beyond the pleura or peritoneum into adipose tissue (Figure 11.35),

lung (Figure 11.36), or other non-serosal tissues. The invasive nature of epithelioid MM with solid or tubulo-papillary growth patterns is usually readily recognizable on pleural biopsies, as these histopathologic features are usually not seen in normal serosa, reactive mesothelial hyperplasia, or atypical mesothelial hyperplasia. However, it may be difficult to diagnose the presence of pleural invasion in epithelioid exhibiting a predominantly trabecular growth pattern (Figure 11.37). In MM with trabecular growth pattern the invasive epithelioid cells are distributed haphazardly throughout the pleura and tend to involve the entire pleural thickness (Figure 11.38), while reactive mesothelial cells are distributed more densely in areas closer to the pleural surface with maturation toward the deeper pleura (Figure 11.39). The presence of epithelioid mesothelial cells arranged in trabeculae that are parallel and more mature toward the pleural surface, the so-called zonation

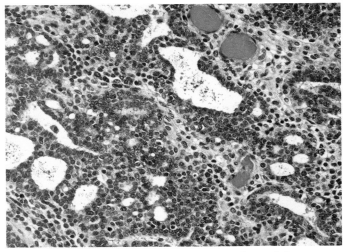

Figure 11.30 Epithelioid malignant mesothelioma with growth features similar to adenoid cystic carcinoma. The tumor shows multiple tubules with cribriform growth pattern. However, the tumor cells do not exhibit immunoreactivity for myoepithelial markers and react with mesothelial markers (H&E, ×200).

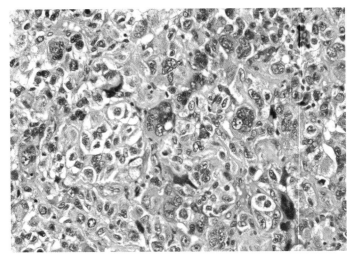

Figure 11.33 Epithelioid pleomorphic mesothelioma with solid growth features and marked cytologic atypia (H&E, ×200).

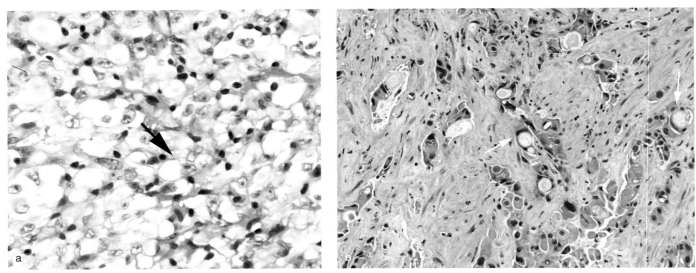

Figure 11.31 (a) Epithelioid mesothelioma with clear cell features and signet-ring cells (arrow). The neoplasm shows more numerous clear cells than those seen in the tumor shown in Figure 11.24. The signet-ring cells show a large, clear, intracytoplasmic vacuole that displaces the peripheral nuclei without usually producing nuclear indentation (H&E, ×400). The signet-ring cell adenocarcinoma shown in (b) shows similar cells, but in contrast to mesothelioma the intracytoplasmic vacuoles in the malignant epithelial cells generally indent the displaced peripheral nuclei (arrows) (H&E, ×400).

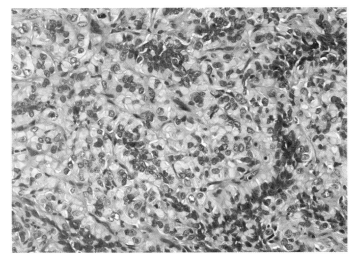

Figure 11.32 Malignant mesothelioma with rhabdoid cells showing round nuclei, focally prominent nucleoli, and abundant eosinophilic cytoplasm (H&E, ×400).

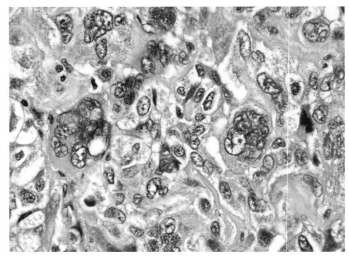

Figure 11.34 The tumor cells of pleomorphic mesotheliomas show marked anisocytosis, hyperchromasia, prominent nucleoli, and multinucleated forms (H&E, ×400).

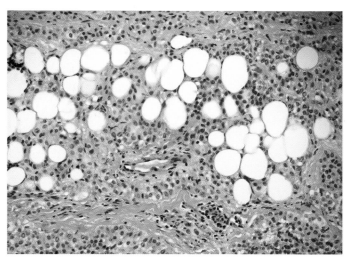

Figure 11.35 Invasion of the parietal pleura adipose tissue by an epithelioid mesothelioma (H&E, ×100).

effect, is in our experience a useful histopathologic feature to diagnose non-neoplastic reactive mesothelial proliferations (Figure 11.40). It probably results from the deposition of successive layers of reactive mesothelial cells as a reaction to a fibrinous pleuritis, and in some cases extracellular fibrin can be seen between the mesothelial cell layers. In contrast, the cells

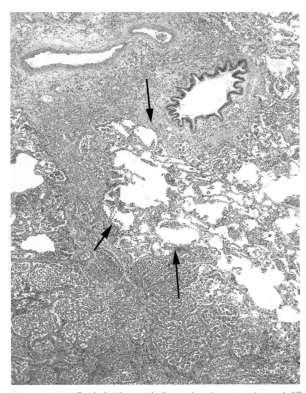

Figure 11.36 Epithelioid mesothelioma showing extensive and diffuse involvement of the visceral pleura with focal invasion of lung tissue (arrows). The tumor tends to spread into septa and/or push into the alveolated lung parenchyma rather than infiltrating it in the diffuse manner usually seen in carcinomas.

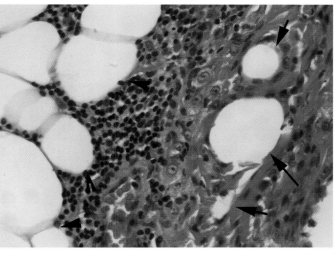

Figure 11.37 Biopsy of epithelioid mesothelioma showing neoplastic cells with trabecular growth features. It can be difficult to distinguish true invasion in these cases. The biopsy shows large spaces that probably represent tissue artifacts (arrows) ("fake fat") while the adipose tissue (arrowheads) shows no unequivocal invasion (H&E, ×100).

of malignant mesothelioma grow into adipose tissue (Figure 11.41) or other structures in a haphazard growth pattern. Reactive pleuritis also often show the presence of neovascularization near the serous membrane surface, with growth of branching capillaries in a perpendicular distribution to the serosal surface (Figure 11.42).

The presence of histopathologic features of stromal invasion are best seen at low-power microscopy (Figure 11.43a). However, the distinction between invasion by malignant cells and pseudoinvasion resulting from the exuberant proliferation of benign mesothelial cells can be very difficult to recognize with certainty by examination of only the pleura and it is important

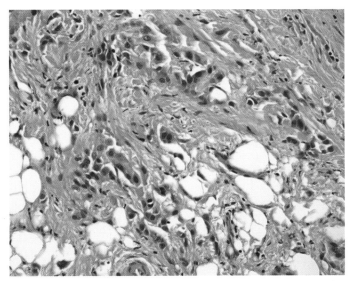

Figure 11.38 Epithelioid mesothelioma showing adipose tissue invasion. The invasive tumor cells are distributed haphazardly and in cords throughout the tissue (H&E, ×200).

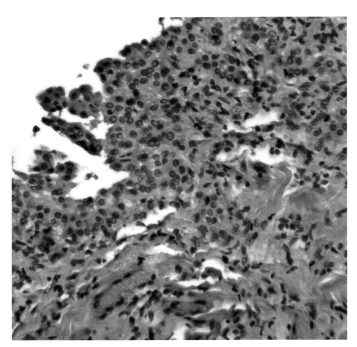

Figure 11.39 Pleural biopsy from a patient with chronic pleuritis showing focal atypical mesothelial hyperplasia. The reactive mesothelial cells show some anisocytosis and focal areas of possible invasion. It is very difficult to distinguish these atypical repair changes from an epithelioid mesothelioma in the absence of adipose tissue or lung tissue invasion (H&E, ×200).

for pathologists to attempt to identify the presence of tumor cells in adipose tissue, lung, or other extrapleural structures before an unequivocal diagnosis of MM is rendered. Detection of the presence of tumor extension into adipose tissue is a par-

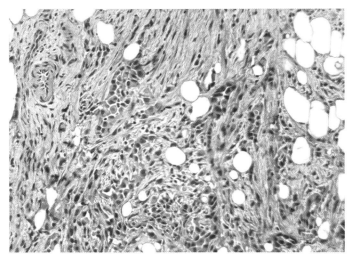

Figure 11.41 Epithelioid mesothelioma with extensive invasion of adipose tissue (H&E, ×100).

ticularly helpful diagnostic feature to confirm the diagnosis of MM and can be established only in pleural biopsies that include adipose tissue. Indeed, thoracic surgeons need to become aware of the need to include subpleural adipose tissue while performing biopsies under VATS thoracoscopy. The identification of adipose invasion by MM often requires careful examination of tissues at ×20 or ×40 (Figure 11.43b), as the histopathologic finding of invasion can be very subtle in cases where few tumor cells infiltrate imperceptibly along adipocytes without eliciting an inflammatory or desmoplastic reaction. Immunostains for pancytokeratin (e.g., keratin AE1/AE3, OSCAR, other)

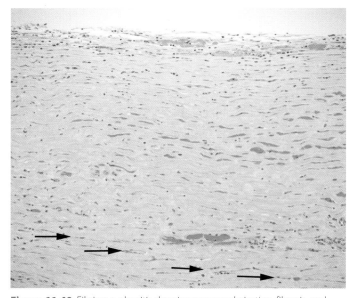

Figure 11.40 Fibrinous pleuritis showing neovascularization, fibrosis, and proliferation of mesothelial cells in parallel layers (the so-called zonation effect) (arrows) (H&E, ×40). The latter features can be helpful to distinguish reactive mesothelial proliferations from mesotheliomas characterized by the more haphazard growth pattern of the neoplastic cells.

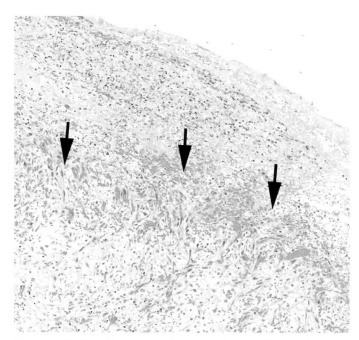

Figure 11.42 Organizing pleuritis showing multiple branching capillaries that grow perpendicular to the pleural surface (arrows) (H&E, ×40).

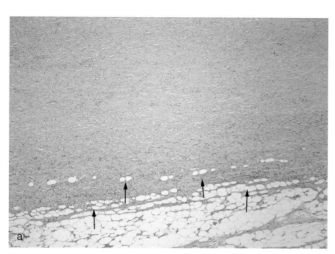
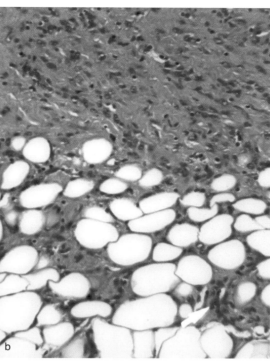

Figure 11.43 (a) Examination of pleural biopsies at low power microscopy can be helpful to identify invasion of adipose tissue (arrows) or other structures. (b) The finding needs to be confirmed by higher power microscopy showing the presence of neoplastic cells admixed with adipocytes (arrow) (H&E, ×40).

(Figure 11.44) and calretinin (Figure 11.45) or other mesothelial markers discussed in one of the next sections are very helpful to help visualize the presence of adipose tissue invasion. Skeletal muscle invasion by epithelioid MM (Figure 11.46) is seldom seen in pleural biopsies and is more frequent in pleurectomy and EPP specimens. Direct invasion of the lung parenchyma from the visceral pleura is an unusual finding in pleural biopsies from MM.

Histochemical Stains

Mucicarmine and D-PAS stains have been used for many years prior to the advent of immunohistochemistry to help distinguish epithelioid MM from adenocarcinomas, but they have

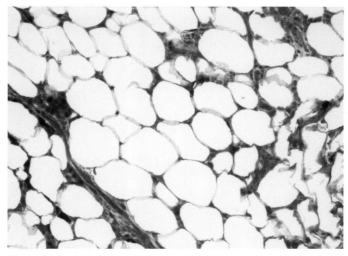

Figure 11.44 Epithelioid mesothelioma showing cytoplasmic immunoreactivity for keratin AE1/AE3. This feature can be very helpful to assist in the diagnosis of mesothelioma and in the identification of tissue invasion (Pap, ×200).

Figure 11.45 Epithelioid mesothelioma showing nuclear and cytoplasmic immunoreactivity for calretinin. The finding helps identify tumor cells within adipose tissue (Pap, ×100).

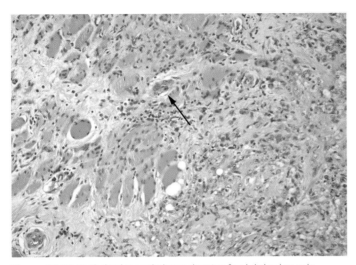

Figure 11.46 Epithelioid mesothelioma showing focal skeletal muscle invasion (arrow) (H&E, ×100).

Alcian blue and colloidal iron stains, but the reactivity is not removed by pretreatment of the sections with hyaluronidase (172).

The histochemical findings need to be considered in context with morphology and immunophenotype, because rare MM can show intracytoplasmic mucicarmine-positive vacuoles and MM can show intracytoplasmic acid mucins that are not removed by hyaluronidase pretreatment, probably as the result of crystallization of the proteoglycans (2,3). In general, histochemical stains are not currently recommended for the diagnosis of MM (2,3).

Immunohistochemical Stains

The definitive diagnosis of MM currently requires evaluation with various immunostains (3,211,212). The selection of antibodies varies according to the subtype of mesothelioma and its histopathological features, the location of the tumor in the pleura, peritoneum or other serosal membranes, and, in selected cases, the clinical history of another known malignancy. There are no consensus or evidence-based guidelines recommended for the minimum percentage of tumor cells that need to exhibit immunoreactivity for a particular antibody. Use of arbitrary 5 percent or 10 percent minimal thresholds for immunoreactivity to be considered as positive is probably not used by practicing pathologists, as immunoreactivity depends on fixation, tumor morphology, and other factors.

The diagnosis of epithelioid MM is relatively straightforward in most cases and requires the use of immunostains for pancytokeratin and other markers that help establish mesothelial differentiation and exclude epithelial differentiation (2,3,211). Pancytokeratin antibodies such as AE1/AE3, OSCAR (Figure 11.49) and CAM5.2 (1–3,168) are very useful for the diagnosis of all subtypes of MM. Practically all epithelioid MM are positive for at least one of the pancytokeratin antibodies, but 5–10 percent of sarcomatoid mesothelioma can

only limited current applicability (2,172,210). The tumor cells of epithelioid MM generally stain negatively for neutral mucin with mucicarmine and D-PAS stains (Figure 11.47a), in contrast with adenocarcinomas that often show intracytoplasmic vacuoles with these stains (Figure 11.47b). Cytoplasmic staining for D-PAS is more specific than mucicarmine stain for the diagnosis of adenocarcinoma, but can be rarely seen in MM.

The neoplastic cells of epithelioid MM also show intracytoplasmic vacuoles containing acid mucopolysaccharides such as hyaluronic acid and proteoglycans that stain with Alcian blue and colloidal iron stains (Figure 11.48a) (172). Characteristically, this reactivity is seen in spaces that are larger than the intracytoplasmic vacuoles seen in adenocarcinomas and it can be removed with pretreatment of the sections with hyaluronidase (Figure 11.48b). Adenocarcinomas can also show intracytoplasmic acid mucins that stain positively with

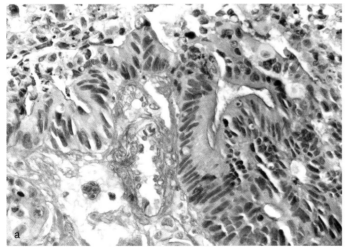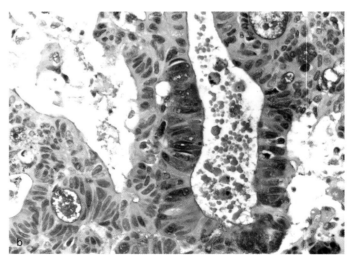

Figure 11.47 (a) The tumor cells of epithelioid mesothelioma usually stain negatively with diastase PAS (D-PAS stain, ×200). (b) In contrast, adenocarcinomas usually show intracytoplasmic staining (D-PAS stain, ×200).

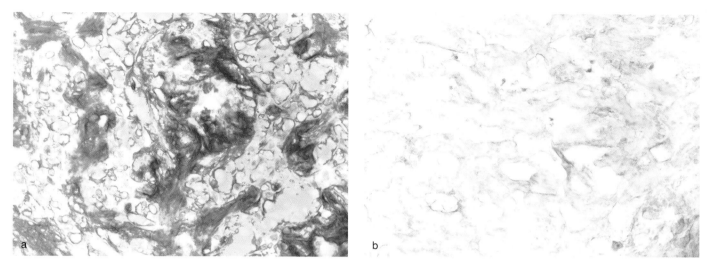

Figure 11.48 (a) The tumor cells of epithelioid mesothelioma often stain with acid mucin stains such as colloidal iron stain. (b) The material is removed by hyaluronidase pretreatment of the sections.

be negative (152,168). The presence of diffuse pancytokeratin in a tumor excludes the diagnosis of tumors that can mimic MM, such as epithelioid hemangioendothelioma, angiosarcoma, lymphomas, and metastatic melanoma. However, the presence of focal pancytokeratin immunoreactivity needs to be interpreted with caution, as angiosarcomas, melanomas, and other tumors can exhibit this feature. Current best practice is to evaluate for the presence of immunoreactivity using a minimum of two mesothelial and two epithelial markers (3). How-

ever, it is important not to rely on a single antibody for the diagnosis of epithelioid MM. Paradoxically, the use of a large number of immunostains also creates diagnostic problems, as none of the markers of mesothelial or epithelial differentiation are 100 percent specific or sensitive and can show false positive findings resulting in diagnostic errors (213,214). For example, one of us (AM) showed that considerably better odds ratio for the differential diagnosis between epithelioid MM vs. adenocarcinoma can be obtained using fewer selected antibodies than 15 immunostains, supporting the notion that "more is not necessarily better" (212).

Table 11.4 lists the five most useful mesothelial markers and their sensitivity and specificity for the differential diagnosis between epithelioid MM and adenocarcinoma originating at various sites (3,169,172,215). Calretinin immunostain shows the presence of both nuclear and cytoplasmic reactivity in MM (Figure 11.50). Wilms' tumor-1 immunostain shows the presence of nuclear immunoreactivity (Figure 11.51). D2–40 (podoplanin) (Figure 11.52) and HBME-1 (Figure 11.53) immunostains show the presence of membrane immunoreactivity. Cytokeratin 5/6 immunostain shows the presence of cytoplasmic immunoreactivity (Figure 11.54).

Table 11.5 lists the five most useful epithelial markers to exclude the diagnosis of epithelioid MM and their

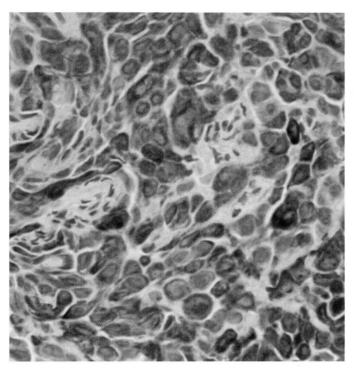

Figure 11.49 Tumor cells of epithelioid mesothelioma showing cytoplasmic immunoreactivity for pancytokeratin OSCAR (Pap, ×200).

Table 11.4 "Mesothelial markers" that are most useful for the differential diagnosis between epithelioid malignant mesothelioma and pulmonary adenocarcinoma

	Sensitivity (%)	Specificity (%)
Calretinin	>90	>90
Wilms' tumor-1 (WT-1)	75–100	>90
D2–40 (podoplanin)	90–100	85
CK5/6	75–100	80–90
HBME-1	75–100	>90

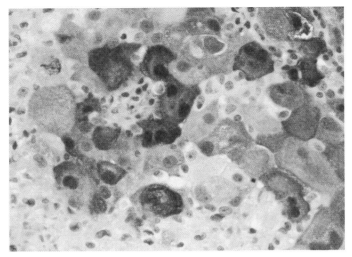

Figure 11.50 Tumor cells of epithelioid mesothelioma showing nuclear and cytoplasmic immunoreactivity for calretinin (Pap, ×400).

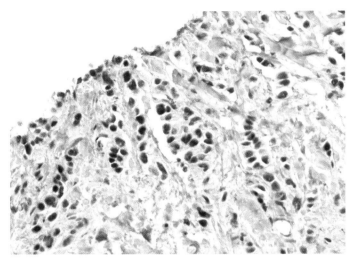

Figure 11.51 Tumor cells of epithelioid mesothelioma showing nuclear immunoreactivity for Wilms' tumor-1 antigen (Pap, ×200).

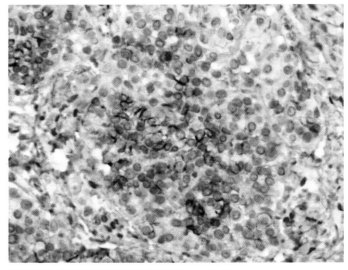

Figure 11.52 Tumor cells of epithelioid mesothelioma showing membrane immunoreactivity for podoplanin (D2–40) (Pap, ×400).

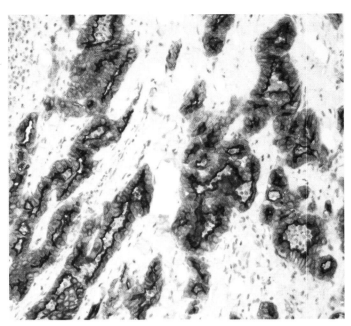

Figure 11.53 Tumor cells of epithelioid mesothelioma showing membrane immunoreactivity for HBME-1 (Pap, ×100).

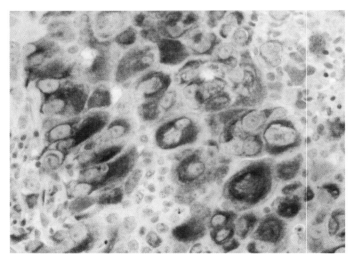

Figure 11.54 Tumor cells of epithelioid mesothelioma showing nuclear and cytoplasmic immunoreactivity for CK5/6 (Pap, ×400).

Table 11.5 "Epithelial markers" that are most useful for the differential diagnosis between epithelioid malignant mesothelioma and adenocarcinoma

	Sensitivity (%)	Specificity (%)
Ber-EP4	> 95	85–98
BG8 (Lewis Y)	> 90	93–97
MOC31	> 95	85–98
Monoclonal CEA	> 80	> 95
B72.3	> 70	50–70
Claudin-4	> 90	100

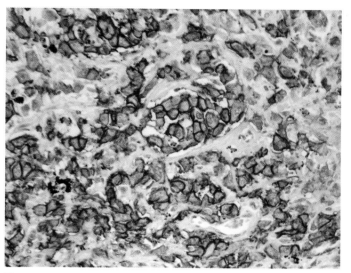

Figure 11.55 Tumor cells of adenocarcinoma showing membrane immunoreactivity for Ber-EP4 (Pap, ×400).

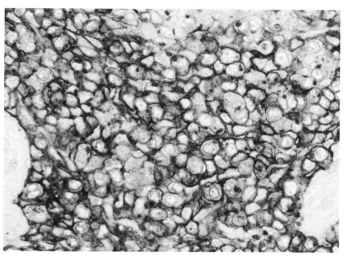

Figure 11.57 Tumor cells of adenocarcinoma showing membrane and focal cytoplasmic immunoreactivity for BG8 (Pap, ×400).

sensitivity and specificity for the differential diagnosis between epithelioid MM and adenocarcinoma originating at various sites. Ber-EP4 immunostain shows the presence of membrane immunoreactivity in adenocarcinomas (Figure 11.55). Monoclonal CEA (Figure 11.56), BG8 (Lewis Y) (Figure 11.57), MOC31 (Figure 11.58), and B72.3 show cytoplasmic and/or membrane immunoreactivity. More recently, claudin-4 has been proposed as a highly specific and sensitive immunohistochemical marker for distinguishing epithelioid MM and metastatic carcinomas to the serosal membranes (216–222).

Claudin-4 is a transmembrane protein that is located in the tight junctions of the epithelial cells, adenocarcinomas, desmoplastic small round cell tumors, and biphasic synovial sarcomas with an epithelioid component, but it is absent in mesothelial cells and epithelioid MM. Claudin-4 is absent in 100 percent of epithelioid MM and exhibits membrane immunoreactivity in > 90 percent of carcinomas (Figure 11.59). The marker is not useful to distinguish sarcomatoid MM from synovial sarcomas, solitary fibrous tumor, melanomas, and other lesions composed of spindle cells because claudin-4 is also negative in these lesions (218).

The selection of mesothelial and epithelial markers most useful for the diagnosis of an epithelioid MM needs to be based on the clinical history, imaging findings, and other clinical data specific for a particular patient, as the antibodies listed in Tables 11.4 and 11.5 may have limitations in certain

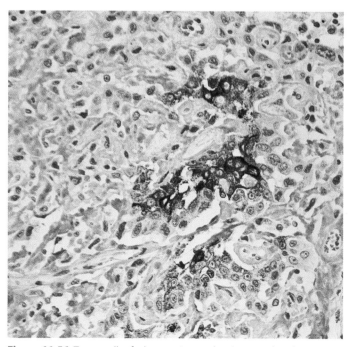

Figure 11.56 Tumor cells of adenocarcinoma showing cytoplasmic immunoreactivity for monoclonal CEA (Pap, ×400).

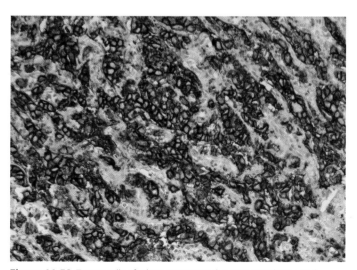

Figure 11.58 Tumor cells of adenocarcinoma showing membrane and cytoplasmic immunoreactivity for MOC-31 (Pap, ×400).

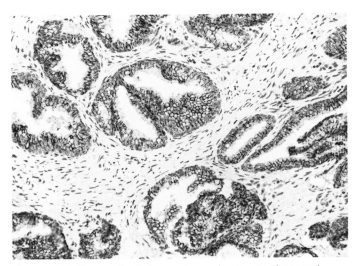

Figure 11.59 Tumor cells of adenocarcinoma showing membrane and cytoplasmic immunoreactivity for claudin-4 (Pap, ×200).

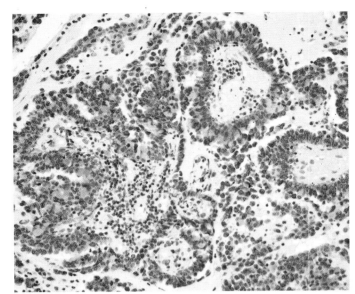

Figure 11.61 Tumor cells of pulmonary adenocarcinoma showing cytoplasmic immunoreactivity for Napsin A (Pap, ×200).

differential diagnoses. For example, if a diagnosis of pulmonary adenocarcinoma metastatic to the pleura is suspected clinically, TTF-1 (Figure 11.60) and Napsin A (Figure 11.61) are the best two epithelial markers to be used in this differential diagnosis (Table 11.6). TTF-1 shows nuclear immunoreactivity and Napsin A shows nuclear cytoplasmic immunoreactivity in over 80 percent of pulmonary adenocarcinomas and in less than 5 percent of epithelioid MM. However, if the differential diagnosis includes MM and squamous cell carcinoma of pulmonary or other origin, the epithelial markers discussed above are not particularly helpful, as squamous cell carcinomas can be best confirmed by the presence of nuclear immunoreactivity for p40 (Figure 11.62) or p63 and/or cytoplasmic immunoreactivity for desmoglein. In this differential diagnosis, the mesothe-

lial marker CK5/6 is also not helpful, as it can show cytoplasmic immunoreactivity in both MM and squamous cell carcinomas.

Table 11.6 lists epithelial markers that can be helpful for the differential diagnosis of carcinomas of breast, gastrointestinal, gynecologic, prostate, and renal origin. It also lists antibodies that are helpful to diagnose epithelioid hemangioendothelioma (EHE) and malignant melanoma, tumors that can result in diffuse pleural or peritoneal metastases that can simulate MM.

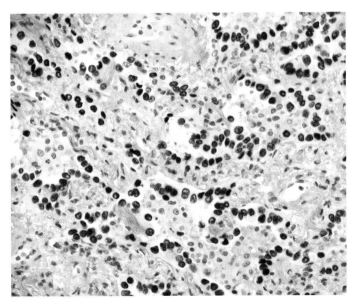

Figure 11.60 Tumor cells of pulmonary adenocarcinoma showing nuclear immunoreactivity for TTF-1 (Pap, ×400).

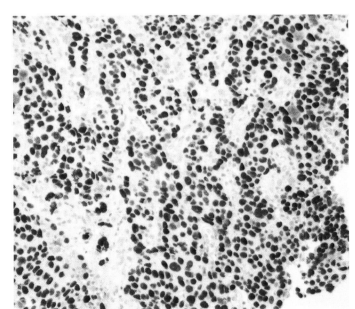

Figure 11.62 Tumor cells of metastatic squamous cell carcinoma showing nuclear immunoreactivity for p40 (Pap, ×200).

Table 11.6 Other "epithelial markers" that can be useful for the differential diagnosis between epithelioid malignant mesothelioma and other epithelioid neoplasms

Epithelial marker	Lung adenocarcinoma	Mesothelioma
TTF-1	Positive	Negative
Napsin A	Positive	Negative
	Breast carcinoma	**Mesothelioma**
GATA-3	Positive	Can be positive
Mammaglobin	Positive	Negative
Estrogen receptor	Positive	Negative
GCDFP15	Positive	Negative
	Squamous cell carcinoma	**Mesothelioma**
P40	Positive	Negative
P63	Positive	Negative
Desmoglein	Positive	Negative
	Renal cell carcinoma	**Mesothelioma**
PAX-8	Positive	Negative
PAX-2	Positive	Negative
RCC	Positive	Negative
	GI adenocarcinoma	**Mesothelioma**
CK20	Positive in colon cancer Negative in upper GI tumors	Negative
CDX-2	Positive in colon cancer	Negative
	Gynecologic adenocarcinoma	**Mesothelioma**
PAX-8	Positive	Negative
PAX-2	Positive	Negative
	Prostatic adenocarcinoma	**Mesothelioma**
PSA	Positive	Negative
PSMA	Positive	Negative
NK3.1	Positive	Negative
	Epithelioid hemangioendothelioma	**Mesothelioma**
CD33	Positive	Negative
CD34	Positive	Negative
ERG	Positive	Negative
FLI1	Positive	Negative
	Malignant melanoma	**Mesothelioma**
HBM45	Positive	Negative
Melan A	Positive	Negative
S100	Positive	Negative
MITF	Positive	Negative
SOX10	Positive	Negative

Sarcomatoid Malignant Mesothelioma

Sarcomatoid MM appear on imaging studies and grossly as diffuse neoplasms of the pleura, peritoneum, pericardium, or other serosal surfaces (1,37,39,168,203,223–228). They are composed of spindle cells that at low-power magnification show a diffuse growth pattern and are usually arranged in discohesive solid sheets (Figure 11.63), fascicles (Figure 11.64), or in a storiform, so-called patternless growth pattern (Figure 11.65) (4). Sarcomatoid MM exhibit variable cellularity, with some lesions showing relatively scanty spindle cells admixed with a densely collagenized stromal matrix (Figure 11.66), while others show diffuse (Figure 11.67) or patchy (Figure 11.68) hypercellular areas. Sarcomatoid mesotheliomas can be difficult to distinguish from reactive fibrous pleuritis (fibrous pleurisy), as this condition can also show fairly diffuse proliferation of spin-

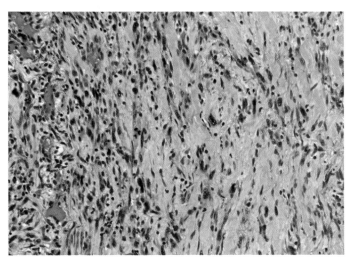

Figure 11.63 Sarcomatoid mesothelioma composed of solid sheets of spindle cells showing hyperchromatic nuclei with modest anisocytosis. Note the variable cellularity with low cellularity in the right portion of the tumor and increased cellularity in the left portion of the photomicrograph (H&E, ×100).

dle cells (Figure 11.69). The reactive spindle mesothelial cells are usually more prominent near the serosal membrane surface and tend to be organized in fascicles that are parallel to the serosal surface, but can extend deep into a thickened pleura simulating a neoplasm. The tumor cells of a sarcomatoid MM infiltrate into adipose tissue, skeletal muscle, bone (Figure 11.70) and other tissues, a finding that is very helpful for the diagnosis of malignancy.

At high-power magnification, the spindle cells of sarcomatoid MM exhibit a variety of nuclear features. Some have large, plump nuclei with variable degrees of hyperchromasia

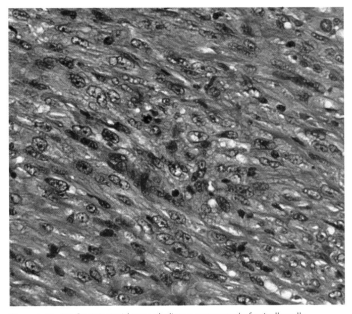

Figure 11.64 Sarcomatoid mesothelioma composed of spindle cells arranged in fascicles. The spindle cells show moderate anisocytosis and small nucleoli (H&E, ×200).

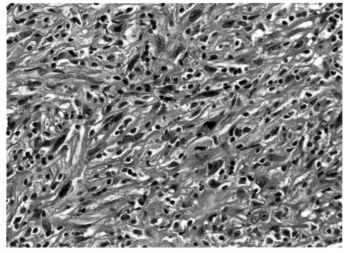

Figure 11.65 Sarcomatoid mesothelioma composed of spindle cells showing a disorganized, "patternless" growth feature (H&E, ×200).

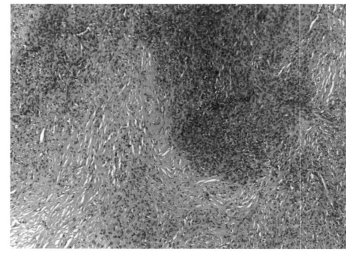

Figure 11.68 Sarcomatoid mesothelioma with patchy cellularity showing relatively hypocellular and fibrotic areas and highly cellular spindle cell areas (H&E, ×40).

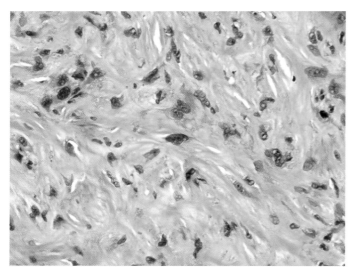

Figure 11.66 Sarcomatoid mesothelioma with densely fibrotic stroma between atypical spindle cells (H&E, ×400).

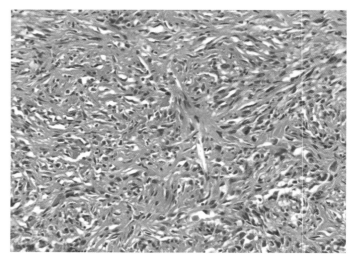

Figure 11.69 Fibrous pleurisy showing proliferation of spindle cells showing a disorganized growth pattern. The spindle cells can show variable atypia. They tend to be more cellular near the pleural surface and, in contrast to sarcomatoid mesothelioma, the spindle cells do not infiltrate into adipose tissue or other structures (H&E, ×100).

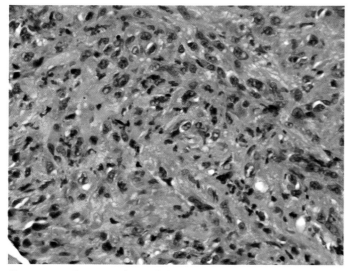

Figure 11.67 Sarcomatoid mesothelioma with highly cellular spindle cell area (H&E, ×400).

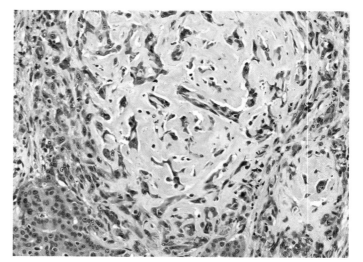

Figure 11.70 Bone invasion by sarcomatoid mesothelioma (H&E, ×100).

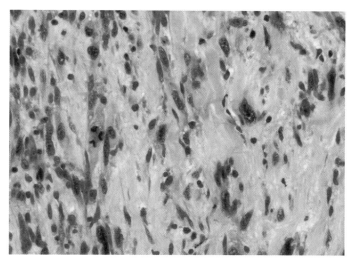

Figure 11.71 Sarcomatoid mesothelioma at high-power microscopy showing pleomorphic spindle cells with plump, hyperchromatic nuclei (H&E, ×400).

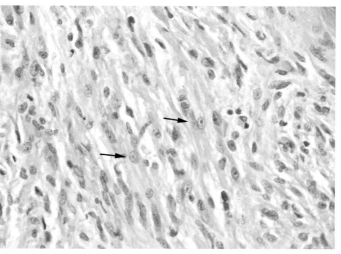

Figure 11.73 Spindle cells of sarcomatoid mesothelioma showing focally prominent nucleoli (arrows) (H&E, ×400).

(Figure 11.71), while others exhibit long, thin nuclei without overt cytologic features of malignancy (Figure 11.72). The cytoplasm of the malignant spindle cells of sarcomatoid MM is usually amphophilic with variable N:C ratios. The degree of nuclear anisocytosis, hyperchromasia, prominent nucleoli (Figure 11.73), necrosis (Figure 11.74), and mitotic activity (Figure 11.75) is variable. Atypical mitoses can be seen in

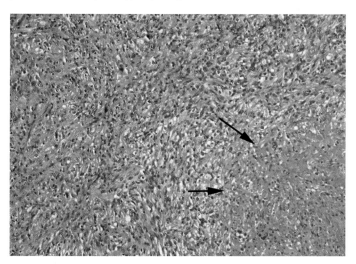

Figure 11.74 Sarcomatoid MM composed of solid sheets of spindle cells. Note the presence of extensive necrosis (arrows) (H&E, ×200).

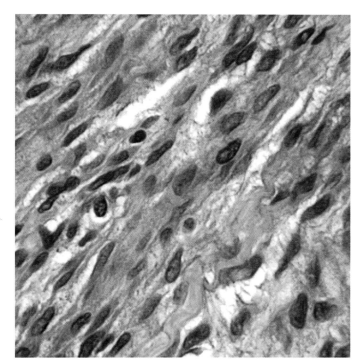

Figure 11.72 Sarcomatoid mesothelioma at high-power microscopy showing less pleomorphic spindle cells with minimal anisocytosis and slight hyperchromasia. Better-differentiated lesions such as this can be difficult to distinguish from fibrous pleurisy (H&E, ×400).

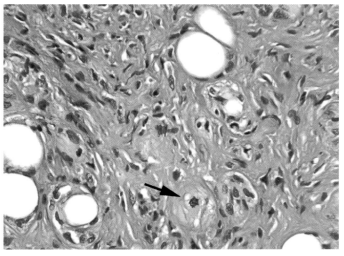

Figure 11.75 Sarcomatoid mesothelioma with mitosis (arrow) (H&E, ×400).

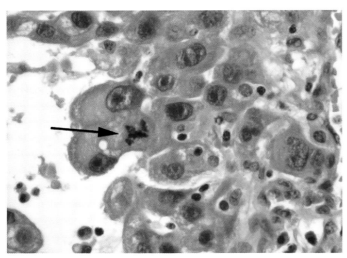

Figure 11.76 Pleomorphic mesothelioma with atypical mitosis (arrow) (H&E, ×400).

sarcomatoid and epithelioid MM and strongly support the diagnosis of malignancy (Figure 11.76).

Less frequently, sarcomatoid MM show the presence of so-called heterologous elements, such as the presence of rhabdomyosarcoma, osteosarcoma, or chondrosarcoma (229–231). Rhabdomyosarcoma elements are characterized by the presence of scattered large cells with round nuclei, prominent nucleoli, and eosinophilic cytoplasm that often shows cross-striations (Figure 11.77). They need to be distinguished from epithelioid MM with rhabdoid features. Osteosarcoma elements are composed of large osteoblastic cells showing round nuclei, prominent nucleoli, basophilic cytoplasm, and variable anisocytosis. They form variable amount of mineralized bony extracellular material (Figure 11.78). Chondrosarcoma elements show cartilage with large, pleomorphic chondroblasts present in hypercellular groups with more than one nucleus in each cartilaginous lacuna (Figure 11.79).

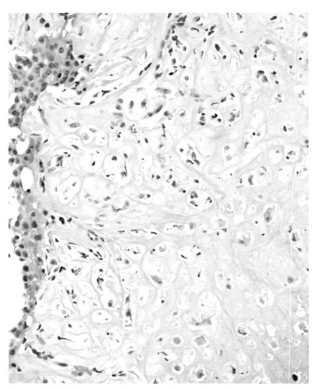

Figure 11.78 Sarcomatoid mesothelioma with malignant osteoid formation. The tumor cells are surrounded by densely eosinophilic and focally mineralized stroma (H&E, ×200).

Rarely, sarcomatoid MM are composed of solid sheets of markedly atypical cells with multinucleation, hyperchromatic nuclei, prominent nucleoli, numerous mitoses, atypical mitoses, and/or necrosis. These sarcomatoid tumors are often difficult to distinguish from pleomorphic epithelioid MM or high-grade sarcomas, not otherwise classified (NOS).

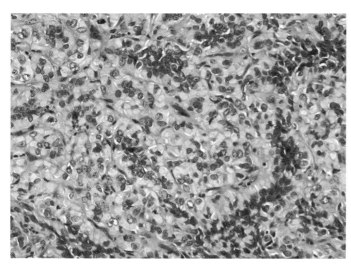

Figure 11.77 Rhabdomyosarcomatous elements (H&E, ×200).

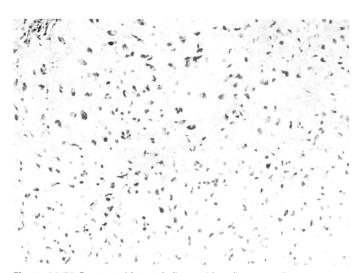

Figure 11.79 Sarcomatoid mesothelioma with malignant cartilage formation. The tumor cells are surrounded by densely basophilic matrix and exhibit features consistent with malignant chondrocytes (H&E, ×200).

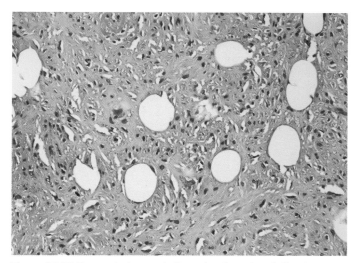

Figure 11.80 Desmoplastic mesothelioma showing a densely fibrotic matrix and atypical spindle cells arranged in a disorganized growth pattern (H&E, ×200).

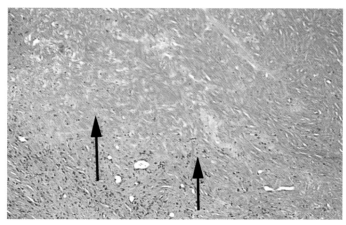

Figure 11.82 Desmoplastic mesothelioma with area of "bland necrosis" (arrows) (H&E, ×100).

Desmoplastic Malignant Mesothelioma

Desmoplastic MM is an unusual variant of sarcomatoid MM characterized by the presence of extensive hyalinized fibrous stroma in at least 50 percent of the lesion (168,229,232–240). The spindle tumor cells are relatively sparse in cellularity and are organized in a so-called patternless growth pattern (Figure 11.80). The tumor cells often exhibit minimal cytologic atypia with only focal hypercellular nodular areas composed of larger spindle cells with hyperchromatic nuclei and moderate anisocytosis (Figure 11.81). The tumors can also exhibit bland necrosis (Figure 11.82). The most reliable diagnostic feature of desmoplastic MM is the presence of invasion into adipose tissue (Figure 11.83), lung, or other extrapleural structures. A somewhat less-reliable but useful diagnostic feature is the presence

of cellular stromal nodules that are interspersed among acellular areas exhibiting hyalinized fibrous stroma that may exhibit focal areas of bland necrosis.

Patients with desmoplastic MM have a particularly poor prognosis with bone and other metastases developing more frequently than in other MM subtypes (229,234,241). For example, the median survival in the large series reported by Klebe et al. was only 3.5 months (229).

Histochemical and Immunohistochemical Stains in the Diagnosis of Sarcomatoid Malignant Mesothelioma

Immunohistochemical stains are often less helpful for the diagnosis of sarcomatoid MM than of epithelioid MM (152). As explained above, the most sensitive and useful

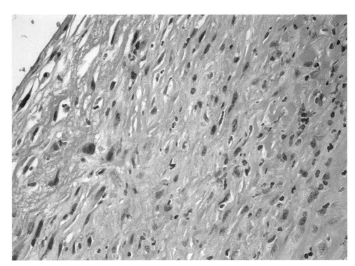

Figure 11.81 Desmoplastic mesothelioma showing nodular densely fibrotic, sparsely cellular areas alternating with more cellular areas composed of slightly atypical spindle cells (H&E, ×100).

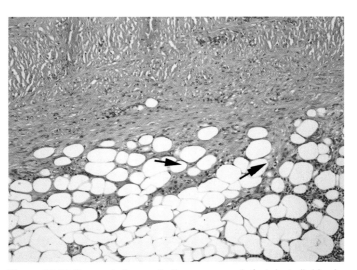

Figure 11.83 Desmoplastic mesothelioma composed of cytologically bland spindle cells admixed with collagenous stroma. However, note that the spindle cells focally infiltrate adipose tissue (arrows), a feature that is not seen in fibrous pleurisy (H&E, ×200).

Figure 11.84 Sarcomatoid mesothelioma with scattered spindle cells showing focal cytoplasmic immunoreactivity for pancytokeratin AE1/AE3. The immunostain is particularly helpful in biopsies that exhibit considerable chronic inflammation, as shown in this photomicrograph (H&E, ×200).

immunostains for the initial workup of a suspected MM are various broad spectrum antikeratin antibody cocktails, including pancytokeratin such as AE1/AE3, OSCAR, or CAM 5.2. These antibodies usually stain (Figure 11.84), over 90 percent of sarcomatoid MM. Most sarcomatoid MM exhibit fairly diffuse keratin immunoreactivity (Figure 11.85), although some tumors exhibit only focal immunoreactivity. Immunoreactivity for pancytokeratin needs to be interpreted with caution, particularly if expressed only focally, as these antibodies also stain reactive, benign epithelioid or spindle mesothelial cells,

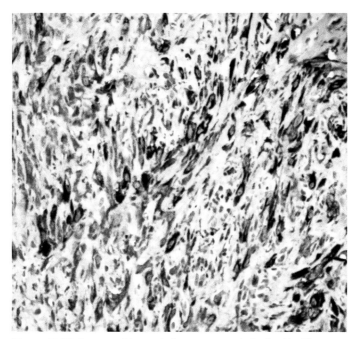

Figure 11.85 Sarcomatoid mesothelioma composed of cells with diffuse cytoplasmic immunoreactivity for pancytokeratin AE1/AE3 (Pap, ×200).

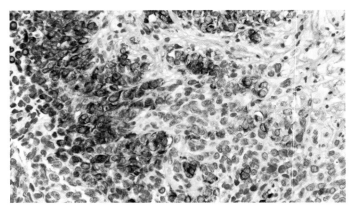

Figure 11.86 Sarcomatoid mesothelioma composed of cells with focal cytoplasmic immunoreactivity for keratin CK5/6 (Pap, ×200).

sarcomatoid carcinomas of lung or renal cell origin, primary, and metastatic synovial sarcomas, melanomas, and other tumors. Correlation of the histopathological findings and immunophenotype with the imaging findings is important, as sarcomas and sarcomatoid carcinomas usually present as localized masses rather than as diffuse tumor involving a serosal surface, although some metastatic lesions can present with diffuse pleural thickening, and/or multinodularity. Negative immunoreactivity for keratin in a sarcomatoid serosal tumor generally suggests the diagnosis of sarcoma or other neoplasms, but not all sarcomatoid MM exhibit positive keratin immunoreactivity.

Mesothelial markers are less sensitive than keratins for the diagnosis of sarcomatoid MM. Immunoreactivity for relatively non-specific mesothelial markers, such as keratin CK5/6 (Figure 11.86) needs to be interpreted with caution and considered in conjunction with the distribution and morphological features of the immunoreactive cells as they stain benign,

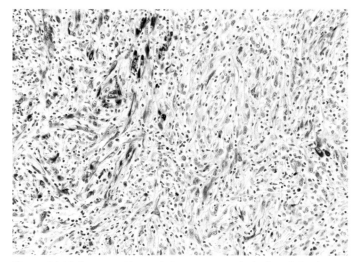

Figure 11.87 Sarcomatoid mesothelioma composed of cells with focal nuclear and cytoplasmic immunoreactivity for calretinin. The finding needs to be correlated with the morphological features of the lesion, as reactive mesothelial cells can exhibit an identical immunophenotype (Pap, ×200).

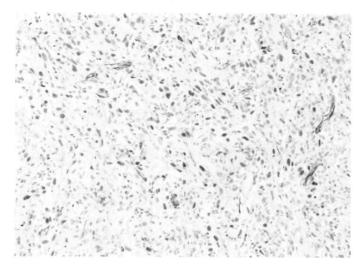

Figure 11.88 Sarcomatoid mesothelioma composed of cells with nuclear immunoreactivity for WT-1. Although WT-1 is more specific than calretinin as a mesothelial marker, this finding also needs to be correlated with the morphological features of the lesion, as reactive mesothelial cells can exhibit an identical immunophenotype (Pap, ×100).

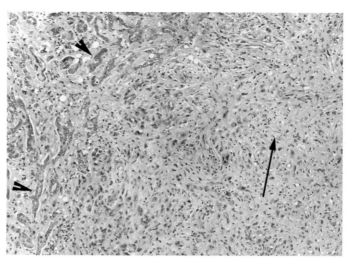

Figure 11.90 Biphasic mesothelioma at low power microscopy showing sarcomatoid elements (arrow) and epithelioid elements showing trabecular growth features (arrowheads) (H&E, ×100).

reactive epithelioid or spindle mesothelial cells. In our experience, calretinin (Figure 11.87) has limited utility in the diagnosis of sarcomatoid as immunoreactivity is seen in only approximately 30 percent of these lesions and tends to be patchy and/or focal. In addition, calretinin is often positive in sarcomatoid carcinomas, limiting its specificity for the diagnosis of sarcomatoid MM. WT-1 (Figure 11.88) and D2–40 (Figure 11.89) (podoplanin) are the two mesothelial markers that in our experience are most sensitive and specific for the diagnosis of sarcomatoid MM (1,152). D2–40 (podoplanin) immunoreactivity needs to be interpreted with caution as it also stains lymphatic endothelial cells.

Biphasic (Mixed) Malignant Mesotheliomas

Biphasic MM are neoplasms composed of both epithelioid and sarcomatoid elements (Figure 11.90). The sarcomatoid elements are composed of atypical spindle cells, as described above, and become admixed with variable amounts of epithelioid mesothelioma with solid (Figure 11.91), trabecular, tubulopapillary, and other growth features (168). The recent WHO book on tumors of the lung, pleura, and other intrathoracic structures arbitrarily defined an MM as biphasic if the second neoplastic component involves at least 10 percent of the tumor (169).

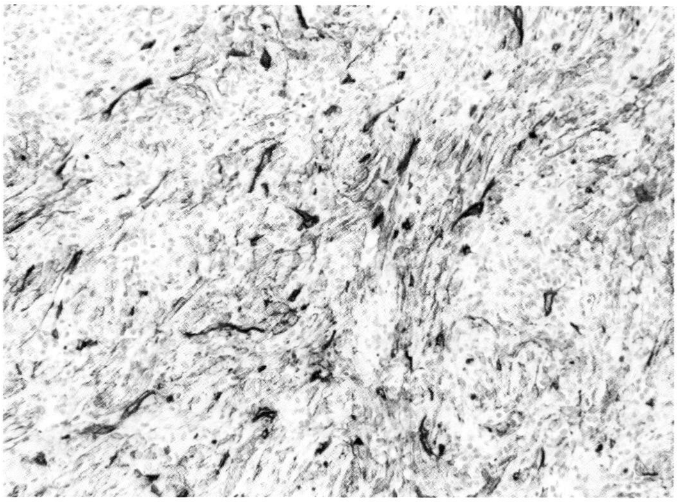

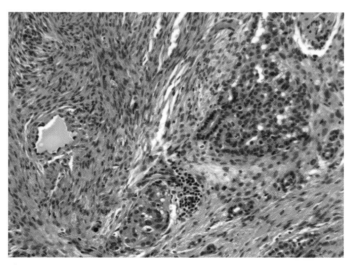

Figure 11.91 Biphasic mesothelioma at high-power microscopy showing the malignant cells of the sarcomatoid component admixed with epithelioid elements (H&E, ×200).

Figure 11.89 Sarcomatoid mesothelioma composed of cells with membrane immunoreactivity for D2–40 (podoplanin) (Pap, ×100).

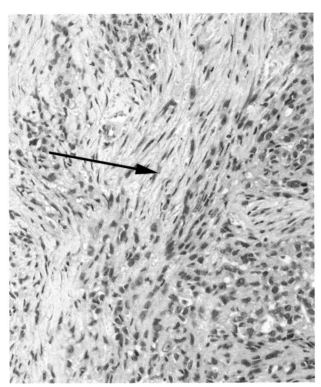

Figure 11.92 Malignant epithelioid mesothelioma shown in the right portion of the photomicrograph, composed of solid sheets of polygonal cells. The arrow marks the presence of reactive spindle stromal cells showing moderate pleomorphism. They can be difficult to distinguish from the sarcomatoid component of a biphasic mesothelioma. However, the spindle cells of a sarcomatoid mesothelioma tend to form more cellular areas and exhibit cytological features of malignancy. Immunostains are not helpful for this distinction, as both neoplastic and reactive spindle cells can exhibit keratin immunoreactivity and/or react with mesothelial markers (H&E, ×200).

Comparison of Reactive Stromal Changes with Neoplastic Proliferations in Sarcomatoid and Biphasic Mesotheliomas

The stroma of epithelioid and sarcomatoid MM often exhibits reactive changes that can result in difficult diagnostic problems, such as the distinction between fibrosis and desmoplastic mesothelioma, or between epithelioid MM and biphasic lesions. MM often exhibit the proliferation of spindle-shaped myofibroblasts arranged in haphazard solid nests that surround the epithelioid neoplastic elements (Figure 11.92). The reactive nature of the spindle cell proliferation can be difficult to distinguish from the sarcomatoid elements of a biphasic/mixed MM. In general, the benign processes are less cellular and usually less pleomorphic than seen in sarcomatoid neoplasms and lack significant nuclear hyperchromasia (Figure 11.93a,b). Some MM exhibit a mostly acellular, sometimes hyalinized, collagenized stroma that can be difficult to distinguish from the stromal nodules of desmoplastic mesothelioma (Figure 11.94). Myxoid change can be a conspicuous stromal finding in 5–10 percent of epithelioid MM and shows pools of amorphous, basophilic stromal material (Figure 11.95) admixed with usually round epithelioid cells with bland cytologic features and abundant, vacuolated cytoplasm (242,243). The stroma of MM can also exhibit focal areas of osseous metaplasia, with mature bone spicules showing no nuclear atypia (Figure 11.96) that need to be distinguished from osteosarcoma elements of a sarcomatoid MM.

Immunohistochemistry can be helpful to distinguish benign from malignant spindle-shaped mesothelial cells, although there are no entirely specific antibodies (152,233,244–250). Immunostains for pancytokeratin (e.g., keratin AE1/AE3, OSCAR, others) and mesothelial markers (e.g., calretinin,

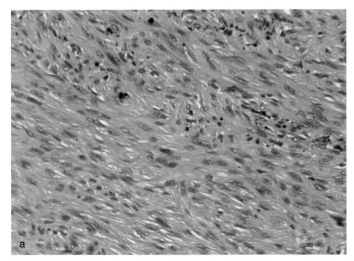

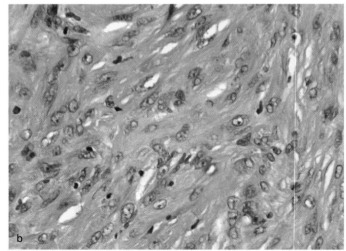

Figure 11.93 (a) Reactive spindle cells in fibrous pleurisy. They are admixed with a collagenized stroma and show only mild cytologic atypia (H&E, ×200). (b) In contrast, a sarcomatoid mesothelioma shows spindle cells with greater anisocytosis and focal nucleoli (H&E, ×400). The distinction between these two entities is often difficult in biopsies that do not show invasion of adipose tissue or other structures. Immunostains for keratin or mesothelial markers are not helpful in the differential diagnosis, as reactive and neoplastic spindle cells can exhibit identical immunophenotype.

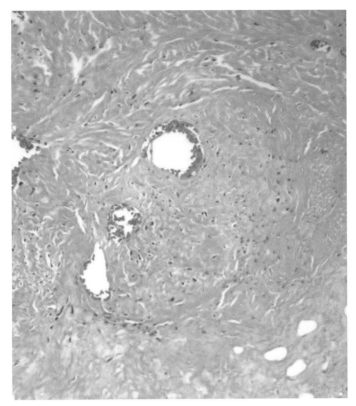

Figure 11.94 Sarcomatoid mesothelioma showing extensive fibrosis and hyalinization of the stroma. Biopsies showing this feature can be very difficult to distinguish from a fibrous pleurisy (H&E, ×40).

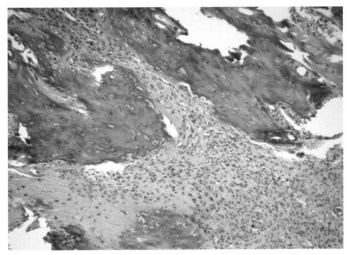

Figure 11.96 Sarcomatoid mesothelioma showing extensive areas of osteoid metaplasia. Note that the bone spicules resemble woven bone and do not exhibit malignant features (H&E, ×40).

WT-1, others) are not very useful in the differential diagnosis between reactive stromal cells and sarcomatoid MM, as both the benign and malignant mesothelial lesions exhibit immunoreactivity for these markers. Other markers that have been proposed as helpful for this differential diagnosis have included desmin, EMA, insulin-like growth factor 2 messenger RNA

binding protein 3 (IMP3), glucose transporter 1 (GLUT1), and h-caldesmon (233,250–252). Desmin is a marker of myofibroblastic cells that also often shows cytoplasmic immunoreactivity in reactive mesothelial cells and some MM (Figure 11.97) (245). IMP3, GLUT1, and EMA stain most epithelioid MM, but they have low expression in sarcomatoid MM, the lesions that are often difficult to distinguish from benign, reactive spindle cell proliferations, so a negative finding does not exclude a MM (244). H-caldesmon is also usually quite insensitive for the diagnosis of sarcomatoid MM (233,248,250,251,253).

Grading of Epithelioid Malignant Mesothelioma

As patients with MM generally have a dismal prognosis, there have been relatively few studies attempting to develop prognostic grading systems for these neoplasms (254). Multiple

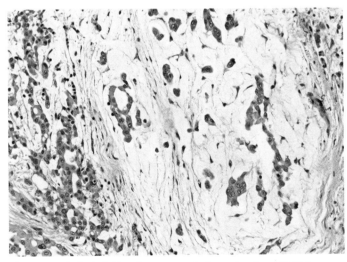

Figure 11.95 Epithelioid malignant mesothelioma showing extensive myxoid stromal changes (H&E, ×100).

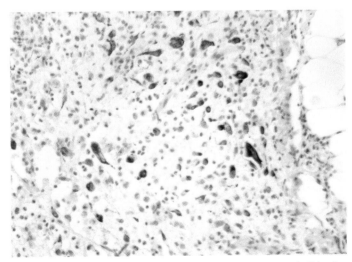

Figure 11.97 Pleural biopsy showing pleomorphic reactive mesothelial cells with cytoplasmic immunoreactivity for desmin (Pap, ×200).

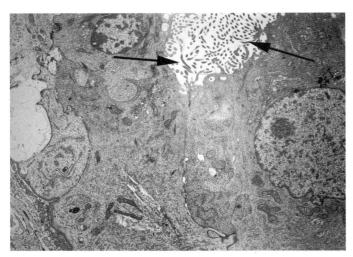

Figure 11.98 Electron micrograph of epithelioid mesotheliomas showing characteristic long and thin microvilli (arrows). It has been proposed that villi with a length/width ratio > 11 support the diagnosis of epithelioid mesothelioma.

studies have shown that patients with tumors with a sarcomatoid component, either sarcomatoid or biphasic (mixed) MM, have worse prognosis than those with epithelioid MM (3,225,255–257).

Kadota et al. have suggested a relatively simple three-tiered grading score for pleural diffuse epithelioid MM based on degree of nuclear atypia and mitotic activity (258). Nuclear atypia is scored as 1 for mild, 2 for moderate, and 3 for severe. Mitotic counts are scored as 1 (0–1 mitoses/10 HPF), 2 (2–4 mitoses/10 HPF) and 3 ($\geq$ 5 mitoses/10 HPF). A total score is calculated by adding the nuclear atypia and mitotic count scores and resulting in three grades: grade I with total scores of up to 2, grade II with total scores of 3 or 4, and grade III with total scores of 5 or 6. Median overall survival for patients with

tumors graded with this system were 28 months, 14 months, and 5 months for MM grades I to III, respectively. The study reported good interobserver reproducibility among different pathologists applying this grading system.

Diagnostic Utility of Electron Microscopy in the Diagnosis of Malignant Mesothelioma

Electron microscopy is currently not routinely used for the diagnosis of MM since the advent of various immunostains that can help resolve most diagnostic problems in a more rapid and less-expensive manner (3,179,204,207,237,259–261). It is recommended in cases that are difficult to diagnose due to a totally negative or equivocal immunophenotype (262). Care must be taken during the examination of serosal neoplasms under electron microscopy, as benign mesothelial cells admixed with the tumor cannot be reliably distinguished ultrastructurally from neoplastic cells, underscoring the importance of properly selecting tumor areas prior to examination.

The neoplastic cells of epithelioid MM exhibit characteristic ultrastructural features that include the presence of nuclear polarity, long and thin microvilli, glycogen granules, junctional structures, tonofilaments, intracellular vacuoles, and basement membrane material. These features are best seen in well-differentiated epithelioid MM and are progressively lost in less-differentiated epithelioid and sarcomatoid MM (263–265).

The presence of long and thin microvilli present on the surface of MM cells is a particularly helpful diagnostic feature for this tumor (Figure 11.98). In contrast to MM, the villi of adenocarcinomas are short and stubby with glycocalyx. Burns et al. have proposed that the presence of villi with a length/width ratio greater than 11 supports the diagnosis of epithelioid MM (266).

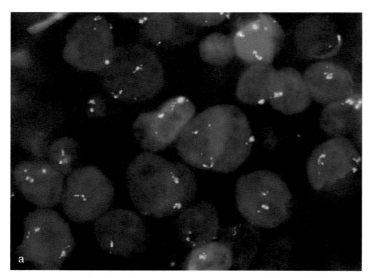
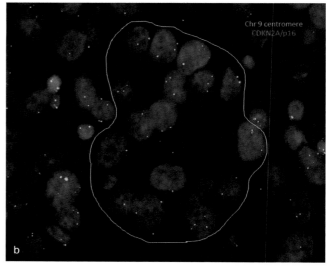

Figure 11.99 Malignant mesothelioma evaluated with p16 FISH. (a) Normal cells exhibit red signals in addition to green signals, while (b) the malignant mesothelial cells have lost the red signal.

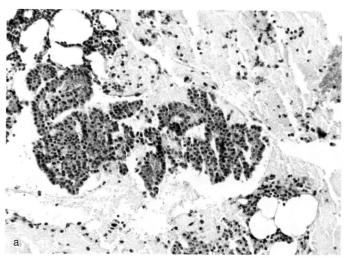
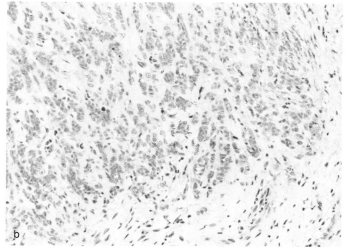

Figure 11.100 The cells of epithelioid mesothelioma often lack nuclear immunoreactivity for BAP-1. (a) The reactive mesothelial cells (Pap, ×200) show nuclear immunoreactivity in a similar staining pattern to normal cells. This finding can also be seen in approximately 1/3 of epithelioid MM, limiting the sensitivity of this marker to distinguish benign from malignant mesothelial proliferations. (b) The epithelioid mesothelioma (Pap, ×200) shows the characteristic loss of BAP-1 nuclear immunoreactivity, a finding that is almost 100 percent specific for the diagnosis of mesothelioma in this context. Note the presence of few lymphocytes with nuclear immunoreactivity providing a useful internal positive control for the immunostain.

Genetic Profile and Molecular Changes in Malignant Mesothelioma

MM have a variety of molecular alterations that are discussed in detail in Chapter 10. The potential diagnostic and prognostic value of the molecular alterations is the subject of intense investigation. Homozygous deletion of the 9p21 locus within a cluster of genes that includes cyclin-dependent kinase inhibitor (CDKN) 2A, CDKN2B, and methylthioadenosinephosphorylase is the molecular alteration that has been studied most extensively for diagnostic purposes (157,159–161,267–269). It can be detected by FISH (Figure 11.99a,b) and polymerase chain reaction (PCR)-based molecular methods in up to 70 percent of pleural epithelioid MM and 90 percent of sarcomatoid MM (169,210). Interestingly, p16/CDKN2A deletions are seen in only 25 percent of peritoneal mesotheliomas.

BRCA-1-associated protein 1 (BAP-1) somatic and germline mutations are also being studied with great interest, as they can be detected with immunohistochemistry in sporadic and hereditary MM (166,267,270–273). Normal or reactive mesothelial cells exhibit nuclear immunoreactivity for BAP-1 (Figure 11.100a), while MM cells frequently but not always lack this finding (Figure 11.100b). It is important for the interpretation of low BAP-1 immunoreactivity in MM cells to detect the presence of normal lymphocytes or other benign cells that exhibit nuclear immunoreactivity, as built-in positive controls for the immunostain. A recent study by Cicognetti et al. reported that all benign cases exhibited nuclear BAP-1 immunoreactivity, while 69 percent of epithelioid MM and 15 percent of sarcomatoid MM lacked this finding. Their findings suggest 100 percent specificity for a diagnosis of malignancy in cases that exhibit BAP-1 loss of immunoreactivity in tissue samples. Cytologic samples exhibited slightly lower specificity, as BAP-1 nuclear expression was lost in 5 percent of non-neoplastic cases.

BAP-1 mutation has also been shown to be associated with better prognosis in MM patients (118,270). For example, a recent study by Farzin et al. detected negative staining for BAP-1, as defined by completely absent nuclear staining in the presence of positive internal controls in non-neoplastic cells, in 46.3 percent of 229 MM (270). Patients in this study showing BAP-1 loss had a 16.11 median survival vs. a 6.34 median survival for patients that lacked this mutation. BAP-1 mutation also significantly correlated with younger age at onset and epithelioid differentiation.

Familial Mesotheliomas and BAP-1 Mutations

The presence of familial cases of MM was described many years ago (112–117,119,274–282). Some of these cases are probably asbestos-related in families with household or environmental exposure, as demonstrated by the presence of asbestos fibers in lung tissues (282–285). However, the presence of MM clustering in certain families and the fact that only a very small fraction of individuals exposed to asbestos develop MM has raised questions regarding the presence of genetic predisposing factors in at least some MM patients. Testa et al. reported the presence of BAP-1 germline mutations in neoplasms from patients from two families with high incidence of MM and somatic mutations and in 26 sporadic MM, and proposed that germline BAP-1 mutations predispose to MM (123). Interestingly, the two patients with germline BAP-1-associated MM also had uveal melanomas. More recently, Alakus demonstrated the frequent presence of somatic BAP-1 mutations in patients with peritoneal MM, and Nasu et al. reported a 63.5 percent incidence of BAP-1 alterations in biopsies from MM patients (271,272).

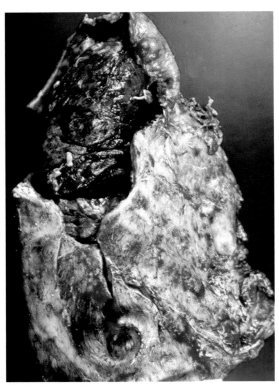

Figure 11.101 Extrapleural pneumonectomy specimen. The entire lung, parietal pleura, and portion of diaphragm have been resected.

Malignant Mesothelioma in Children

MM is very rare in childhood and adolescence and it has been reported in multiple case reports and small case series (99–104,106–108,110,286–293). Patients have had an extremely poor prognosis. A rare association with ataxia telangiectasia and previous Wilms' tumor has been described (103,291). Interestingly, a majority of MM in children have been peritoneal lesions (100,287,289,294).

Nishioka and Paterson have reported rare patients with congenital MM (295,296).

Some children and adolescents with MM have had a history of asbestos exposure, but as they were younger than the usual 15 years latency period of asbestos-associated MM, genetic mechanisms have been suspected in the tumor pathogenesis. Taylor et al. have reported a 16-year-old patient with peritoneal MM and *BAP-1* mutation (100).

Pathologic Evaluation of Extrapleural Pneumonectomy Specimens

Most patients with MM are treated with decortication, pleurectomy, radical pleurectomy, radiation therapy, and/or chemotherapy, with poor results, as described in Chapter 12. Extrapleural pneumonectomy has been proposed for the treatment of selected patients with epithelioid MM (Figure 11.101) (151,156,297).

EPP is an extremely complex and advanced procedure for malignant mesothelioma and that is more uncommonly used for other neoplasms involving the pleura, like carcinoma of the lung or other diffusely involving pleural malignancies. The lung with the ipsilateral diaphragm is resected together with the surrounding parietal and mediastinal pleura and with a segment of the pericardium. EPP specimens can present the surgical pathologists with diagnostic challenges during gross and microscopic evaluation, particularly as these cases are unusual except for selected medical centers.

An essential step in the evaluation of the extrapleural pneumonectomy pathology specimens is careful examination and recording of the specimen parameters for pathologic staging and identification of the various structures resected, such as the lung, pericardium, and hemidiaphragm. Multiple sections are taken from these various structures in an effort to document the extent of involvement and all the various features important for staging. As the entire parietal surface is a margin (the parietal pleura is blindly dissected and removed from the underlying chest wall soft tissue), taking multiple sections of resection margins (after selective inking), with underlying tumor margins and superficial lung parenchyma perpendicular to the pleural surface, is essential. In the usual cases where there is extensive fusion of parietal and visceral pleurae, it is extremely important to take approximately 10–12 sections including margins of parietal pleura to demonstrate the closest approach of the tumor to the resection margin (apical, anterior, lateral, posterior, and medial pleura), tumor and diaphragm, tumor and lung (with potential lung invasion), and tumor in the most thickened areas. Additional sections will be taken to demonstrate different other lesions like hyaline pleural plaques, and talc granulomas. Two to three sections are taken from the pericardial surface, showing the deepest penetration of the pericardium by tumor with the closest margin. Additional sections will be provided from the diaphragmatic margins, perpendicular inked sections from the anterior lateral posterior and medial margins, demonstrating also the deepest penetration of the tumor into the diaphragm. Sampling the uninvolved lung in separate cassettes would be important to evaluate the severity of emphysema and/or determining the exposure to asbestos. Bronchial resection margin is usually taken as a frozen section slide during the intraoperative pathologic examination. Sampling of the hilar lymph nodes is essential to demonstrate the lymph node involvement for adequacy of staging. If the extrapleural pneumonectomy specimen is submitted with additional segments of ribs, submission of the bone marrow samples is also important.

It has been shown in selected studies that EPP is associated with a better prognosis in patients with malignant mesothelioma, while other studies and recent review with meta-analysis have shown no survival differences over pleurectomy (151,156,297). However, it is still unclear if this is because of a careful selection of the cohort of patients who undergo this procedure or the benefits of the therapeutic surgical technique. These patients tend to be younger, with limited disease, and have a better performance status.

Table 11.7 TNM staging of pleural malignant mesothelioma

Staging T descriptors
TX: Primary tumor cannot be assessed
T0: No evidence of primary tumor
T1: Tumor limited to the ipsilateral parietal pleura with or without involvement of – visceral pleura – mediastinal pleura – diaphragmatic pleura
T2: Tumor involving each of the ipsilateral pleural surfaces with at least one of the following features – involvement of diaphragmatic muscle – extension of tumor from visceral pleura into the underlying pulmonary parenchyma
T3: Describes locally advanced but potentially resectable tumor involving all the ipsilateral pleural surfaces with at least one of the following features – involvement of the endothoracic fascia – extension into the mediastinal fat – solitary, completely resectable focus of tumor extending into the soft tissues of the chest wall – nontransmural involvement of the pericardium
T4: Describes locally advanced technically unresectable tumor extending beyond T3

Table 11.9 TNM staging of pleural malignant mesothelioma

Stage groupings	
Stage IA	T1a, N0, M0
Stage IB	T1b, N0, M0
Stage II	T2, N0, M0
Stage III	T1 or T2 with either N1 or N2 and M0 T3 with any nodal status and M0
Stage IV	T4 with any nodal status N3 with any T status M1, any T and any N

Table 11.9 shows the four staging groups. Median survival for MM patients in stages I–IV are 21, 19, 16, and 12 months, respectively (315). Women with MM have a better prognosis than men (316). For example, a recent study by Taioli et al. has shown a threefold increase in five-year survival for women (13.4 percent) vs. men (4.5 percent) with MM (316).

Recent studies have proposed the need to adjust the TNM pathologic staging criteria of patients with epithelioid MM undergoing EPP. The median survival for patients with MM, epithelioid in most instances, who underwent EPP were 51, 26, 15, and 9 months for stages I, II, III, and IV, respectively (317).

TNM Staging and Prognosis of Patients with Pleural Malignant Mesothelioma

The current T status of a pleural mesothelioma is determined by the presence of the tumor in the visceral pleura, parietal pleura, and other thoracic structures, as shown in Table 11.7. Classification of nodal status is considerably simpler than for lung cancer and is shown in Table 11.8. Metastatic status is classified as M0 when distant metastases are absent and M1 when present. MM usually metastasize to mediastinal lymph nodes and the lungs, but bone, liver, brain, and other metastases can rarely occur (174,298–308). In patients with biphasic MM either the epithelioid component or both the epithelioid and sarcomatoid components can spread to the N2 mediastinal lymph nodes, although spread of only the sarcomatoid component is unusual. Rarely, MM can metastasize to unusual places such as the skin, salivary glands, and central nervous system, or present with widespread lung metastases with a miliary pattern (298,305,306,309–314). Purek recently reported two patients with miliary spread of MM and 36 and 41 months survival following multimodality treatment (311).

Pathology of Peritoneal Diffuse Malignant Mesothelioma

Peritoneal MM usually presents as a diffuse or multifocal intra-abdominal neoplasm associated with severe ascites (35,318–325). Patients exhibit diffuse omental involvement (Figure 11.102), and/or multiple nodules of variable size covering the diaphragmatic surface, colon, and other intra-abdominal sites (Figure 11.103). Histologically, peritoneal MM shows identical features to its pleural counterpart, although biphasic MM are less frequent than in the thorax, and sarcomatoid peritoneal

Table 11.8 TNM staging of pleural malignant mesothelioma

N regional lymph node involvement
NX: Cannot be assessed
N0: Absent
N1: Ipsilateral hilar or bronchopulmonary lymph nodes
N2: Subcarinal and/or ipsilateral mediastinal or internal mammary lymph nodes
N3: Ipsilateral or contralateral supraclavicular or scalene lymph nodes and any other contralateral lymph node

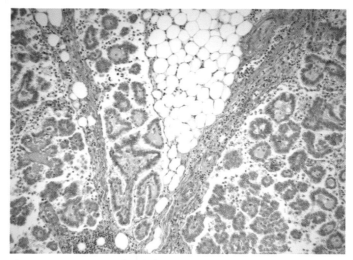

Figure 11.102 Peritoneal epithelioid mesothelioma with extensive involvement of omental adipose tissue (H&E, ×100).

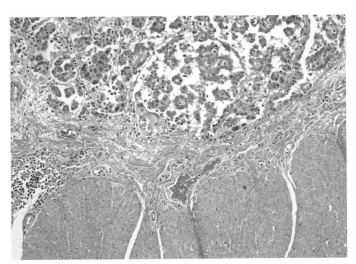

Figure 11.103 Peritoneal MM involving diaphragmatic surface or colonic surface (H&E, ×100).

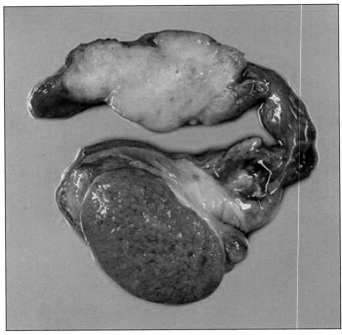

Figure 11.104 Gross tunica vaginalis MM. Adapted from Park YJ, et al. *Korean J Urol.* 2011;52:225–29.

MM are rare (3,168). Patients with biphasic peritoneal MM have a worse prognosis than those with epithelioid morphology. Biphasic peritoneal MM are so infrequent that there are no expert-opinion or evidence-based guidelines available to support the use of a minimum of 10 percent of spindle cells to classify a peritoneal MM as biphasic. The presence of any amount of neoplastic spindle cell proliferation should probably be used to classify a peritoneal MM as biphasic (3).

The differential diagnosis of peritoneal epithelioid MM usually includes neoplasms that less frequently present with multiple pleural metastasis simulating a mesothelial neoplasm, particularly in women where the differential diagnosis of Müllerian tumors needs to be considered. As explained above, calretinin and possibly D2–40 need to be used with caution in this particular differential diagnosis, as they can stain a number of primary peritoneal carcinomas, particularly papillary serious carcinomas of ovarian and fallopian tube origin (3). Nuclear immunoreactivity for PAX-8, a marker that is often positive in Müllerian tumors, is also helpful in this differential diagnosis as MM are consistently negative (215,226,253). Estrogen receptor (ER), another marker that is often positive in Müllerian tumors, should not be used in the differential diagnosis with MM, as nuclear ER immunoreactivity is present in some MM and is associated with poor prognosis (326). The use of other markers in cases when the differential diagnosis includes renal cell carcinoma, carcinomas of GI origin and others has been described in the previous section.

Pathology of Diffuse Malignant Mesothelioma of the Pericardium and the Tunica Vaginalis

The vast majority of MM develop in the pleura and less frequently in the peritoneum. However, MM can rarely arise in the pericardium or the tunica vaginalis (7,36,38–41,44,171, 327–336).

Primary pericardial MM needs to be distinguished from the more common pericardial involvement seen in patients with advanced pleural MM. Patients with primary pericardial lesions present with acute pericarditis, constrictive pericarditis, or superior vena cava syndrome (36,37,171,332,334, 337,338).

Primary MM of the tunica vaginalis (Figure 11.104) needs to be distinguished from peritoneal MM extending into this location. Indeed, peritoneal MM can extend directly into the tunica vaginalis or masquerade as hernia sacs (339–341). Patients with primary MM of the tunica vaginalis present with testicular, paratesticular, and/or scrotal masses (42,328,342).

Primary MM of the pericardium and tunica vaginalis show identical histopathological features to their pleural and peritoneal counterparts and can exhibit epithelioid, sarcomatoid, or biphasic features. Epithelioid MM in these locations need to be distinguished from florid mesothelial hyperplasia (Figure 11.105), a lesion that can be particularly prominent in the pericardium and the tunica vaginalis (343). Patients with florid mesothelial hyperplasia of the tunica vaginalis can present with hydrocele and exhibit the presence of horizontally oriented, non-branching elongated tubules, small solid nests, and cords that are well spaced apart in an inflamed and often fibrotic serosal membrane. A FISH test can be helpful to investigate for the presence of homologous p16 deletion, indicative of a MM. BAP-1 immunostains can also be helpful in the differential diagnosis, as negative immunoreactivity in the presence of positive internal controls supports the diagnosis of MM (343).

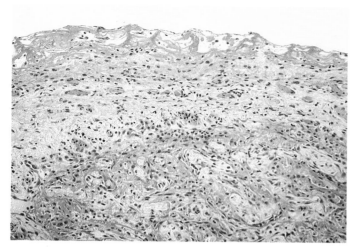

Figure 11.105 Fibrinous pericarditis with florid mesothelial hyperplasia that simulates an infiltrating mesothelioma in the lower portion of the photomicrograph. Caution should be exerted when evaluating biopsies showing fibrinous exudates, as they are often associated with considerable mesothelial hyperplasia composed of epithelioid cells that exhibit variable cytologic atypia. Evaluation for the presence of invasion of adipose tissue or other structures is often necessary to render a diagnosis of mesothelioma (H&E, ×200).

Differential Diagnosis Between Malignant Mesothelioma and Benign Conditions

Epithelioid and Biphasic MM vs. Atypical Mesothelial Hyperplasia

Distinguishing epithelioid and biphasic (mixed) MM from benign mesothelial cell proliferations can be very difficult in selected cases, particularly in small biopsies that do not include adipose tissue or other extrapleural tissues to evaluate for the presence of invasion. Non-neoplastic epithelioid and/or spindle mesothelial cells can grow exuberantly and develop cytologic atypia in response to acute and chronic pleuritis in patients with infections, collagen vascular diseases, drug reactions, pulmonary infarcts, pneumothorax, surgery, trauma, and pulmonary or metastatic extrapleural neoplasms (2,227,344–346). Atypical mesothelial proliferation (Figure 11.106) can be seen in the pleura, pericardium, and peritoneum, and, in our experience, tends to be particularly exuberant in the pericardium and the tunica vaginalis. The reactive mesothelial cells can show features often seen in MM, such as high cellularity, mitoses, focal necrosis, and papillary growth pattern and can also show changes simulating serosal membrane invasion as a result of entrapment of mesothelial cells within fibrotic tissues (347). Atypical mesothelial hyperplasia tends to be more prominent in reaction to active fibrinous pleuritis (Figure 11.105), pericarditis, or peritonitis, so pathologists need to be cautious about diagnosing an MM in the presence of an exuberant fibrinous exudate covering the serosal membrane and/or a prominent inflammatory reaction.

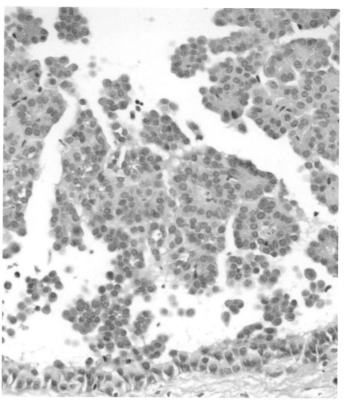

Figure 11.106 Atypical mesothelial hyperplasia showing mesothelial cells with moderate anisocytosis and focally prominent nucleoli, forming pseudopapillary structures on the pericardial surface (H&E, ×200). No stromal invasion was seen. It is often difficult to exclude the possibility of an epithelioid mesothelioma that was not adequately sampled in biopsies showing these features. Immunostains for BAP-1 and/or FISH for CDKN2A/16 deletions can be very helpful tests to confirm a diagnosis of malignancy.

Histopathological features that favor a non-neoplastic mesothelial cell proliferation include absence of adipose tissue invasion, distribution of reactive mesothelial cells toward the serosal membrane surface (Figure 11.107), with growth of cords, solid or small solid nests that are generally parallel to the serosal surface and are more cellular toward the surface, the so-called zonation effect (Figure 11.108), simple papillae lined by single cell layers without prominent cellular stratification (Figure 11.09), and the presence of capillaries that are perpendicular to the serosal surface (Figure 11.110). Necrosis is rare in non-neoplastic mesothelial cell proliferations that are not associated with a granulomatous reaction, so its presence (Figure 11.111) should raise suspicion for MM or other malignancy involving the serosal surface. Other histopathologic features that are usually seen in MM include extensive cellularity without maturation toward the deep portions of the serosal membrane, complex papillae with cellular stratification, and expansile nodules with cellular areas surrounded by fibrotic tissues (3). However, as some of these features can be seen in atypical mesothelial proliferation, demonstration of adipose invasion peripheral lung parenchyma or other organs by the atypical mesothelial cells is the key diagnostic feature to distinguish MM

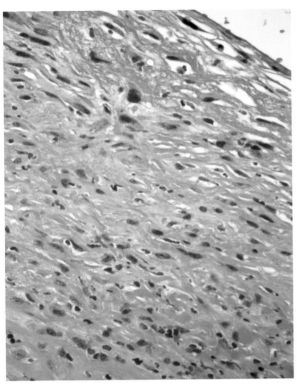

Figure 11.107 Pleural biopsy showing reactive mesothelial hyperplasia. Note that the reactive cells exhibit greater cytologic atypia toward the surface, while the cells present in the deeper portion of the pleura show some zonation with parallel cellular trabecula (H&E, ×200).

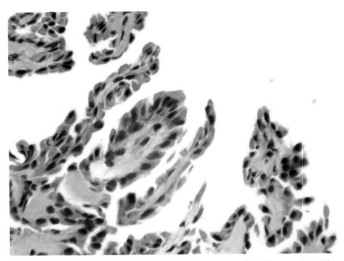

Figure 11.109 Pleural biopsy showing reactive mesothelial hyperplasia. The pleural surface shows focal papillary structures with a fibrovascular core and a single layer of reactive mesothelial cells. No significant stratification of the reactive mesothelial cells is seen on the papillary structures. The biopsy showed no pleural invasion (H&E, ×200).

from non-neoplastic proliferations. It can be highlighted with immunostains for pancytokeratin, calretinin (Figure 11.112), or other mesothelial markers. Finding tissue invasion in a biopsy can be very difficult as the malignant cells of MM often elicit no inflammatory reaction or significant desmoplastic reaction in areas of adipose tissue invasion (Figure 11.113). In MM cases

where the tumor is growing as a solid mass there is no need to find adipose tissue or lung invasion for a diagnosis of malignancy (Figure 11.114).

Histopathologic features that are usually not helpful to distinguish reactive mesothelioma hyperplasia from epithelioid MM include presence of mitoses, as they can be frequent in pleuritis, and cellular atypia, which can be prominent in atypical mesothelial hyperplasia secondary to various inflammatory conditions. Immunohistochemistry also has limited value in the differential diagnosis between atypical mesothelial proliferations and MM. Immunostains that have been proposed for

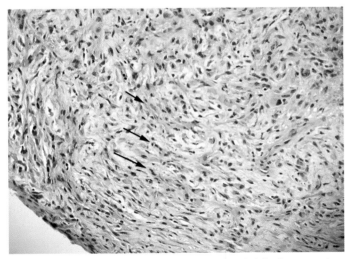

Figure 11.108 Pleural biopsy showing reactive mesothelial cells growing in rows that are parallel to each other and the mesothelial surface (arrows) (H&E, ×100).

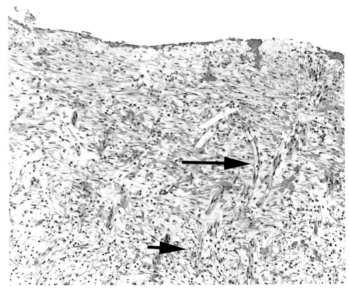

Figure 11.110 Pleural biopsy with pleuritis showing the proliferation of capillaries that are generally oriented at 90 degrees to the pleural surface (arrows) (H&E, ×100).

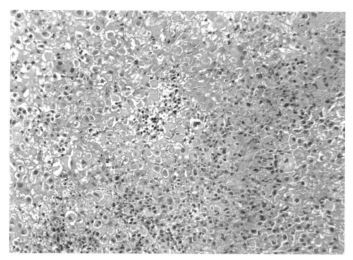

Figure 11.111 Pleural biopsy showing mostly necrotic tissue. The presence of necrosis in the absence of a granulomatous reaction is strongly suspicious for a mesothelioma or other malignancy involving a serosal surface (H&E, ×100).

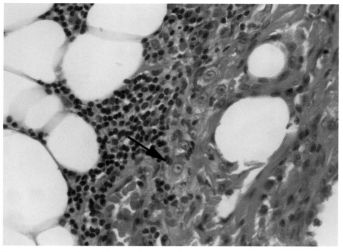

Figure 11.113 Pleural biopsy showing the inconspicuous presence of tumor cells (arrow) next to "fake fat." Adipose tissue was not invaded (H&E, ×400).

this differential diagnosis include EMA, desmin, p53, GLUT-1, IMP3, and h-caldesmon (233,244,250,251,348). Desmin is often positive in benign mesothelial proliferations and while the presence of p53, GLUT-1, and IMP3 immunoreactivity favors a malignant process, none of these markers are 100 percent specific for either a non-neoplastic mesothelial cell proliferation or MM (3,169). For example, the reported sensitivities and specificities of GLUT-1 for the diagnosis of MM are 54 percent and 98 percent, respectively (3,169). IMP3 appears to be more specific with 73 percent of MM and none of the reactive non-neoplastic mesothelial cell proliferations showing immunoreactivity.

Recent studies have shown that FISH- or PCR-based molecular methods for the detection of p16 homozygous deletion and immunostains for the detection of loss of BAP-1

immunoreactivity in MM appear to be very useful in the differential diagnosis between mesothelial malignant tumors and atypical mesothelial proliferations, as discussed earlier in this chapter.

Desmoplastic Malignant Mesothelioma vs. Fibrous Pleurisy

Fibrous pleurisy is a relatively uncommon process characterized by the presence of diffuse pleural thickening resulting from a chronic pleuritis exhibiting marked fibroblastic proliferation and/or collagen deposition resulting in extensive hyalinization (160,233,345,349–352). It can be very difficult to distinguish from a sarcomatoid MM, particularly desmoplastic MM.

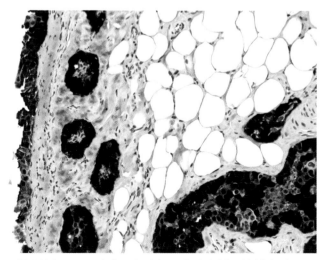

Figure 11.112 Immunostain for calretinin can be helpful to highlight the presence of a mesothelioma invading adipose tissue (Pap, ×40).

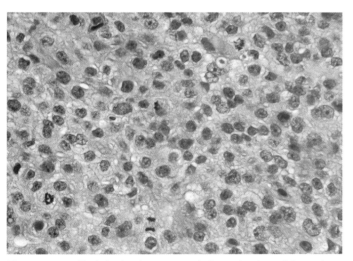

Figure 11.114 Epithelioid malignant mesothelioma showing solid growth feature. In biopsies showing this feature there is no need to find invasion of adipose tissue, lung or other structures to render a diagnosis of mesothelioma (H&E, ×100).

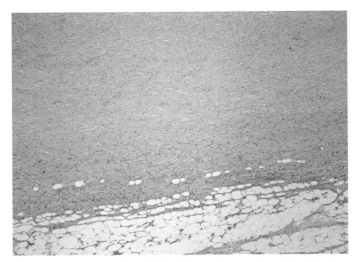

Figure 11.115 Desmoplastic MM with inconspicuous adipose tissue invasion (H&E, ×40).

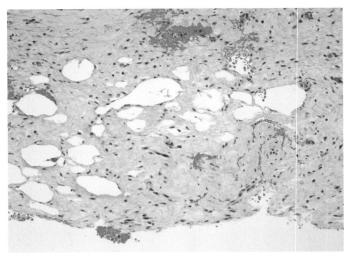

Figure 11.117 Higher magnification of an area of "fake fat" showing that tumor cells appear to grow in a direction parallel to the pleural surface, shown in the lower portion of the photomicrograph (H&E, ×40).

Presence of tumor invasion into adipose tissue (Figure 11.115) or lung is the most reliable histopathologic finding to distinguish fibrous pleurisy from desmoplastic MM as the other histopathologic features that distinguish fibrous pleurisy from desmoplastic MM can be difficult to interpret with certainty. Recognition of invasion requires availability of biopsies that include subpleural adipose tissue or lung tissue. Immunostains for keratin and mesothelial markers are particularly helpful to demonstrate adipose tissue invasion, a feature that can be quite inconspicuous on H&E-stained slides. The presence of true invasion of adipose tissue by an MM needs to be distinguished from the presence of artefactual spaces in adipose-tissue ("fake fat") encountered within the parietal pleura in cases of organizing pleuritis (Figure 11.116) (353). In these artefactual spaces the reactive cells, which can be highlighted by cytokeratin or

mesothelial markers, tend to be oriented in a horizontal distribution parallel to the pleural surface (Figure 11.117), while truly invasive neoplastic cells grow in a vertical or other haphazard distribution into adipose tissue (Figure 11.118). Immunostains for S100 (Figure 11.119), laminin, and collagen IV stain adipocytes and can be used to confirm the presence of tumor in "true" adipose tissue.

Histopathologic features that favor a fibrous pleurisy include the absence of storiform growth pattern and necrosis and presence of uniform pleural thickness, increased cellularity that is more prominent near the serosal surface (Figure 11.107) with maturation into deeper areas of the pleura (the so-called zonation effect) (Figure 11.108) and capillaries that are perpendicularly oriented toward the surface (Figure 11.110) (3,347).

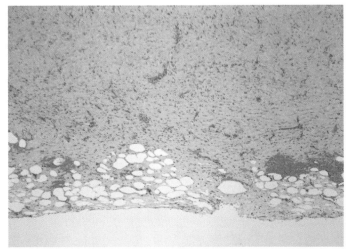

Figure 11.116 Pleural biopsy showing artefactual changes that simulate adipose tissue (so-called "fake fat") and that can lead to an erroneous diagnosis of invasion. The spaces shown in the photograph are located near the pleural surface, seen in the lower portion of the photomicrograph (H&E, ×40).

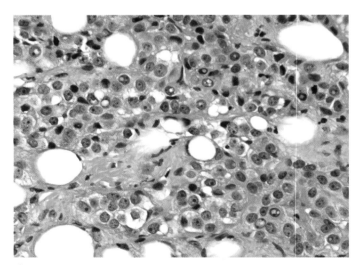

Figure 11.118 Mesothelioma cells grow in a haphazard growth pattern around adipose tissue, in contrast to the features usually seen around "fake fat" (H&E, ×200).

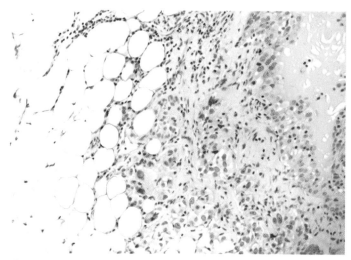

Figure 11.119 S100 immunostain stains in red the cytoplasm of fat cells. This immunostain can be helpful to confirm the presence of invasion into adipose tissue by a mesothelioma (Pap, ×200).

Histopathologic features that favor desmoplastic MM include a prominent storiform growth pattern (Figure 11.81), bland necrosis that is paucicellular and admixed with collagenized tissue (Figure 11.82), irregular pleural thickness, and increased cellularity that has random distribution within the pleura (3,347).

The presence of cytologic atypia in proliferating spindle cells is not helpful for the differential diagnosis, as reactive fibroblasts can exhibit anisocytosis, prominent nucleoli and mitotic activity in fibrous pleurisy, while the neoplastic cells of desmoplastic mesotheliomas are usually cytologically bland with minimal atypia.

Immunostains that have been used in an attempt to distinguish fibrous pleurisy from desmoplastic mesothelioma include desmin, that stains mostly benign cells, and GLUT-1 that stains MM and is negative in benign proliferations. However, a recent collaborative international study reported that all five desmoplastic MM in their cohort were negative for GLUT-1, limiting the usefulness of this marker for the differential diagnosis with fibrous pleurisy (349). As described above, a FISH test to evaluate for homozygous deletion of p16 and BAP-1 immunostains can be helpful to distinguish benign mesothelial proliferations from MM, although the sensitivity and specificity of these methods for the differential diagnosis between fibrous pleurisy and desmoplastic MM needs to be evaluated in future studies.

Differential Diagnosis Between Malignant Mesothelioma and Other Neoplasms

Epithelioid Mesothelioma vs. Adenocarcinoma

Epithelioid mesotheliomas can show histopathologic features that are very similar to those of adenocarcinomas, requiring immunohistochemistry for this differential diagnosis. Because there are no markers that are 100 percent specific for either diagnosis, diagnostic panels that include "epithelial" and "mesothelial" markers are needed, as explained before. There is no consensus about the number of antibodies and which antibodies are required for a standardized diagnosis of epithelioid mesothelioma, but most publications recommend the use of two mesothelial markers and two "epithelial" markers (3,211,215). The International Mesothelioma Interest Group (IMIG) recommended the following epithelial markers for this differential diagnosis based on their sensitivity and specificity: MOC-31, Ber-EO4, CAE, and Lewis (y) antigen blood group 8 (BG8) (3). More recent studies have also recommended the use of claudin-4 as a highly specific marker to differentiate adenocarcinomas from epithelioid MM, as the marker is positive in most carcinomas and uniformly negative in MM and benign mesothelial proliferations (216–222). As explained above, claudin-4 is not helpful in the diagnosis of sarcomatoid neoplasms, as it can be negative in a variety of neoplasms. In patients where the differential diagnosis includes a pulmonary adenocarcinoma, TTF-1 and Napsin A claudin-4 are particularly helpful as they are negative in MM.

Epithelioid Mesothelioma vs. Squamous Cell Carcinoma

Squamous cell carcinomas can be difficult to distinguish from epithelioid mesotheliomas with solid pleomorphic growth patterns (3,215,354–357). In this differential diagnosis, CK5/6 is not helpful and the most useful "epithelial" markers are p63, p40, and desmoglein, although other "epithelial" markers such as MOC-31 can be positive (358,359). In this differential diagnosis, WT-1 is probably the best "mesothelial" marker, as it is absent in squamous cell carcinomas. Calretinin is not a useful "mesothelial" marker in this differential diagnosis, as it stains a significant number of squamous cell carcinomas.

Epithelioid Mesothelioma vs. Renal Cell, Breast, GYN, GI, and Other Primary Origins

Other epithelial markers can often be helpful when included in the differential diagnosis between epithelioid MM and carcinomas of extrapulmonary origin. For example, in patients with a history of breast carcinoma, GATA-3, mammaglobin, and estrogen receptor (ER) can be positive in metastatic lesions (3,215,360). PAX-8, PAX-2, and RCC are helpful for the diagnosis of metastatic renal cell carcinoma, although the latter has low sensitivity for the diagnosis of this malignancy (217).

In patients with a history of endometrial, ovarian or other adenocarcinomas of gynecologic origin, PAX-8, PAX-2, and ER can be helpful for diagnosis (215,253,361). WT-1 is not a useful "mesothelial" marker in this differential diagnosis, as it often stains ovarian and other adenocarcinomas of Müllerian origin.

Epithelioid MM needs to be considered in the diagnosis of serosal membrane neoplasms composed of signet-ring

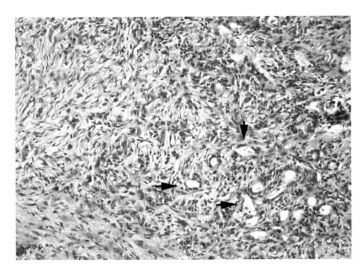

Figure 11.120 Sarcomatoid mesothelioma showing adipose tissue invasion. Note that the tumor cells grow in variable direction around the scanty remnants of adipose tissue (arrows) (H&E, ×100).

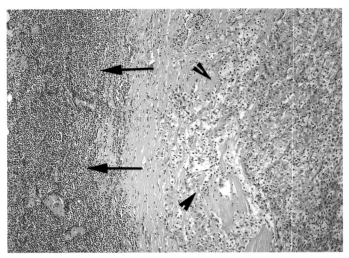

Figure 11.121 The pleura can be rarely simultaneously involved by a lymphoma and a malignant mesothelioma. The photomicrograph shows a low-grade lymphoma (arrows) colliding with an epithelioid mesothelioma (arrowheads) (H&E, ×40).

cells (202,204,205). Mucicarmine and D-PAS stains and immunostains for CK20 and CDX-2 are particularly useful in this differential diagnosis.

Rarely, epithelioid MM can exhibit an adenoid cystic growth pattern and need to be distinguished from metastatic adenoid cystic carcinomas (169). A complete clinical history and review of imaging studies is useful for diagnosis. Positive immunoreactivity for "mesothelial" markers can confirm the diagnosis of MM.

Pleomorphic Epithelioid Mesothelioma and Sarcomatoid MM vs. Sarcomatoid Carcinomas

Sarcomatoid carcinomas of the lung are currently classified by WHO as pleomorphic and spindle cell carcinomas (169). They usually present as localized lesions, but can metastasize to multiple sites in the pleura, presenting with multifocal nodules and pleural thickening. They are usually composed of solid sheets of pleomorphic polygonal cells with variable numbers of spindle cells, closely simulating the histopathologic features of pleomorphic, sarcomatoid, or biphasic MM (Figure 11.120).

"Epithelial markers" can be helpful in the differential diagnosis between sarcomatoid MM and sarcomatoid carcinomas. For example, immunohistochemical stains TTF-1 and Napsin A can occasionally confirm a pulmonary origin, while immunoreactivity for p63, p40, and/or desmoglein can favor squamous differentiation (3). However, these markers are often negative in both pleomorphic and MM, limiting their usefulness. Approximately 45 percent of sarcomatoid carcinomas of the kidney exhibit nuclear immunoreactivity for PAX-8, but this marker has not been adequately studied in sarcomatoid MM to assess its specificity in this differential diagnosis.

"Mesothelial markers" have also limited applicability in the differential diagnosis between metastatic sarcomatoid carci-

noma and sarcomatoid MM as they are often negative in most sarcomatoid MM. Moreover, immunoreactivity for CK5/6, calretinin, and D2–40 has been evaluated only in a few renal cell carcinomas.

Molecular studies may be helpful, as pulmonary sarcomatoid carcinomas can exhibit *KRAS* mutation in 20–30 percent of cases of rare EGFR mutations, but their clinical applicability in the differential diagnosis between sarcomatoid carcinomas and MM has not been investigated (2,169,362).

Pleomorphic MM and Lymphohistiocytoid MM vs. Malignant Lymphoma

Selected cases of pleomorphic MM and lymphohistiocytoid MM can be difficult to distinguish from large-cell lymphomas and other lymphomas (229,363–367). Use of keratin antibodies and "mesothelial" markers and lymphoid markers such as CD3, CD20, CD45, and others are helpful in this differential diagnosis. Rare cases exhibiting both a MM and pleural involvement by malignant lymphomas can be seen (Figure 11.121).

Malignant Mesothelioma vs. Metastatic Melanoma

Metastatic melanoma needs to be included in the differential diagnosis of all epithelioid or spindle-cell malignant neoplasms (122,125). Use of appropriate "epithelial" markers and melanocytic markers such as HMB45, S100 protein, Melan A, and microphthalmia transcription factor (MITF) allow for differential diagnosis (368,369). Metastatic clear-cell melanomas are particularly difficult to differentiate on H&E-stained preparations from an epithelioid MM with prominent clear-cell growth pattern until appropriate antibodies are used.

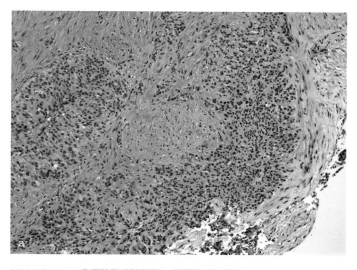
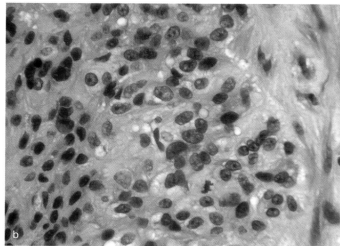
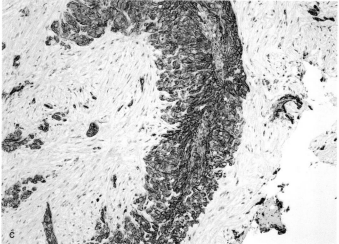

Figure 11.122 Primary epithelioid hemangioendothelioma of the pleura that was initially misdiagnosed as epithelioid mesothelioma. (a) The tumor presented as a diffuse pleural tumor composed of solid sheets of epithelioid cells with round nuclei and slightly eosinophilic cytoplasm (H&E, ×100). (b) The tumor cells at higher power, demonstrating the presence of focal cytoplasmic vacuoles (H&E, ×400). (c) The tumor cells showed diffuse immunoreactivity for CD31 and other vascular markers (Pap, ×100). It is important to consider epithelioid hemangioendothelioma in the differential diagnosis of epithelioid mesothelioma. This tumor showed extensive cytoplasmic immunoreactivity for pancytokeratin AE1/AE, but immunostains for mesothelial markers were negative.

Malignant Mesothelioma vs. Epithelioid Hemangioendothelioma

Epithelioid hemangioendothelioma (EHE) and angiosarcomas can grow diffusely in the pleura, closely resembling the imaging and gross pathology features of MM (370–374). EHE are composed of epithelioid cells with round nuclei, small nucleoli, and amphophilic or eosinophilic cytoplasm arranged in cords or pseudo-glandular spaces on H&E-stained sections (Figure 11.122a,b). The tumor cells can exhibit intracytoplasmic vacuoles that resemble early vascular spaces and often exhibit keratin intracytoplasmic and CD31 immunoreactivity (Figure 11.122b).

The possibility of a vascular tumor needs to be considered in epithelioid lesions that stain with pancytokeratin antibodies but are negative for mesothelial markers. Immunohistochemi-cal stains for vascular markers such as CD31 (Figure 11.122c), CD34, Factor VIII, INI-1, and/or ERG will help establish a correct diagnosis (375–379). D2–40 can be misleading in the differential diagnosis between epithelioid MM and vascular lesions, as it also stains lymphatic endothelial cells.

Sarcomatoid and Desmoplastic Malignant Mesothelioma vs. Solitary Fibrous Tumor

Solitary fibrous tumor (SFT) needs to be considered in the differential diagnosis of sarcomatoid MM and desmoplastic MM in biopsy specimens, as both neoplasms are composed of spindle cells (380–383). Information about the imaging characteristics of the tumor is very helpful for the differential diagnosis, as SFT present as a single or multiple localized mass rather than a diffuse pleural process. Microscopically, SFT is

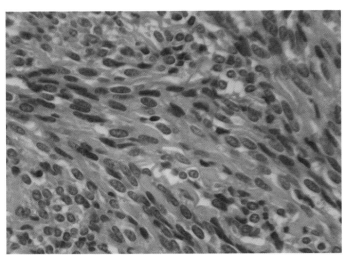

Figure 11.123 Solitary fibrous tumor composed of interlacing bundles of spindle cells. This tumor showed no significant cytologic atypia and very low mitotic activity. However, solitary fibrous tumors can exhibit variable cellularity and nuclear atypia and can be difficult to distinguish from a sarcomatoid mesothelioma. It is important to correlate histopathological findings with the imaging findings and gross pathology, as solitary fibrous tumors present as localized neoplasms rather than diffuse lesions (H&E, ×400).

composed of spindle cells that usually exhibit minimal pleomorphism, no necrosis, rare mitoses, and are arranged among collagenous bands (Figure 11.123). However, they can exhibit cellular areas that can mimic a sarcomatoid MM. Lesions with extensive fibrosis can be difficult to distinguish from a desmoplastic MM in the absence of clinical information.

Immunohistochemistry is often useful in this differential diagnosis. SFT are usually negative for keratins, with rare cases showing focal immunoreactivity and mesothelial markers, and exhibit cytoplasmic immunoreactivity for CD34 (Figure 11.124), BCL-2, and/or STAT6 (381,382). FISH tests can show the presence of NAB2-STAT6 translocation in STF, a finding that is absent in MM.

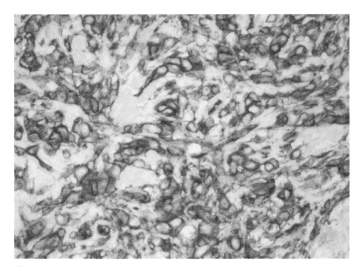

Figure 11.124 Solitary fibrous tumor cells showing characteristic CD34 cytoplasmic immunoreactivity (Pap, ×200).

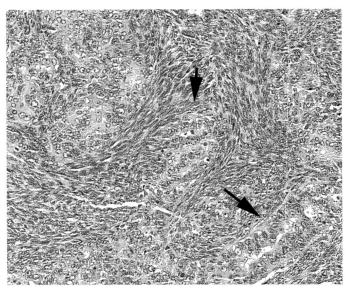

Figure 11.125 Biphasic synovial sarcoma showing epithelioid elements forming solid nests and pseudoglandular spaces (arrows) admixed with hyperchromatic spindle cells (H&E, ×100).

Sarcomatoid and Biphasic Malignant Mesothelioma vs. Synovial Sarcoma

Synovial sarcomas can be primary in the pleura or metastatic from extremities, head and neck, or other soft-tissue sites (384,385). Their diagnosis can be suspected in neoplasms composed of highly cellular, hyperchromatic spindle cells with scanty cytoplasm resulting in nuclear overlap and focal hemangiopericytoma-like growth features. Synovial sarcomas can also exhibit biphasic morphology, with epithelioid cells forming solid nests or pseudoacini admixed with hyperchromatic spindle cells and/or heterologous elements (Figure 11.125). The cells of synovial sarcomas usually exhibit keratin immunoreactivity, but the extent of expression is more limited than in sarcomatoid MM. Immunohistochemistry has limited value in distinguishing sarcomatoid MM from synovial sarcomas as both neoplasms can exhibit cytoplasmic immunoreactivity for pancytokeratin antibodies, although immunoreactivity is usually more diffuse in MM. "Mesenchymal markers" such as desmin, STAT6, smooth muscle actin (SMA), muscle-specific actin (HHF-35), myoglobin, and S100 can focally stain some sarcomatoid MM.

A FISH test to evaluate for the presence of the synovial sarcoma translocation t(X;18)(SYT-SSX) (Figure 11.126) is very useful in this differential diagnosis as it is diagnostic of this sarcoma and negative in sarcomatoid MM (386).

Peritoneal Malignant Mesothelioma vs. Benign Multicystic Mesothelioma

Benign multicystic mesothelioma is a rare entity that has been reported in about 150 cases, mostly women (225,387–395). Most cases have been described in the peritoneum with

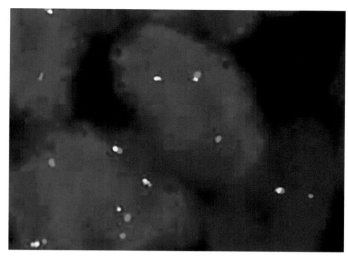

Figure 11.126 FISH test showing a t(X;18)(SYT-SSX) translocation. The test uses a break-apart probe, so the red and green signals are separate from each other within the nucleus (×1000).

rare pleural lesions (396). It is controversial whether benign multicystic mesothelioma is neoplastic or reactive post-inflammatory. No association with asbestos exposure has been demonstrated.

Grossly, benign multicystic mesothelioma is characterized by the presence of multiple mesothelial lined cysts in the peritoneum and, very rarely, in the pleura (387–389,391,393). In contrast with malignant epithelioid MM and well-differentiated papillary mesothelioma, the cysts of benign multicystic mesothelioma are lined by a single layer of mesothelial cells that lack cytologic atypia, anisocytosis, nuclear stratifications, and papillary structures (Figure 11.127a,b). Benign multicystic mesotheliomas are cured by resection in most patients, but can recur within the peritoneal cavity (390,397).

Reproducibility of the Diagnosis of Malignant Mesothelioma

The diagnosis of MM can usually be rendered without much difficulty in cases of epithelioid and sarcomatoid lesions exhibiting the various histopathologic features and immunophenotypes described in this chapter. However, some MM can be very difficult to distinguish from atypical mesothelial hyperplasia or fibrous pleurisy, and poorly differentiated MM can be difficult to distinguish from the other neoplasms described above. Various mesothelioma review panels of expert pathologists have been developed in different countries to help pathologists diagnose difficult cases and/or confirm the diagnosis of this relatively rare neoplasm. In North America, the US–Canadian Mesothelioma panel, currently chaired by Dr. Andrew Churg, has been providing this service for several decades (398). The French Mesopath panel chaired by one of us (FGS) reviews all presumed MM diagnosed in France and periodically finds diagnostic discrepancies between submitted diagnoses and those of the experienced pathologists working at the center (2,27,364,399).

Interestingly, the diagnosis of certain cases of MM can be controversial even among experts. Reports from various groups have reported approximately 70–80 percent agreement rates among different expert pathologists for the diagnosis of MM and its differential diagnosis with reactive lesions (3,398,400–402). However, the studies evaluating interobserver variability among pathologists for the diagnosis of MM are over 10 years old and it is possible that they may have improved as a result of the reporting of newer diagnostic tools such as immunostains for claudin-4, BAP-1 and others, and the FISH test to evaluate for the presence of homozygous p16 deletions.

Well-differentiated Papillary Mesothelioma

Well-differentiated papillary mesothelioma (WDPM) is a very rare neoplasm characterized by the presence of multifocal

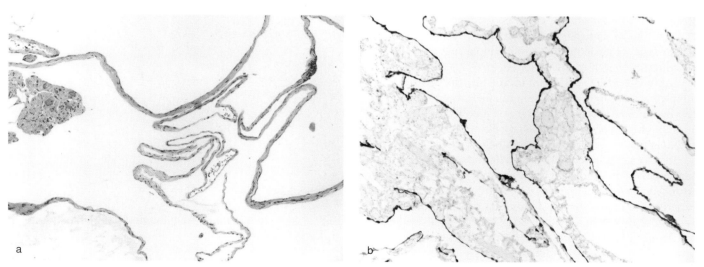

Figure 11.127 (a) Multicystic mesothelioma composed of multiple spaces lined by bland cuboidal mesothelial cells that lack anisocytosis, nucleoli, and other cytological features of malignancy (H&E, ×100). (b) The cells of this lesion exhibit calretinin immunoreactivity (Pap, ×100).

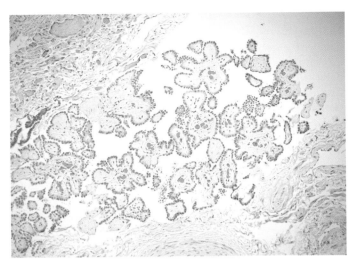

Figure 11.128 Well-differentiated papillary mesothelioma of the peritoneum showing multiple papillary structures on the serosal surface. There is no stromal invasion (H&E, ×100).

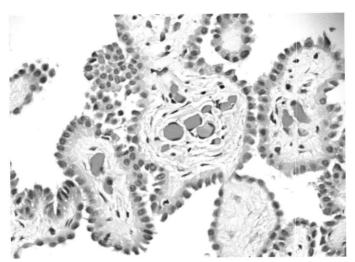

Figure 11.129 Papillary structures of well-differentiated papillary mesothelioma of the peritoneum, composed of a fibrovascular core covered by a single layer of cuboidal epithelioid cells that lack cytologic atypia and nuclear stratification (H&E, ×200).

papillary structures (20,121,226,403–410). Fewer than 50 cases have been described, mostly involving the peritoneum and the pleura in a handful of patients. It has been described in various age groups, with a predominance in the seventh decade of life. The etiology of WDPM is unknown and an association with asbestos exposure has not been reported.

Patients present with abdominal pain or distention, dyspnea, chest pain, or other symptoms (226). Imaging studies show the presence of ascites or pleural effusion without visible nodularity (411,412). Grossly, the lesions are usually multiple, although they can be localized and appear as multiple small, soft nodules on laparoscopy or thoracoscopy.

Microscopically, WDPM is characterized by the presence of simple papillae without secondary structures, composed of a vascularized connective tissue core lined by a single layer of mesothelial cells which exhibit no cytologic atypia (Figure 11.128). The mesothelial cells have small, round nuclei that lack prominent nucleoli, and exhibit ample amphophilic cytoplasm resulting in low N:C ratios (Figure 11.129). Mitoses are rarely present. WDPM does not invade into the peritoneum or the pleura, although very focal and superficial stromal invasion has been reported in some cases (Figure 11.130) (413). The immunophenotype of the epithelial cells of WDPM is identical to that of benign or malignant mesothelial cells.

The diagnosis of WDPM should be rendered with caution, particularly in patients with bulky peritoneal disease that could be undersampled or with pleural lesions that are extremely rare. Superficial biopsies from patients that exhibit what appears as a well-differentiated epithelioid MM with papillary growth pattern need to be diagnosed with caution, as malignant MM with papillary growth features can closely resemble WDPM if the materials are insufficient to evaluate for the presence of invasion. The presence of diffuse or multinodular, grossly

apparent tumor, stratification of epithelial cells lining papillary structures, presence of prominent nucleoli and anisocytosis, formation of tubules, solid, cribriform, and/or complex papillae and stromal invasion are pathologic features that help distinguish a malignant epithelioid MM with prominent papillary growth pattern and WDPM (Figure 11.131a,b). The value of p16 FISH and BAP1 immunostain in the differential diagnosis between WDPM and papillary MM is unknown. Five cases of WDPM tested with FISH showed no p16 homozygous deletion (413).

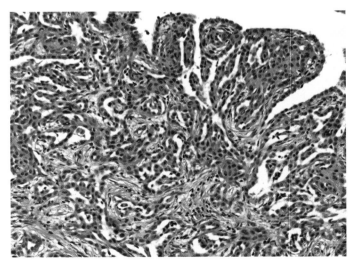

Figure 11.130 Well-differentiated papillary mesothelioma of the peritoneum showing focal stromal invasion. Looking at this microscopic field it is very difficult to distinguish the lesion from a malignant epithelioid mesothelioma. However, this was the only focus of invasion in a tumor that showed extensive papillary features as shown in Figure 11.129 (H&E, ×200).

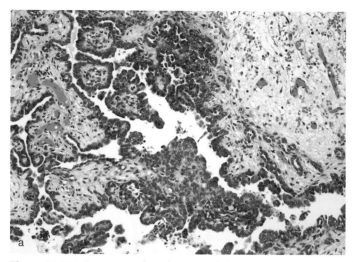 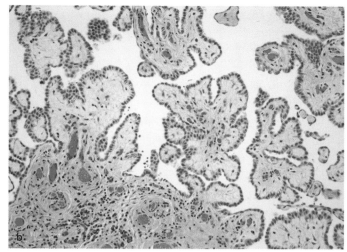

Figure 11.131 Comparison of a malignant epithelioid mesothelioma with papillary growth features with a well-differentiated papillary mesothelioma. (a) A malignant lesion with papillary structures lined by tumor cells with minimal cytologic atypia. However, the papillae are somewhat irregular and complex and the tumor cells show nuclear stratification (H&E, ×200). (b) In contrast, the well-differentiated papillary mesothelioma is composed of fairly regular papillae lined by a single layer of tumor cells (H&E, ×200).

The prognosis of patients with WDPM is excellent and most patients are cured by surgical resection. However, recurrences have been described in patients with WDPM and at least one well-documented case reported by Churg et al. died with disseminated intraperitoneal disease 8 years after initial diagnosis (408,413,414).

Localized Malignant Mesothelioma

A characteristic growth feature of epithelioid, biphasic, and sarcomatoid MM is the presence of diffuse disease involving the pleura, peritoneum, or other serosal surfaces. However, MM can rarely present as localized tumor masses usually involving the pleura and rarely other serosal membranes such as pericardium and tunica vaginalis (415–429). Patients are in their seventh decade of life, with a slight male predominance. It remains uncertain whether asbestos exposure causes localized MM with asbestos exposure. At least some asbestos exposure has been reported in few localized MM patients, but it has been poorly characterized by fiber type, dose, and time from exposure to disease. To our knowledge, there are no epidemiologic studies demonstrating an increased risk for localized malignant mesothelioma in patients with a history of asbestos exposure (428).

Patients with localized MM present with dyspnea, chest wall pain, fever, and/or other non-specific features. CT scans show the presence of a well-circumscribed pleural-based mass. Pleural effusion is uncommon and should raise the suspicions of other lesions present in a multifocal MM presenting on imaging studies with a predominant mass.

Grossly, localized MM are well-circumscribed, non-encapsulated with a gray mass of variable consistency attached to a serosal membrane (Figure 11.132). Microscopically, they

show identical histopathologic features and immunophenotype to diffuse MM. Most reported localized lesions have been epithelioid MM, but a small number of localized sarcomatoid and biphasic MM have been described (243,415,416,418–421,423,425,428,430–434).

The prognosis of patients with localized MM is considerably better than those with diffuse MM, and some patients have been cured with surgical resection, particularly when complete resection with negative margins could be obtained. Galvez-Zapata et al. recently performed a systematic literature review and encountered descriptions of survivals ranging from 0 to 11 years, with a median survival of 29 months in patients with pleural localized MM (417).

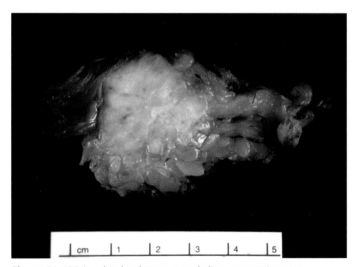

Figure 11.132 Localized malignant mesothelioma presenting as an ill-circumscribed, yellow–gray, firm mass. Histologically, the lesion showed identical features to those illustrated for diffuse epithelioid mesothelioma.

References

1. Churg A, Roggli V, Chirieac LR, Galateau-Sallé F, Burczuk A, Dacic S, et al. Sarcomatoid, desmoplastic, and biphasic mesothelioma. In: Travis WD, Brambilla E, Burke AP, Marx A, Nicholson AG, editors. *WHO classification of tumors of the lung, pleura, thymus and heart.* Lyon: IARC Press, 2015.

2. Galateau-Sallé F, Churg A, Roggli V, Chirieac LR, Burczuk A, Cagle P, et al. Mesothelial tumors. Diffuse malignant mesothelioma. Epithelioid mesothelioma. In: Travis WD, Brambilla E, Burke AP, Marx A, Nicholson AG, editors. *WHO classification of tumors of the lung, pleura, thymus and heart.* Lyon: IARC Press, 2015.

3. Husain AN, Colby T, Ordonez N, Krausz T, Attanoos R, Beasley MB, et al. Guidelines for pathologic diagnosis of malignant mesothelioma: 2012 update of the consensus statement from the International Mesothelioma Interest Group. *Arch Pathol Lab Med.* 2013;137;647–67.

4. Roggli V, Borczuk A, Chirieac LR, Churg A, Dacic S, Galateau-Sallé F, et al. Sarcomatoid, desmoplastic, and biphasic mesothelioma. In: Travis WD, Brambilla E, Burke AP, Marx A, Nicholson AG, editors. *WHO classification of tumors of the lung, pleura, thymus and heart.* Lyon: IARC Press, 2015.

5. de Klerk DP, Nime F. Adenomatoid tumors (mesothelioma) of testicular and paratesticular tissue. *Urology.* 1975;6:635–41.

6. Amin W, Parwani AV. Adenomatoid tumor of testis. *Clin Med Pathol.* 2009;2:17–22.

7. Gkentzis A, Sawalem K, Husain J. An unusual case of paratesticular mesothelioma on the site of previously excised epididymal adenomatoid tumour. *Int J Surg Case Rep.* 2013;4:460–62.

8. Hatano Y, Hirose Y, Matsunaga K, Kito Y, Yasuda I, Moriwaki H, et al. Combined adenomatoid tumor and well differentiated papillary mesothelioma of the omentum. *Pathol Int.* 2011;61:681–85.

9. Makkar M, Dayal P, Gupta C, Mahajan N. Adenomatoid tumor of testis: a rare cytological diagnosis. *J Cytol.* 2013;30:65–67.

10. Minato H, Nojima T, Kurose N, Kinoshita E. Adenomatoid tumor of the pleura. *Pathol Int.* 2009;59:567–71.

11. Bisset DL, Morris JA, Fox H. Giant cystic adenomatoid tumour (mesothelioma) of the uterus. *Histopathology.* 1988;12:555–58.

12. Chan JK, Fong MH. Composite multicystic mesothelioma and adenomatoid tumour of the uterus: different morphological manifestations of the same process? *Histopathology.* 1996;29:375–77.

13. Katsube Y, Mukai K, Silverberg SG. Cystic mesothelioma of the peritoneum: a report of five cases and review of the literature. *Cancer.* 1982;50:1615–22.

14. Kawai T, Kawashima K, Serizawa H, Miura H, Kyeongil K. Adenomatoid mesothelioma with intranuclear inclusion bodies: a case report with cytological and histological findings. *Diagn Cytopathol.* 2014;42:436–40.

15. Kurisu Y, Tsuji M, Shibayama Y, Yamada T, Ohmichi M. Multicystic mesothelioma caused by endometriosis: 2 case reports and review of the literature. *Int J Gynecol Pathol.* 2011;30:163–66.

16. Sawada K, Inoue K, Ishihara T, Kurabayashi A, Moriki T, Shuin T. Multicystic malignant mesothelioma of the tunica vaginalis with an unusually indolent clinical course. *Hinyokika Kiyo.* 2004;50:511–13.

17. Sheng B, Zhang YP, Wei HH, Ma M, Nan X. Primary adenomatoid tumor of the testis: report of a case and review of literature. *Int J Clin Exp Pathol.* 2015;8:5914–18.

18. Terry NE, Fowler CL. Benign cystic mesothelioma in a child. *J Pediatr Surg.* 2009;44:e9–11.

19. Weiss SW, Tavassoli FA. Multicystic mesothelioma. An analysis of pathologic findings and biologic behavior in 37 cases. *Am J Surg Pathol.* 1988;12:737–46.

20. Chen X, Sheng W, Wang J. Well-differentiated papillary mesothelioma: a clinicopathological and immunohistochemical study of 18 cases with additional observation. *Histopathology.* 2013;62:805–13.

21. Hanrahan JB. A combined papillary mesothelioma and adenomatoid tumor of the omentum; report of a case. *Cancer.* 1963;16:1497–500.

22. Zamecnik M, Gomolcak P. Composite multicystic mesothelioma and adenomatoid tumor of the ovary: additional observation suggesting common histogenesis of both lesions. *Cesk Patol.* 2000;36:160–62.

23. Abratt RP, White NW, Vorobiof DA. Epidemiology of mesothelioma – a South African perspective. *Lung Cancer.* 2005;49(Suppl 1):S13–15.

24. Andersson M, Olsen JH. Trend and distribution of mesothelioma in Denmark. *Br J Cancer.* 1985;51:699–705.

25. Armstrong BK, Musk AW, Baker JE, Hunt JM, Newall CC, Henzell HR, et al. Epidemiology of malignant mesothelioma in Western Australia. *Med J Aust.* 1984;141:86–88.

26. Ferguson DA, Berry G, Jelihovsky T, Andreas SB, Rogers AJ, Fung SC, et al. The Australian Mesothelioma Surveillance Program 1979–1985. *Med J Aust.* 1987;147:166–72.

27. Goldberg M, Imbernon E, Rolland P, Gilg Soit Ilg A, Saves M, de Quillacq A, et al. The French National Mesothelioma Surveillance Program. *Occup Environ Med.* 2006;63:390–95.

28. Hinds MW. Mesothelioma in the United States. Incidence in the 1970s. *J Occup Med.* 1978;20:469–71.

29. Leigh J, Driscoll T. Malignant mesothelioma in Australia, 1945–2002. *Int J Occup Environ Health.* 2003;9:206–17.

30. McDonald AD, McDonald JC. Malignant mesothelioma in North America. *Cancer.* 1980;46:1650–56.

31. Peto J, Decarli A, La Vecchia C, Levi F, Negri E. The European mesothelioma epidemic. *Br J Cancer.* 1999;79:666–72.

32. Price B, Ware A. Time trend of mesothelioma incidence in the United States and projection of future cases: an update based on SEER data for 1973 through 2005. *Crit Rev Toxicol.* 2009;39:576–88.

33. Price B, Ware A. Mesothelioma trends in the United States: an update based on Surveillance, Epidemiology, and End Results Program data for 1973 through 2003. *Am J Epidemiol.* 2004;159:107–12.

34. Robinson BM. Malignant pleural mesothelioma: an epidemiological perspective. *Ann Cardiothorac Surg.* 2012;1:491–96.

35. Cao S, Jin S, Cao J, Shen J, Hu J, Che D, et al. Advances in malignant peritoneal mesothelioma. *Int J Colorectal Dis.* 2015;30:1–10.

36. Ramachandran R, Radhan P, Santosham R, Rajendiran S. A rare case of primary malignant pericardial mesothelioma. *J Clin Imaging Sci.* 2014;4:47.

37. Tateishi K, Ikeda M, Yokoyama T, Urushihata K, Yamamoto H, Hanaoka M, et al. Primary malignant sarcomatoid mesothelioma in the pericardium. *Intern Med.* 2013;52:249–53.

38. Kayatta MO, Dineen SP, Sica G, Puskas JD, Pickens A. Primary pericardial mesothelioma in a 19-year-old presenting as pericarditis. *Ann Thorac Surg.* 2013;96:680–81.

39. Jiang D, Kong M, Li J, Qian J. Primary sarcomatoid malignant pericardial mesothelioma. *Intern Med.* 2013;52:157–58.

40. Godar M, Liu J, Zhang P, Xia Y, Yuan Q. Primary pericardial mesothelioma: a rare entity. *Case Rep Oncol Med.* 2013;2013:283601.

41. Akin Y, Bassorgun I, Basara I, Yucel S. Malignant mesothelioma of tunica vaginalis: an extremely rare case presenting without risk factors. *Singapore Med J.* 2015;56:e53–55.

42. Yang LH, Yu JH, Xu HT, Lin XY, Liu Y, Miao Y, et al. Mesothelioma of the tunica vaginalis testis with prominent adenomatoid features: a case report. *Int J Clin Exp Pathol.* 2014;7:7082–87.

43. Rajan V, Nandhakumar R, Shanmugasundaram S, Ravi R, Natarajan S, Mohan G, et al. Paratesticular malignant mesothelioma – a rare case presentation. *Indian J Surg.* 2013;75:174–76.

44. Yen CH, Lee CT, Su CJ, Lo HC. Malignant mesothelioma of the tunica vaginalis testis: a malignancy associated with recurrent epididymitis? *World J Surg Oncol.* 2012;10:238.

45. Mrinakova B, Ondrus D, Kajo K, Kunderlik M, Tkacova M, Ondrusova M. Paratesticular mesothelioma in young age. Case report. *Klin Onkol.* 2012;25:290–93.

46. Mensi C, Pellegatta M, Sieno C, Consonni D, Riboldi L, Bertazzi PA. Mesothelioma of tunica vaginalis testis and asbestos exposure. *BJU Int.* 2012;110:533–37.

47. Corfiati M, Scarselli A, Binazzi A, Di Marzio D, Verardo M, Mirabelli D, et al. Epidemiological patterns of asbestos exposure and spatial clusters of incident cases of malignant mesothelioma from the Italian national registry. *BMC Cancer.* 2015;15:286.

48. Beckett P, Edwards J, Fennell D, Hubbard R, Woolhouse I, Peake MD. Demographics, management and survival of patients with malignant pleural mesothelioma in the National Lung Cancer Audit in England and Wales. *Lung Cancer.* 2015;88:344–48.

49. Kataoka Y, Yamamoto Y, Otsuki T, Shinomiya M, Terada T, Fukuma S, et al. A new prognostic index for overall survival in malignant pleural mesothelioma: the rPHS (regimen, PS, histology or stage) index. *Jpn J Clin Oncol.* 2015;45(6):562–68.

50. Meyerhoff RR, Yang CF, Speicher PJ, Gulack BC, Hartwig MG, D'Amico TA, et al. Impact of mesothelioma histologic subtype on outcomes in the Surveillance, Epidemiology, and End Results database. *J Surg Res.* 2015;196:23–32.

51. Najmi K, Khosravi A, Seifi S, Emami H, Chaibakhsh S, Radmand G, et al. Clinicopathologic and survival characteristics of malignant pleural mesothelioma registered in hospital cancer registry. *Tanaffos.* 2014;13:6–12.

52. Rolland P, Gramond C, Lacourt A, Astoul P, Chamming's S, Ducamp S, et al. Occupations and industries in France at high risk for pleural mesothelioma: a population-based case-control study (1998–2002). *Am J Ind Med.* 2010;53:1207–19.

53. McDonald JC. Epidemiology of malignant mesothelioma – an outline. *Ann Occup Hyg.* 2010;54:851–57.

54. Teta MJ, Mink PJ, Lau E, Sceurman BK, Foster ED. US mesothelioma patterns 1973–2002: indicators of change and insights into background rates. *Eur J Cancer Prev.* 2008;17:525–34.

55. Gibbs GW, Berry G. Mesothelioma and asbestos. *Regul Toxicol Pharmacol.* 2008;52:S223–31.

56. Robinson BW, Lake RA. Advances in malignant mesothelioma. *N Engl J Med.* 2005;353:1591–603.

57. McElvenny DM, Darnton AJ, Price MJ, Hodgson JT. Mesothelioma mortality in Great Britain from 1968 to 2001. *Occup Med (Lond).* 2005;55:79–87.

58. Hodgson JT, McElvenny DM, Darnton AJ, Price MJ, Peto J. The expected burden of mesothelioma mortality in Great Britain from 2002 to 2050. *Br J Cancer.* 2005;92:587–93.

59. Musk AW, de Klerk NH. Epidemiology of malignant mesothelioma in Australia. *Lung Cancer.* 2004;45(Suppl 1):S21–23.

60. Faig J, Howard S, Levine EA, Casselman G, Hesdorffer M, Ohar JA. Changing pattern in malignant mesothelioma survival. *Transl Oncol.* 2015;8:35–39.

61. Neumann V, Loseke S, Nowak D, Herth FJ, Tannapfel A. Malignant pleural mesothelioma: incidence, etiology, diagnosis, treatment, and occupational health. *Dtsch Arztebl Int.* 2013;110:319–26.

62. Frost G. The latency period of mesothelioma among a cohort of British asbestos workers (1978–2005). *Br J Cancer.* 2013;109:1965–73.

63. Bianchi C, Giarelli L, Grandi G, Brollo A, Ramani L, Zuch C. Latency periods in asbestos-related mesothelioma of the pleura. *Eur J Cancer Prev.* 1997;6:162–66.

64. Craighead JE. Epidemiology of mesothelioma and historical background. *Recent Results Cancer Res.* 2011;189:13–25.

65. Berman DW, Crump KS. Update of potency factors for asbestos-related lung cancer and mesothelioma. *Crit Rev Toxicol.* 2008;38(Suppl 1):1–47.

66. McDonald AD, Case BW, Churg A, Dufresne A, Gibbs GW, Sebastien P, et al. Mesothelioma in Quebec chrysotile miners and millers: epidemiology and aetiology. *Ann Occup Hyg.* 1997;41:707–19.

67. McDonald JC. Tremolite, other amphiboles, and mesothelioma. *Am J Ind Med.* 1988;14:247–49.

68. Churg A. Chrysotile, tremolite, and malignant mesothelioma in man. *Chest.* 1988;93:621–28.

69. Churg A. Malignant mesothelioma in British Columbia in 1982. *Cancer.* 1985;55:672–74.

70. Garabrant DH, Alexander DD, Miller PE, Fryzek JP, Boffetta P, Teta MJ, et al. Mesothelioma among motor vehicle mechanics: an updated review and meta-analysis. *Ann Occup Hyg.* 2016;60:8–26.

71. McDonald JC, McDonald AD. The epidemiology of mesothelioma in historical context. *Eur Respir J.* 1996;9:1932–42.

72. Yarborough CM. The risk of mesothelioma from exposure to chrysotile asbestos. *Curr Opin Pulm Med.* 2007;13:334–38.

73. Yarborough CM. Chrysotile as a cause of mesothelioma: an assessment based on epidemiology. *Crit Rev Toxicol.* 2006;36:165–87.

74. Lee D. Genetic basis of mesothelioma – more than asbestos exposure. *J Thorac Oncol.* 2016;11:e27–28.

75. Ohar JA, Cheung M, Talarchek J, Howard SE, Howard TD, Hesdorffer M, et al. Germline *BAP1* mutational landscape of asbestos-exposed malignant mesothelioma patients with family history of cancer. *Cancer Res.* 2016;76:206–15.

76. Abakay A, Tanrikulu AC, Ayhan M, Imamoglu MS, Taylan M, Kaplan MA, et al. High-risk mesothelioma relation to meteorological and geological condition and distance from naturally occurring asbestos. *Environ Health Prev Med.* 2016;21:82–90.

77. Chirieac LR, Barletta JA, Yeap BY, Richards WG, Tilleman T, Bueno R, et al. Clinicopathologic characteristics of malignant mesotheliomas arising in patients with a history of radiation for Hodgkin and non-Hodgkin lymphoma. *J Clin Oncol.* 2013;31:4544–49.

78. Baumann F, Buck BJ, Metcalf RV, McLaurin BT, Merkler DJ, Carbone M. The presence of asbestos in the natural environment is likely related to mesothelioma in young individuals and women from southern Nevada. *J Thorac Oncol.* 2015;10:731–37.

79. Demirer E, Ghattas CF, Radwan MO, Elamin EM. Clinical and prognostic features of erionite-induced malignant mesothelioma. *Yonsei Med J.* 2015;56:311–23.

80. Kanbay A, Ozer Simsek Z, Tutar N, Yilmaz I, Buyukoglan H, Canoz O, et al. Non-asbestos-related malignant pleural mesothelioma. *Intern Med.* 2014;53:1977–79.

81. Carbone M, Baris YI, Bertino P, Brass B, Comertpay S, Dogan AU, et al. Erionite exposure in North Dakota and Turkish villages with mesothelioma. *Proc Natl Acad Sci U S A* 2011;108:13618–23.

82. Metintas M, Hillerdal G, Metintas S, Dumortier P. Endemic malignant mesothelioma: exposure to erionite is more important than genetic factors. *Arch Environ Occup Health.* 2010;65:86–93.

83. Dodson RF, Mark EJ, Poye LW. Biodurability/retention of Libby amphiboles in a case of mesothelioma. *Ultrastruct Pathol.* 2014;38:45–51.

84. Jasani B, Gibbs A. Mesothelioma not associated with asbestos exposure. *Arch Pathol Lab Med.* 2012;136:262–67.

85. Dikensoy O. Mesothelioma due to environmental exposure to erionite in Turkey. *Curr Opin Pulm Med.* 2008;14:322–25.

86. Carbone M, Emri S, Dogan AU, Steele I, Tuncer M, Pass HI, et al. A mesothelioma epidemic in Cappadocia: scientific developments and unexpected social outcomes. *Nat Rev Cancer.* 2007;7:147–54.

87. Emri S, Demir AU. Malignant pleural mesothelioma in Turkey, 2000–2002. *Lung Cancer.* 2004;45(Suppl 1):S17–20.

88. Farioli A, Violante FS, Mattioli S, Curti S, Kriebel D. Risk of mesothelioma following external beam radiotherapy for prostate cancer: a cohort analysis of SEER database. *Cancer Causes Control.* 2013;24:1535–45.

89. De Bruin ML, Burgers JA, Baas P, van 't Veer MB, Noordijk EM, Louwman MW, et al. Malignant mesothelioma after radiation treatment for Hodgkin lymphoma. *Blood.* 2009;113:3679–81.

90. Witherby SM, Butnor KJ, Grunberg SM. Malignant mesothelioma following thoracic radiotherapy for lung cancer. *Lung Cancer.* 2007;57:410–13.

91. Velissaris TJ, Tang AT, Millward-Sadler GH, Morgan JM, Tsang GM. Pericardial mesothelioma following mantle field radiotherapy. *J Cardiovasc Surg (Torino).* 2001;42:425–27.

92. Weissmann LB, Corson JM, Neugut AI, Antman KH. Malignant mesothelioma following treatment for Hodgkin's disease. *J Clin Oncol.* 1996;14:2098–100.

93. Cavazza A, Travis LB, Travis WD, Wolfe JT, 3rd, Foo ML, Gillespie DJ, et al. Post-irradiation malignant mesothelioma. *Cancer.* 1996;77:1379–85.

94. Comar M, Zanotta N, Pesel G, Visconti P, Maestri I, Rinaldi R, et al. Asbestos and SV40 in malignant pleural mesothelioma from a hyperendemic area of north-eastern Italy. *Tumori.* 2012;98:210–14.

95. Price MJ, Darnton AJ, McElvenny DM, Hodgson JT. Simian virus 40 and mesothelioma in Great Britain. *Occup Med (Lond).* 2007;57:564–68.

96. De Rienzo A, Tor M, Sterman DH, Aksoy F, Albelda SM, Testa JR. Detection of SV40 DNA sequences in malignant mesothelioma specimens from the United States, but not from Turkey. *J Cell Biochem.* 2002;84:455–59.

97. Carbone M, Kratzke RA, Testa JR. The pathogenesis of mesothelioma. *Semin Oncol.* 2002;29:2–17.

98. Carbone M, Fisher S, Powers A, Pass HI, Rizzo P. New molecular and epidemiological issues in mesothelioma: role of SV40. *J Cell Physiol.* 1999;180:167–72.

99. Wolff-Bar M, Dujovny T, Vlodavsky E, Postovsky S, Morgenstern SM, Braslavsky D, et al. An 8-year-old child with malignant deciduoid mesothelioma of the abdomen: report of a case and review of the literature. *Pediatr Dev Pathol.* 2015;18(4):327–30.

100. Taylor S, Carpentieri D, Williams J, Acosta J, Southard R. Malignant peritoneal mesothelioma in an adolescent male with *BAP1* deletion. *J Pediatr Hematol Oncol.* 2015;37(5):e323–27.

101. Kobayashi S, Waragai T, Sano H, Mochizuki K, Akaihata M, Ohara Y, et al. Malignant peritoneal mesothelioma in a child: chemotherapy with gemcitabine and platinum was effective for the disease unresponsive to other treatments. *Anticancer Drugs.* 2014;25:1102–05.

102. Sugalski A, Davis M, Prasannan L, Saldivar V, Hung JY, Tomlinson GE. Clinical, histologic, and genetic features of mesothelioma in a 7-year-old child. *Pediatr Blood Cancer.* 2013;60:146–48.

103. Rosas-Salazar C, Gunawardena SW, Spahr JE. Malignant pleural mesothelioma in a child with ataxia–telangiectasia. *Pediatr Pulmonol.* 2013;48:94–97.

104. Khan MA, Puri P, Devaney D. Mesothelioma of tunica vaginalis testis in a child. *J Urol.* 1997;158:198–99.

105. Fraire AE, Cooper S, Greenberg SD, Buffler P, Langston C. Mesothelioma of childhood. *Cancer.* 1988;62:838–47.

106. Armstrong GR, Raafat F, Ingram L, Mann JR. Malignant peritoneal mesothelioma in childhood. *Arch Pathol Lab Med.* 1988;112:1159–62.

107. Berry PJ, Favara BE, Odom LF. Malignant peritoneal mesothelioma in a child. *Pediatr Pathol.* 1986;5:397–409.

108. Kovalivker M, Motovic A. Malignant peritoneal mesothelioma in children: description of two cases and review of the literature. *J Pediatr Surg.* 1985;20:274–75.

109. Wassermann M, Wassermann D, Steinitz R, Katz L, Lemesch C. Mesothelioma in children. *IARC Sci Publ.* 1980;30:253–57.

110. Kauffman SL, Stout AP. Mesothelioma in children. *Cancer.* 1964;17:539–44.

111. Ascoli V, Romeo E, Carnovale Scalzo C, Cozzi I, Ancona L, Cavariani F, et al. Familial malignant mesothelioma: a population-based study in central Italy (1980–2012). *Cancer Epidemiol.* 2014;38:273–78.

112. Kalogeraki AM, Tamiolakis DJ, Lagoudaki ED, Papadakis MN, Papadakis GZ, Agelaki SI, et al. Familial mesothelioma in first degree relatives. *Diagn Cytopathol.* 2013;41:654–57.

113. Serio G, Scattone A, Gentile M, Nazzaro P, Pennella A, Buonadonna AL, et al. Familial pleural mesothelioma with environmental asbestos exposure: losses of DNA sequences by comparative genomic hybridization (CGH). *Histopathology.* 2004;45:643–45.

114. Musti M, Cavone D, Aalto Y, Scattone A, Serio G, Knuutila S. A cluster of familial malignant mesothelioma with del(9p) as the sole chromosomal anomaly. *Cancer Genet Cytogenet.* 2002;138:73–76.

115. Saracci R, Simonato L. Familial malignant mesothelioma. *Lancet.* 2001;358:1813–14.

116. Ascoli V, Scalzo CC, Bruno C, Facciolo F, Lopergolo M, Granone P, et al. Familial pleural malignant mesothelioma: clustering in three sisters and one cousin. *Cancer Lett.* 1998;130:203–07.

117. Risberg B, Nickels J, Wagermark J. Familial clustering of malignant mesothelioma. *Cancer.* 1980;45:2422–27.

118. Baumann F, Flores E, Napolitano A, Kanodia S, Taioli E, Pass H, et al. Mesothelioma patients with germline *BAP1* mutations have 7-fold improved long-term survival. *Carcinogenesis.* 2015;36:76–81.

119. Betti M, Casalone E, Ferrante D, Romanelli A, Grosso F, Guarrera S, et al. Inference on germline *BAP1* mutations and asbestos exposure from the analysis of familial and sporadic mesothelioma in a high-risk area. *Genes Chromosomes Cancer.* 2015;54:51–62.

120. Xu J, Kadariya Y, Cheung M, Pei J, Talarchek J, Sementino E, et al. Germline mutation of *BAP1* accelerates development of asbestos-induced malignant mesothelioma. *Cancer Res.* 2014;74:4388–97.

121. Ribeiro C, Campelos S, Moura CS, Machado JC, Justino A, Parente B. Well-differentiated papillary mesothelioma: clustering in a Portuguese family with a germline *BAP1* mutation. *Ann Oncol.* 2013;24:2147–50.

122. Carbone M, Ferris LK, Baumann F, Napolitano A, Lum CA, Flores EG, et al. *BAP1* cancer syndrome: malignant mesothelioma, uveal and cutaneous melanoma, and MBAITs. *J Transl Med.* 2012;10:179.

123. Testa JR, Cheung M, Pei J, Below JE, Tan Y, Sementino E, et al. Germline *BAP1* mutations predispose to malignant mesothelioma. *Nat Genet.* 2011;43:1022–25.

124. Rusch A, Ziltener G, Nackaerts K, Weder W, Stahel RA, Felley-Bosco E. Prevalence of *BRCA*-1 associated protein 1 germline mutation in sporadic malignant pleural mesothelioma cases. *Lung Cancer.* 2015;87:77–79.

125. Cheung M, Talarchek J, Schindeler K, Saraiva E, Penney LS, Ludman M, et al. Further evidence for germline *BAP1* mutations predisposing to melanoma and malignant mesothelioma. *Cancer Genet.* 2013;206:206–10.

126. Marchevsky AM, Harber P, Crawford L, Wick MR. Mesothelioma in patients with nonoccupational asbestos exposure. An evidence-based approach to causation assessment. *Ann Diagn Pathol.* 2006;10:241–50.

127. Robinson BW, Musk AW, Lake RA. Malignant mesothelioma. *Lancet.* 2005;366:397–408.

128. Choi BY, Yoon MJ, Shin K, Lee YJ, Song YW. Characteristics of pleural effusions in systemic lupus erythematosus: differential diagnosis of lupus pleuritis. *Lupus.* 2015;24:321–26.

129. Dogan M, Utkan G, Hocazade C, Uncu D, Toptas S, Ozdemir N, et al. The clinicopathological characteristics with long-term outcomes in malignant mesothelioma. *Med Oncol.* 2014;31:232.

130. Mott FE. Mesothelioma: a review. *Ochsner J.* 2012;12:70–79.

131. Haber SE, Haber JM. Malignant mesothelioma: a clinical study of 238 cases. *Ind Health.* 2011;49:166–72.

132. Gill RR. Imaging of mesothelioma. *Recent Results Cancer Res.* 2011;189:27–43.

133. Marrannes J, Delvaux S, Verheezen J. Malignant peritoneal mesothelioma: contribution and limitation of imaging for its diagnosis. *JBR-BTR.* 2009;92:248–50.

134. Smith TR. Malignant peritoneal mesothelioma: marked variability of CT findings. *Abdom Imaging.* 1994;19:27–29.

135. Bianchi C, Brollo A, Ramani L, Zuch C. Pleural plaques as risk indicators for malignant pleural mesothelioma: a necropsy-based study. *Am J Ind Med.* 1997;32:445–49.

136. Hillerdal G. Pleural plaques and risk for bronchial carcinoma and mesothelioma. A prospective study. *Chest.* 1994;105:144–50.

137. Borasio P, Berruti A, Bille A, Lausi P, Levra MG, Giardino R, et al. Malignant pleural mesothelioma: clinicopathologic and survival characteristics in a consecutive series of 394 patients. *Eur J Cardiothorac Surg.* 2008;33:307–13.

138. Nickell LT, Jr., Lichtenberger JP, 3rd, Khorashadi L, Abbott GF, Carter BW. Multimodality imaging for characterization, classification, and staging of malignant pleural

mesothelioma. *Radiographics.* 2014;34:1692–706.

139. Truong MT, Viswanathan C, Godoy MB, Carter BW, Marom EM. Malignant pleural mesothelioma: role of CT, MRI, and PET/CT in staging evaluation and treatment considerations. *Semin Roentgenol.* 2013;48:323–34.

140. Larsen BT, Klein JR, Hornychova H, Nuti R, Thirumala S, Leslie KO, et al. Diffuse intrapulmonary malignant mesothelioma masquerading as interstitial lung disease: a distinctive variant of mesothelioma. *Am J Surg Pathol.* 2013;37:1555–64.

141. Amosite asbestos and mesothelioma. *Lancet* 1981;2:1397–98.

142. Boffetta P. Epidemiology of peritoneal mesothelioma: a review. *Ann Oncol.* 2007;18:985–90.

143. Suster S, Moran CA. Applications and limitations of immunohistochemistry in the diagnosis of malignant mesothelioma. *Adv Anat Pathol.* 2006;13:316–29.

144. Hjerpe A, Ascoli V, Bedrossian CW, Boon ME, Creaney J, Davidson B, et al. Guidelines for the cytopathologic diagnosis of epithelioid and mixed-type malignant mesothelioma. Complementary statement from the International Mesothelioma Interest Group, also endorsed by the International Academy of Cytology and the Papanicolaou Society of Cytopathology. *Acta Cytol.* 2015;59:2–16.

145. Kawai T, Hiroshima K, Kamei T. Pulmonary Pathology: SY22-2 diagnosis of mesothelioma by cytology using Japanese criteria. *Pathology.* 2014;46(Suppl 2):S39.

146. Segal A, Sterrett GF, Frost FA, Shilkin KB, Olsen NJ, Musk AW, et al. A diagnosis of malignant pleural mesothelioma can be made by effusion cytology: results of a 20 year audit. *Pathology.* 2013;45:44–48.

147. Paintal A, Raparia K, Zakowski MF, Nayar R. The diagnosis of malignant mesothelioma in effusion cytology: a reappraisal and results of a multi-institution survey. *Cancer Cytopathol.* 2013;121:703–07.

148. Arrossi AV, Lin E, Rice D, Moran CA. Histologic assessment and prognostic factors of malignant pleural mesothelioma treated with extrapleural pneumonectomy. *Am J Clin Pathol.* 2008;130:754–64.

149. Burkholder D, Hadi D, Kunnavakkam R, Kindler H, Todd K, Celauro AD, et al. Effects of extended pleurectomy and decortication on quality of life and pulmonary function in patients with malignant pleural mesothelioma. *Ann Thorac Surg.* 2015;99:1775–80.

150. Cao C, Tian D, Park J, Allan J, Pataky KA, Yan TD. A systematic review and meta-analysis of surgical treatments for malignant pleural mesothelioma. *Lung Cancer.* 2014;83:240–45.

151. Cardillo G, Treasure T. Extrapleural pneumonectomy is not shown to be clinically effective in the treatment of malignant pleural mesothelioma. *Ann Surg.* 2017;265(4):e53.

152. Chirieac LR, Pinkus GS, Pinkus JL, Godleski J, Sugarbaker DJ, Corson JM. The immunohistochemical characterization of sarcomatoid malignant mesothelioma of the pleura. *Am J Cancer Res.* 2011;1:14–24.

153. de Perrot M, McRae K, Anraku M, Karkouti K, Waddell TK, Pierre AF, et al. Risk factors for major complications after extrapleural pneumonectomy for malignant pleural mesothelioma. *Ann Thorac Surg.* 2008;85:1206–10.

154. Gupta V, Krug LM, Laser B, Hudka K, Flores R, Rusch VW, et al. Patterns of local and nodal failure in malignant pleural mesothelioma after extrapleural pneumonectomy and photon-electron radiotherapy. *J Thorac Oncol.* 2009;4:746–50.

155. Sugarbaker DJ, Wolf AS, Chirieac LR, Godleski JJ, Tilleman TR, Jaklitsch MT, et al. Clinical and pathological features of three-year survivors of malignant pleural mesothelioma following extrapleural pneumonectomy. *Eur J Cardiothorac Surg.* 2011;40:298–303.

156. Taioli E, Wolf AS, Flores RM. Meta-analysis of survival after pleurectomy decortication versus extrapleural pneumonectomy in mesothelioma. *Ann Thorac Surg.* 2015;99:472–80.

157. Ito T, Hamasaki M, Matsumoto S, Hiroshima K, Tsujimura T, Kawai T, et al. p16/CDKN2A FISH in differentiation of diffuse malignant peritoneal mesothelioma from mesothelial hyperplasia and epithelial ovarian cancer. *Am J Clin Pathol.* 2015;143:830–38.

158. Hasegawa M, Sakai F, Sato A, Tsubomizu S, Arimura K, Katsura H, et al. FISH analysis of intrapulmonary malignant mesothelioma without a clinically detectable primary pleural lesion: an autopsy case. *Jpn J Clin Oncol.* 2014;44:1239–42.

159. Hwang H, Tse C, Rodriguez S, Gown A, Churg A. p16 FISH deletion in surface epithelial mesothelial proliferations is predictive of underlying invasive mesothelioma. *Am J Surg Pathol.* 2014;38:681–88.

160. Wu D, Hiroshima K, Matsumoto S, Nabeshima K, Yusa T, Ozaki D, et al. Diagnostic usefulness of p16/CDKN2A FISH in distinguishing between sarcomatoid mesothelioma and fibrous pleuritis. *Am J Clin Pathol.* 2013;139:39–46.

161. Matsumoto S, Nabeshima K, Kamei T, Hiroshima K, Kawahara K, Hata S, et al. Morphology of 9p21 homozygous deletion-positive pleural mesothelioma cells analyzed using fluorescence *in situ* hybridization and virtual microscope system in effusion cytology. *Cancer Cytopathol.* 2013;121:415–22.

162. Al-Salam S, Hammad FT, Salman MA, AlAshari M. Expression of Wilms tumor-1 protein and CD 138 in malignant mesothelioma of the tunica vaginalis. *Pathol Res Pract.* 2009;205:797–800.

163. Illei PB, Ladanyi M, Rusch VW, Zakowski MF. The use of CDKN2A deletion as a diagnostic marker for malignant mesothelioma in body cavity effusions. *Cancer.* 2003;99:51–56.

164. Cheng JQ, Jhanwar SC, Klein WM, Bell DW, Lee WC, Altomare DA, et al. p16 alterations and deletion mapping of 9p21-p22 in malignant mesothelioma. *Cancer Res.* 1994;54:5547–51.

165. Hiroshima K, Wu D, Hasegawa M, Koh E, Sekine Y, Ozaki D, et al. Cytologic differential diagnosis of malignant mesothelioma and reactive mesothelial cells with FISH analysis of p16. *Diagn Cytopathol.* 2016;44(7):591–98.

166. Cigognetti M, Lonardi S, Fisogni S, Balzarini P, Pellegrini V, Tironi A, et al. *BAP1* (*BRCA1*-associated protein 1) is a highly specific marker for differentiating mesothelioma from reactive mesothelial proliferations. *Mod Pathol.* 2015;28:1043–57.

167. Walts AE, Hiroshima K, McGregor SM, Wu D, Husain AN, Marchevsky AM. *BAP1* immunostain and *CDKN2A* (p16) FISH analysis: clinical applicability for the diagnosis of malignant mesothelioma in effusions. *Diagn Cytopathol.* 2016;44(7):599–606.

168. Roggli V, Churg A, Chiriac LR, Burczuk A, Dacic S, Hammar S, et al. Sarcomatoid, desmoplastic, and biphasic mesothelioma. In: Travis WD, Brambilla E, Burke AP, Marx A, Nicholson AG, editors. *WHO classification of tumors of the lung, pleura, thymus and heart.* Lyon: IARC Press, 2015.

169. Travis LB, Brambilla E, Burke AP, Marx A, Nicholson AG, editors. *WHO classification of tumours of the lung, pleura, thymus and heart.* Lyon: IARC Press, 2015.

170. Oury TD, Sporn TA, Roggli VL. *Pathology of asbestos-associated diseases.* New York, NY: Springer, 2014.

171. Makarawate P, Chaosuwannakit N, Chindaprasirt J, Ungarreevittaya P, Chaiwiriyakul S, Wirasorn K, et al. Malignant mesothelioma of the pericardium: a report of two different presentations. *Case Rep Oncol Med.* 2013;2013:356901.

172. Churg A, Cagle PT, Roggli V. *Tumors of the serosal membranes.* Washington, DC: American Registry of Pathology, 2006.

173. Brcic L, Jakopovic M, Brcic I, Klaric V, Milosevic M, Sepac A, et al. Reproducibility of histological subtyping of malignant pleural mesothelioma. *Virchows Arch.* 2014;465:679–85.

174. Mogi A, Nabeshima K, Hamasaki M, Uesugi N, Tamura K, Iwasaki A, et al. Pleural malignant mesothelioma with invasive micropapillary component and its association with pulmonary metastasis. *Pathol Int.* 2009;59:874–79.

175. Mark EJ, Shin DH. Diffuse malignant mesothelioma of the pleura: a clinicopathological study of six patients with a prolonged symptom-free interval or extended survival after biopsy and a review of the literature of long-term survival. *Virchows Arch A Pathol Anat Histopathol.* 1993;422:445–51.

176. Weissferdt A, Kalhor N, Suster S. Malignant mesothelioma with prominent adenomatoid features: a clinicopathologic and

immunohistochemical study of 10 cases. *Ann Diagn Pathol.* 2011;15:25–29.

177. Ordonez NG, Myhre M, Mackay B. Clear cell mesothelioma. *Ultrastruct Pathol.* 1996;20:331–36.

178. Ordonez NG, Mackay B. Glycogen-rich mesothelioma. *Ultrastruct Pathol.* 1999;23:401–06.

179. Ordonez NG. Mesothelioma with clear cell features: an ultrastructural and immunohistochemical study of 20 cases. *Hum Pathol.* 2005;36:465–73.

180. Ustun H, Astarci HM, Sungu N, Ozdemir A, Ekinci C. Primary malignant deciduoid peritoneal mesothelioma: a report of the cytohistological and immunohistochemical appearances. *Diagn Cytopathol.* 2011;39:402–08.

181. Tsai LY, Yang YL, Lu MY, Lin DT, Huang HY, Lin KH. Deciduoid mesothelioma of the pleura in an adolescent boy. *Pediatr Hematol Oncol.* 2010;27:132–37.

182. Talerman A. Deciduoid or pseudodecidual mesothelioma. *Am J Surg Pathol.* 2000;24:1179.

183. Shia J, Erlandson RA, Klimstra DS. Deciduoid mesothelioma: a report of 5 cases and literature review. *Ultrastruct Pathol.* 2002;26:355–63.

184. Serio G, Scattone A, Pennella A, Giardina C, Musti M, Valente T, et al. Malignant deciduoid mesothelioma of the pleura: report of two cases with long survival. *Histopathology.* 2002;40:348–52.

185. Santos C, Gamboa F, Fradinho F, Pego A, Carvalho L, Bernardo J. Deciduoid pleural mesothelioma–a rare entity in a young woman. *Rev Port Pneumol.* 2012;18:294–98.

186. Puttagunta L, Vriend RA, Nguyen GK. Deciduoid epithelial mesothelioma of the pleura with focal rhabdoid change. *Am J Surg Pathol.* 2000;24:1440–43.

187. Orosz Z, Nagy P, Szentirmay Z, Zalatnai A, Hauser P. Epithelial mesothelioma with deciduoid features. *Virchows Arch.* 1999;434:263–66.

188. Ordonez NG. Deciduoid mesothelioma: report of 21 cases with review of the literature. *Mod Pathol.* 2012;25:1481–95.

189. Nascimento AG, Keeney GL, Fletcher CD. Deciduoid peritoneal mesothelioma. An unusual phenotype

affecting young females. *Am J Surg Pathol.* 1994;18:439–45.

190. Ordonez NG. Epithelial mesothelioma with deciduoid features: report of four cases. *Am J Surg Pathol.* 2000;24: 816–23.

191. Gloeckner-Hofmann K, Zhu XZ, Bartels H, Feller AC, Merz H. Deciduoid pleural mesothelioma affecting a young female without prior asbestos exposure. *Respiration.* 2000;67:456–58.

192. Desai S, Kane S, Bharde S, Kulkarni JN, Soman CS. Malignant peritoneal mesothelioma deciduoid or anaplastic variant? A point to ponder. *Indian J Pathol Microbiol.* 2000;43:479–83.

193. Okonkwo A, Musunuri S, Diaz L, Jr., Bedrossian C, Stryker S, Rao S. Deciduoid mesothelioma: a rare, distinct entity with unusual features. *Ann Diagn Pathol.* 2001;5:168–71.

194. Monaghan H, Al-Nafussi A. Deciduoid pleural mesothelioma. *Histopathology.* 2001;39:104–06.

195. Henley JD, Loehrer PJ, Sr., Ulbright TM. Deciduoid mesothelioma of the pleura after radiation therapy for Hodgkin's disease presenting as a mediastinal mass. *Am J Surg Pathol.* 2001;25:547–48.

196. Gillespie FR, van der Walt JD, Derias N, Kenney A. Deciduoid peritoneal mesothelioma. A report of the cytological appearances. *Cytopathology.* 2001;12:57–61.

197. Desai S, Kane S, Bharde S, Kulkarni JN, Soman CS. Malignant peritoneal mesothelioma deciduoid or anaplastic variant? Point to ponder. *Indian J Pathol Microbiol.* 2001;44:159–62.

198. Cook HC. Small cell mesothelioma. *Histopathology.* 1993;22:294–95.

199. Tsao AS, Heymach J. Mesothelioma and small cell lung cancer. *J Thorac Oncol.* 2011;6:S1825–26.

200. Takeda T, Saitoh M, Fukita S, Takeda S. Small cell carcinoma presenting with massive pleural spread mimicking malignant pleural mesothelioma. *Intern Med.* 2014;53:613–16.

201. Allen TC. Recognition of histopathologic patterns of diffuse malignant mesothelioma in differential diagnosis of pleural biopsies. *Arch Pathol Lab Med.* 2005;129:1415–20.

202. Cook DS, Attanoos RL, Jalloh SS, Gibbs AR. 'Mucin-positive' epithelial

mesothelioma of the peritoneum: an unusual diagnostic pitfall. *Histopathology*. 2000;37:33–36.

203. Ohnuma-Koyama A, Yoshida T, Takahashi N, Akema S, Takeuchi-Kashimoto Y, Kuwahara M, et al. Malignant peritoneal mesothelioma with a sarcomatoid growth pattern and signet-ring-like structure in a female f344 rat. *J Toxicol Pathol*. 2013;26:197–201.

204. Ordonez NG. Mesothelioma with signet-ring cell features: report of 23 cases. *Mod Pathol*. 2013;26:370–84.

205. Rekhi B, Pathuthara S, Ajit D, Kane SV. "Signet-ring" cells – a caveat in the diagnosis of a diffuse peritoneal mesothelioma occurring in a lady presenting with recurrent ascites: an unusual case report. *Diagn Cytopathol*. 2010;38:435–39.

206. Matsukuma S, Aida S, Hata Y, Sugiura Y, Tamai S. Localized malignant peritoneal mesothelioma containing rhabdoid cells. *Pathol Int*. 1996;46:389–91.

207. Ordonez NG. Mesothelioma with rhabdoid features: an ultrastructural and immunohistochemical study of 10 cases. *Mod Pathol*. 2006;19:373–83.

208. Ordonez NG. Pleomorphic mesothelioma: report of 10 cases. *Mod Pathol*. 2012;25:1011–22.

209. Kadota K, Suzuki K, Sima CS, Rusch VW, Adusumilli PS, Travis WD. Pleomorphic epithelioid diffuse malignant pleural mesothelioma: a clinicopathological review and conceptual proposal to reclassify as biphasic or sarcomatoid mesothelioma. *J Thorac Oncol*. 2011;6:896–904.

210. Husain AN, Colby TV, Ordonez NG, Krausz T, Borczuk A, Cagle PT, et al. Guidelines for pathologic diagnosis of malignant mesothelioma: a consensus statement from the International Mesothelioma Interest Group. *Arch Pathol Lab Med*. 2009;133:1317–31.

211. Marchevsky AM. Application of immunohistochemistry to the diagnosis of malignant mesothelioma. *Arch Pathol Lab Med*. 2008;132:397–401.

212. Marchevsky AM, Wick MR. Evidence-based guidelines for the utilization of immunostains in diagnostic pathology: pulmonary adenocarcinoma versus mesothelioma. *Appl Immunohistochem Mol Morphol*. 2007;15:140–44.

213. Yaziji H, Battifora H, Barry TS, Hwang HC, Bacchi CE, McIntosh MW, et al. Evaluation of 12 antibodies for distinguishing epithelioid mesothelioma from adenocarcinoma: identification of a three-antibody immunohistochemical panel with maximal sensitivity and specificity. *Mod Pathol*. 2006;19:514–23.

214. Battifora H, Kopinski MI. Distinction of mesothelioma from adenocarcinoma. An immunohistochemical approach. *Cancer*. 1985;55:1679–85.

215. Ordonez NG. Application of immunohistochemistry in the diagnosis of epithelioid mesothelioma: a review and update. *Hum Pathol*. 2013;44:1–19.

216. Jo VY, Cibas ES, Pinkus GS. Claudin-4 immunohistochemistry is highly effective in distinguishing adenocarcinoma from malignant mesothelioma in effusion cytology. *Cancer Cytopathol*. 2014;122:299–306.

217. Ordonez NG. Value of PAX8, PAX2, napsin A, carbonic anhydrase IX, and claudin-4 immunostaining in distinguishing pleural epithelioid mesothelioma from metastatic renal cell carcinoma. *Mod Pathol*. 2013;26:1132–43.

218. Ordonez NG. Value of claudin-4 immunostaining in the diagnosis of mesothelioma. *Am J Clin Pathol*. 2013;139:611–19.

219. Ohta Y, Sasaki Y, Saito M, Kushima M, Takimoto M, Shiokawa A, et al. Claudin-4 as a marker for distinguishing malignant mesothelioma from lung carcinoma and serous adenocarcinoma. *Int J Surg Pathol*. 2013;21:493–501.

220. Facchetti F, Lonardi S, Gentili F, Bercich L, Falchetti M, Tardanico R, et al. Claudin 4 identifies a wide spectrum of epithelial neoplasms and represents a very useful marker for carcinoma versus mesothelioma diagnosis in pleural and peritoneal biopsies and effusions. *Virchows Arch*. 2007;451:669–80.

221. Facchetti F, Gentili F, Lonardi S, Bercich L, Santin A. Claudin-4 in mesothelioma diagnosis. *Histopathology*. 2007;51:261–63.

222. Soini Y, Kinnula V, Kahlos K, Paakko P. Claudins in differential diagnosis between mesothelioma and metastatic adenocarcinoma of the pleura. *J Clin Pathol*. 2006;59:250–54.

223. Kimura T, Doi Y, Nakashima T, Imano N, Katsuta T, Takahashi S, et al. Clinical experience of volumetric modulated arc therapy for malignant pleural mesothelioma after extrapleural pneumonectomy. *J Radiat Res*. 2015;56:315–24.

224. Tsukamoto Y, Hao H, Kajimoto N, Katayama A, Suzuki C, Terada T, et al. Sarcomatoid pleural mesothelioma with osteosarcomatous, chondrosarcomatous and rhabdomyoblastic elements: an extremely rare autopsy case. *Pathol Int*. 2015;65:51–53.

225. Liu S, Staats P, Lee M, Alexander HR, Burke AP. Diffuse mesothelioma of the peritoneum: correlation between histological and clinical parameters and survival in 73 patients. *Pathology*. 2014;46:604–09.

226. Lee M, Alexander HR, Burke A. Diffuse mesothelioma of the peritoneum: a pathological study of 64 tumours treated with cytoreductive therapy. *Pathology*. 2013;45:464–73.

227. Henderson DW, Reid G, Kao SC, van Zandwijk N, Klebe S. Challenges and controversies in the diagnosis of malignant mesothelioma: Part 2. Malignant mesothelioma subtypes, pleural synovial sarcoma, molecular and prognostic aspects of mesothelioma, *BAP1*, aquaporin-1 and microRNA. *J Clin Pathol*. 2013;66:854–61.

228. Nakamura M, Kobashikawa K, Uchima N, Hirata T. Sarcomatoid peritoneal malignant mesothelioma. *Intern Med*. 2011;50:2045.

229. Klebe S, Brownlee NA, Mahar A, Burchette JL, Sporn TA, Vollmer RT, et al. Sarcomatoid mesothelioma: a clinical-pathologic correlation of 326 cases. *Mod Pathol*. 2010;23:470–79.

230. Salgado RA, Corthouts R, Parizel PM, Germonpre P, Carp L, Van Schil P, et al. Malignant pleural mesothelioma with heterologous osteoblastic elements: computed tomography, magnetic resonance, and positron emission tomography imaging characteristics of a rare tumor. *J Comput Assist Tomogr*. 2005;29:653–56.

231. Chave G, Chalabreysse L, Picaud G, Blineau N, Loire R, Thivolet F, et al. Malignant pleural mesothelioma with osteoblastic heterologous elements: CT and MR imaging findings. *AJR Am J Roentgenol*. 2002;178:949–51.

232. Badak B, Turk O, Ates E, Arik D. Desmoplastic malignant mesothelioma of the peritoneum. *Oxf Med Case Reports*. 2014;2014:49–51.

233. Horiuchi T, Ogata S, Tominaga S, Hiroi S, Kawahara K, Hebisawa A, et al. Immunohistochemistry of cytokeratins 7, 8, 17, 18, and 19, and GLUT-1 aids differentiation of desmoplastic malignant mesothelioma from fibrous pleuritis. *Histol Histopathol*. 2013;28: 663–70.

234. Baccioglu A, Kaba E, Ozmen SA, Demirci M. Desmoplastic malignant mesothelioma. *J Bronchology Interv Pulmonol*. 2013;20:155–58.

235. Takamaru H, Arimura Y, Shinomura Y. Desmoplastic malignant mesothelioma originating from the peritoneum. *Med Oncol*. 2012;29:3155–56.

236. Ishikawa R, Kikuchi E, Jin M, Fujita M, Itoh T, Sawa H, et al. Desmoplastic malignant mesothelioma of the pleura: autopsy reveals asbestos exposure. *Pathol Int*. 2003;53:401–06.

237. Hirano H, Maeda H, Sawabata N, Okumura Y, Takeda S, Maekura R, et al. Desmoplastic malignant mesothelioma: two cases and a literature review. *Med Electron Microsc*. 2003;36:173–78.

238. Colby TV. The diagnosis of desmoplastic malignant mesothelioma. *Am J Clin Pathol*. 1998;110:135–36.

239. Thomas JS, Burnett RA. Desmoplastic mesothelioma. *Thorax*. 1988;43:584.

240. Cantin R, Al-Jabi M, McCaughey WT. Desmoplastic diffuse mesothelioma. *Am J Surg Pathol*. 1982;6:215–22.

241. Yamamoto J, Ueta K, Takenaka M, Takahashi M, Nishizawa S. Sarcomatoid malignant mesothelioma presenting with intramedullary spinal cord metastasis: a case report and literature review. *Global Spine J*. 2014;4:115–20.

242. Goldova B, Dundr P, Zikan M, Tomancova V. Myxoid variant of peritoneal epithelioid malignant mesothelioma. A case report. *Cesk Patol*. 2014;50:149–51.

243. Yang GZ, Li J, Ding HY. Localized malignant myxoid anaplastic mesothelioma of the pericardium. *J Clin Med Res*. 2009;1:115–18.

244. Minato H, Kurose N, Fukushima M, Nojima T, Usuda K, Sagawa M, et al. Comparative immunohistochemical analysis of IMP3, GLUT1, EMA, CD146, and desmin for distinguishing malignant mesothelioma from reactive mesothelial cells. *Am J Clin Pathol*. 2014;141:85–93.

245. Hyun TS, Barnes M, Tabatabai ZL. The diagnostic utility of D2–40, calretinin, CK5/6, desmin and MOC-31 in the differentiation of mesothelioma from adenocarcinoma in pleural effusion cytology. *Acta Cytol*. 2012;56:527–32.

246. Hasteh F, Lin GY, Weidner N, Michael CW. The use of immunohistochemistry to distinguish reactive mesothelial cells from malignant mesothelioma in cytologic effusions. *Cancer Cytopathol*. 2010;118:90–96.

247. Geyer SJ. The use of immunohistochemistry to distinguish reactive mesothelial cells from malignant mesothelioma in cytologic effusions. *Cancer Cytopathol*. 2010;118:225; author reply 225.

248. Takeshima Y, Amatya VJ, Kushitani K, Kaneko M, Inai K. Value of immunohistochemistry in the differential diagnosis of pleural sarcomatoid mesothelioma from lung sarcomatoid carcinoma. *Histopathology*. 2009;54:667–76.

249. Salman WD, Eyden B, Shelton D, Howat A, Al-Dawoud A, Twaij Z. An EMA negative, desmin positive malignant mesothelioma: limitations of immunohistochemistry? *J Clin Pathol*. 2009;62:651–52.

250. Comin CE, Dini S, Novelli L, Santi R, Asirelli G, Messerini L. h-Caldesmon, a useful positive marker in the diagnosis of pleural malignant mesothelioma, epithelioid type. *Am J Surg Pathol*. 2006;30:463–69.

251. Comin CE, Saieva C, Messerini L. h-Caldesmon, calretinin, estrogen receptor, and Ber-EP4: a useful combination of immunohistochemical markers for differentiating epithelioid peritoneal mesothelioma from serous papillary carcinoma of the ovary. *Am J Surg Pathol*. 2007;31:1139–48.

252. Shi M, Fraire AE, Chu P, Cornejo K, Woda BA, Dresser K, et al. Oncofetal protein IMP3, a new diagnostic biomarker to distinguish malignant mesothelioma from reactive mesothelial proliferation. *Am J Surg Pathol*. 2011;35:878–82.

253. Laury AR, Hornick JL, Perets R, Krane JF, Corson J, Drapkin R, et al. *PAX8* reliably distinguishes ovarian serous tumors from malignant mesothelioma. *Am J Surg Pathol*. 2010;34:627–35.

254. Butnor KJ, Sporn TA, Ordonez NG, Association of Directors of Anatomic and Surgical Pathology (ADASP). Recommendations for the reporting of pleural mesothelioma. *Hum Pathol*. 2007;38:1587–89.

255. Davidson B. Prognostic factors in malignant pleural mesothelioma. *Hum Pathol*. 2015;46:789–804.

256. Scherpereel A, Astoul P, Baas P, Berghmans T, Clayson H, de Vuyst P, et al. Guidelines of the European Respiratory Society and the European Society of Thoracic Surgeons for the management of malignant pleural mesothelioma. *Eur Respir J*. 2010;35:479–95.

257. Chirieac LR, Corson JM. Pathologic evaluation of malignant pleural mesothelioma. *Semin Thorac Cardiovasc Surg*. 2009;21:121–24.

258. Kadota K, Suzuki K, Colovos C, Sima CS, Rusch VW, Travis WD, et al. A nuclear grading system is a strong predictor of survival in epithelioid diffuse malignant pleural mesothelioma. *Mod Pathol*. 2012;25:260–71.

259. Yang GC. Long microvilli of mesothelioma are conspicuous in pleural effusions processed by Ultrafast Papanicolaou stain. *Cancer*. 2003;99:17–22.

260. Zu Y, Sidhu GS, Wieczorek R, Cassai ND. Ultrastructurally "invasive" microvilli in an aggressively metastasizing biphasic malignant mesothelioma. *Ultrastruct Pathol*. 2002;26:403–09.

261. Coleman M, Henderson DW, Mukherjee TM. The ultrastructural pathology of malignant pleural mesothelioma. *Pathol Annu*. 1989; 24(Pt 1):303–53.

262. Oczypok EA, Oury TD. Electron microscopy remains the gold standard for the diagnosis of epithelial malignant mesothelioma: a case study. *Ultrastruct Pathol*. 2015;39:153–58.

263. Suzuki Y. Pathology of human malignant mesothelioma – preliminary analysis of 1,517 mesothelioma cases. *Ind Health*. 2001;39:183–85.

264. Suzuki Y. Pathology of human malignant mesothelioma. *Semin Oncol*. 1981;8:268–82.

265. Suzuki Y, Kannerstein M. Ultrastructure of human malignant diffuse mesothelioma. *Am J Pathol.* 1976;85:241–62.

266. Burns TR, Greenberg SD, Mace ML, Johnson EH. Ultrastructural diagnosis of epithelial malignant mesothelioma. *Cancer.* 1985;56:2036–40.

267. Guo G, Chmielecki J, Goparaju C, Heguy A, Dolgalev I, Carbone M, et al. Whole-exome sequencing reveals frequent genetic alterations in *BAP1*, *NF2*, *CDKN2A*, and *CUL1* in malignant pleural mesothelioma. *Cancer Res.* 2015;75:264–69.

268. Sekido Y. Molecular pathogenesis of malignant mesothelioma. *Carcinogenesis.* 2013;34:1413–19.

269. Chung CT, Santos Gda C, Hwang DM, Ludkovski O, Pintilie M, Squire JA, et al. FISH assay development for the detection of p16/CDKN2A deletion in malignant pleural mesothelioma. *J Clin Pathol.* 2010;63:630–34.

270. Farzin M, Toon CW, Clarkson A, Sioson L, Watson N, Andrici J, et al. Loss of expression of *BAP1* predicts longer survival in mesothelioma. *Pathology.* 2015;47:302–07.

271. Alakus H, Yost SE, Woo B, French R, Lin GY, Jepsen K, et al. *BAP1* mutation is a frequent somatic event in peritoneal malignant mesothelioma. *J Transl Med.* 2015;13:122.

272. Nasu M, Emi M, Pastorino S, Tanji M, Powers A, Luk H, et al. High incidence of somatic *BAP1* alterations in sporadic malignant mesothelioma. *J Thorac Oncol.* 2015;10:565–76.

273. Arzt L, Quehenberger F, Halbwedl I, Mairinger T, Popper HH. *BAP1* protein is a progression factor in malignant pleural mesothelioma. *Pathol Oncol Res.* 2014;20:145–51.

274. de Klerk N, Alfonso H, Olsen N, Reid A, Sleith J, Palmer L, et al. Familial aggregation of malignant mesothelioma in former workers and residents of Wittenoom, Western Australia. *Int J Cancer.* 2013;132:1423–28.

275. Bianchi C, Bianchi T. Pleural mesothelioma in a couple of brothers. *Indian J Occup Environ Med.* 2013;17:122–23.

276. Bianchi C, Brollo A, Ramani L, Bianchi T, Giarelli L. Familial mesothelioma of the pleura – a report of 40 cases. *Ind Health.* 2004;42:235–39.

277. Ascoli V, Mecucci C, Knuutila S. Genetic susceptibility and familial malignant mesothelioma. *Lancet.* 2001;357:1804.

278. Heineman EF, Bernstein L, Stark AD, Spirtas R. Mesothelioma, asbestos, and reported history of cancer in first-degree relatives. *Cancer.* 1996;77:549–54.

279. Bianchi C, Brollo A, Zuch C. Asbestos-related familial mesothelioma. *Eur J Cancer Prev.* 1993;2:247–50.

280. Hammar SP, Bockus D, Remington F, Freidman S, LaZerte G. Familial mesothelioma: a report of two families. *Hum Pathol.* 1989;20:107–12.

281. Lynch HT, Katz D, Markvicka SE. Familial mesothelioma: review and family study. *Cancer Genet Cytogenet.* 1985;15:25–35.

282. Li FP, Lokich J, Lapey J, Neptune WB, Wilkins EW, Jr. Familial mesothelioma after intense asbestos exposure at home. *JAMA.* 1978;240:467.

283. Orenstein MR, Schenker MB. Environmental asbestos exposure and mesothelioma. *Curr Opin Pulm Med.* 2000;6:371–77.

284. Dawson A, Gibbs A, Browne K, Pooley F, Griffiths M. Familial mesothelioma. Details of 17 cases with histopathologic findings and mineral analysis. *Cancer.* 1992;70:1183–87.

285. Li FP, Dreyfus MG, Antman KH. Asbestos-contaminated nappies and familial mesothelioma. *Lancet.* 1989;1:909–10.

286. Abratt RP, Vorobiof DA, White N. Asbestos and mesothelioma in South Africa. *Lung Cancer.* 2004;45(Suppl 1):S3–6.

287. Haliloglu M, Hoffer FA, Fletcher BD. Malignant peritoneal mesothelioma in two pediatric patients: MR imaging findings. *Pediatr Radiol.* 2000;30: 251–55.

288. Goyal M, Swanson KF, Konez O, Patel D, Vyas PK. Malignant pleural mesothelioma in a 13-year-old girl. *Pediatr Radiol.* 2000;30:776–78.

289. Niggli FK, Gray TJ, Raafat F, Stevens MC. Spectrum of peritoneal mesothelioma in childhood: clinical and histopathologic features, including DNA cytometry. *Pediatr Hematol Oncol.* 1994;11:399–408.

290. Kelsey A. Mesothelioma in childhood. *Pediatr Hematol Oncol.* 1994;11:461–62.

291. Antman KH, Ruxer RL, Jr., Aisner J, Vawter G. Mesothelioma following Wilms' tumor in childhood. *Cancer.* 1984;54:367–69.

292. Brenner J, Sordillo PP, Magill GB. Malignant mesothelioma in children: report of seven cases and review of the literature. *Med Pediatr Oncol.* 1981;9:367–73.

293. Kumar R, Chitkara NL. Peritoneal malignant mesothelioma in children. *Indian J Cancer.* 1966;3:190–97.

294. Arora SK, Srinivasan R, Nijhawan R, Bansal D, Menon P. Malignant biphasic peritoneal mesothelioma in a child: fine-needle aspiration cytology, histopathology, and immunohistochemical features along with review of literature. *Diagn Cytopathol.* 2012;40:1112–15.

295. Paterson A, Grundy R, de Goyet Jde V, Raafat F, Beath S, McCarthy A. Congenital malignant peritoneal mesothelioma. *Pediatr Radiol.* 2003;33:73–74.

296. Nishioka H, Furusho K, Yasunaga T, Tanaka K, Yamanouchi A, Yokota T, et al. Congenital malignant mesothelioma. A case report and electron-microscopic study. *Eur J Pediatr.* 1988;147:428–30.

297. Hountis P, Chounti M, Matthaios D, Romanidis K, Moraitis S. Surgical treatment for malignant pleural mesothelioma: extrapleural pneumonectomy, pleurectomy/decortication or extended pleurectomy? *J BUON.* 2015;20:376–80.

298. Elbahaie AM, Kamel DE, Lawrence J, Davidson NG. Late cutaneous metastases to the face from malignant pleural mesothelioma: a case report and review of the literature. *World J Surg Oncol.* 2009;7:84.

299. Wagner D, Bourne PA, Yang Q, Goldman BI, Lewis JS, Jr., Xu H. Unusual features of malignant pleural mesothelioma metastatic to the mediastinal lymph nodes. *Appl Immunohistochem Mol Morphol.* 2008;16:301–07.

300. Muljono A, Ng T, McMaster J, Dexter M. Choroid plexus metastases from pleural sarcomatoid mesothelioma. *Pathology.* 2008;40:530–32.

301. Lester T, Xu H. Malignant pleural mesothelioma with osseous metastases

and pathologic fracture of femoral neck. *Appl Immunohistochem Mol Morphol.* 2008;16:507–09.

302. Abdel Rahman AR, Gaafar RM, Baki HA, El Hosieny HM, Aboulkasem F, Farahat EG, et al. Prevalence and pattern of lymph node metastasis in malignant pleural mesothelioma. *Ann Thorac Surg.* 2008;86:391–95.

303. Teh AY, Ball D, O'Day J, Cassumbhoy R. Bilateral choroidal metastases from mesothelioma. *J Thorac Oncol.* 2006;1:712–13.

304. Cimbaluk D, Kasuganti D, Kluskens L, Reddy V, Gattuso P. Malignant biphasic pleural mesothelioma metastatic to the liver diagnosed by fine-needle aspiration. *Diagn Cytopathol.* 2006;34:33–36.

305. Tho LM, O'Rourke NP. Unusual metastases from malignant pleural mesothelioma. *Clin Oncol (R Coll Radiol).* 2005;17:293.

306. Patel T, Bansal R, Trivedi P, Modi L, Shah MJ. Subcutaneous metastases of sarcomatoid mesothelioma with its differential diagnosis on fine needle aspiration – a case report. *Indian J Pathol Microbiol.* 2005;48:482–84.

307. Mah E, Bittar RG, Davis GA. Cerebral metastases in malignant mesothelioma: case report and literature review. *J Clin Neurosci.* 2004;11:917–18.

308. Lumb PD, Suvarna SK. Metastasis in pleural mesothelioma. Immunohistochemical markers for disseminated disease. *Histopathology.* 2004;44:345–52.

309. Ambroggi M, Orlandi E, Foroni RP, Cavanna L. Malignant pleural mesothelioma metastatic to the submandibular salivary gland, simulating glandular hypertrophy, diagnosed by fine-needle aspiration biopsy: a case report and literature review. *World J Surg Oncol.* 2014;12:129.

310. Miller AC, Miettinen M, Schrump DS, Hassan R. Malignant mesothelioma and central nervous system metastases. Report of two cases, pooled analysis, and systematic review. *Ann Am Thorac Soc.* 2014;11:1075–81.

311. Purek L, Laroumagne S, Dutau H, Maldonado F, Astoul P. Miliary mesothelioma: a new clinical and radiological presentation in mesothelioma patients with prolonged survival after trimodality therapy. *J Thorac Oncol.* 2011;6:1753–56.

312. Musk AW. More cases of miliary mesothelioma. *Chest.* 1995;108:587.

313. Huncharek M. Miliary mesothelioma. *Chest.* 1994;106:605–06.

314. Musk AW, Dewar J, Shilkin KB, Whitaker D. Miliary spread of malignant pleural mesothelioma without a clinically identifiable pleural tumour. *Aust N Z J Med.* 1991;21:460–62.

315. Mazurek JM, Syamlad G, Wood JM, Hendricks SA, Weston A. Malignant mesothelioma mortality – United States, 1999–2015. *MMWR Mortal Wkly Rep.* 2017;66(8):214–18.

316. Taioli E, Wolf AS, Camacho-Rivera M, Flores RM. Women with malignant pleural mesothelioma have a threefold better survival rate than men. *Ann Thorac Surg.* 2014;98:1020–24.

317. Richards WG, Godleski JJ, Yeap BY, Corson JM, Chirieac LR, Zellos L, et al. Proposed adjustments to pathologic staging of epithelial malignant pleural mesothelioma based on analysis of 354 cases. *Cancer.* 2010;116:1510–17.

318. Miura JT, Johnston FM, Gamblin TC, Turaga KK. Current trends in the management of malignant peritoneal mesothelioma. *Ann Surg Oncol.* 2014;21:3947–53.

319. Magge D, Zenati MS, Austin F, Mavanur A, Sathaiah M, Ramalingam L, et al. Malignant peritoneal mesothelioma: prognostic factors and oncologic outcome analysis. *Ann Surg Oncol.* 2014;21:1159–65.

320. Shih CA, Ho SP, Tsy FW, Lai KH, Hsu PI. Diffuse malignant peritoneal mesothelioma. *Kaohsiung J Med Sci.* 2013;29:642–45.

321. Chua TC, Chong CH, Morris DL. Peritoneal mesothelioma: current status and future directions. *Surg Oncol Clin N Am.* 2012;21:635–43.

322. Hassan R, Alexander R, Antman K, Boffetta P, Churg A, Coit D, et al. Current treatment options and biology of peritoneal mesothelioma: meeting summary of the first NIH peritoneal mesothelioma conference. *Ann Oncol.* 2006;17:1615–19.

323. Andrici J, Jung J, Sheen A, D'Urso L, Sioson L, Pickett J, et al. Loss of *BAP1* expression is very rare in peritoneal and gynecologic serous adenocarcinomas and can be useful in the differential diagnosis with abdominal mesothelioma. *Hum Pathol.* 2016;51:9–15.

324. Judge S, Thomas P, Govindarajan V, Sharma P, Loggie B. Malignant peritoneal mesothelioma: characterization of the inflammatory response in the tumor microenvironment. *Ann Surg Oncol.* 2016;23:1496–500.

325. Hubert J, Thiboutot E, Dube P, Cloutier AS, Drolet P, Sideris L. Cytoreductive surgery and hyperthermic intraperitoneal chemotherapy with oxaliplatin for peritoneal mesothelioma: preliminary results and survival analysis. *Surg Oncol.* 2015;24:41–46.

326. Pillai K, Pourgholami MH, Chua TC, Morris DL. Oestrogen receptors are prognostic factors in malignant peritoneal mesothelioma. *J Cancer Res Clin Oncol.* 2013;139:987–94.

327. Hsu LN, Sung MT, Chiang PH. Paratesticular malignant mesothelioma in a patient exposed to asbestos for more than 50 years. *Kaohsiung J Med Sci.* 2014;30:537–38.

328. Manganiello M, Cassalman C, Dugan J, Bennett N. Scrotal mesothelioma. *Can J Urol.* 2014;21:7163–65.

329. Busto Martin L, Portela Pereira P, Sacristan Lista F, Busto Castanon L. Mesothelioma of the tunica vaginalis. Case report. *Arch Esp Urol.* 2013;66:384–88.

330. Shelton D, Dalal N. Mesothelioma of the tunica vaginalis with BerEp4 and LeuM1 expression: identification of cytoplasmic tonofilaments by electron microscopy is a key diagnostic feature. *J Clin Pathol.* 2012;65:958–59.

331. Priester P, Kopecky J, Prosvicova J, Petera J, Zoul Z, Slovacek L. Cutaneous recurrence of malignant mesothelioma of the tunica vaginalis testis: a rare case report. *Onkologie.* 2012;35:46–48.

332. Belli E, Landolfo K. Primary pericardial mesothelioma: a rare cause of constrictive pericarditis. *Asian Cardiovasc Thorac Ann.* 2015;23:599–600.

333. Gong W, Ye X, Shi K, Zhao Q. Primary malignant pericardial mesothelioma – a rare cause of superior vena cava thrombosis and constrictive pericarditis. *J Thorac Dis.* 2014;6:E272–75.

334. Oc M, Oc B, Dogan R. Unexpected malignant pericardial mesothelioma presenting as pericardial constriction. *Bratisl Lek Listy*. 2012;113:620–21.

335. Feng X, Zhao L, Han G, Khalil M, Green F, Ogilvie T, et al. A case report of an extremely rare and aggressive tumor: primary malignant pericardial mesothelioma. *Rare Tumors*. 2012;4:e21.

336. Kamiya M, Eimoto T. Malignant mesothelioma of the tunica vaginalis. *Pathol Res Pract*. 1990;186:680–84; discussion 685–86.

337. Sardar MR, Kuntz C, Patel T, Saeed W, Gnall E, Imaizumi S, et al. Primary pericardial mesothelioma unique case and literature review. *Tex Heart Inst J*. 2012;39:261–64.

338. Choi WS, Im MS, Kang JH, Kim YG, Hwang IC, Lee JM, et al. Primary malignant pericardial mesothelioma presenting as acute pericarditis. *J Cardiovasc Ultrasound*. 2012;20:57–59.

339. Tsuruya K, Matsushima M, Nakajima T, Fujisawa M, Shirakura K, Igarashi M, et al. Malignant peritoneal mesothelioma presenting umbilical hernia and Sister Mary Joseph's nodule. *World J Gastrointest Endosc*. 2013;5:407–11.

340. Chakravartty S, Singh JC, Jayamanne H, Shah V, Williams GL, Stephenson BM. Peritoneal mesothelioma masquerading as an inguinal hernia. *Ann R Coll Surg Engl*. 2012;94:e111–12.

341. Chakravartty S, Singh JC, Jayamanne H, Shah V, Williams GL, Stephenson BM. Peritoneal mesothelioma masquerading as an inguinal hernia. *Ann R Coll Surg Engl*. 2011;93:e107–08.

342. Stradella A, Conde-Gallego E, Escalera-Almendros CA, Duran-Martinez I. Malignant mesothelioma of tunica vaginalis. *Actas Urol Esp*. 2014;38:68–69.

343. Lee S, Illei PB, Han JS, Epstein JI. Florid mesothelial hyperplasia of the tunica vaginalis mimicking malignant mesothelioma: a clinicopathologic study of 12 cases. *Am J Surg Pathol*. 2014;38:54–59.

344. Henderson DW, Reid G, Kao SC, van Zandwijk N, Klebe S. Challenges and controversies in the diagnosis of mesothelioma: Part 1. Cytology-only diagnosis, biopsies, immunohistochemistry, discrimination between mesothelioma and reactive mesothelial hyperplasia, and biomarkers. *J Clin Pathol*. 2013;66:847–53.

345. Mangano WE, Cagle PT, Churg A, Vollmer RT, Roggli VL. The diagnosis of desmoplastic malignant mesothelioma and its distinction from fibrous pleurisy: a histologic and immunohistochemical analysis of 31 cases including p53 immunostaining. *Am J Clin Pathol*. 1998;110:191–99.

346. Henderson DW, Shilkin KB, Whitaker D. Reactive mesothelial hyperplasia vs mesothelioma, including mesothelioma *in situ*: a brief review. *Am J Clin Pathol*. 1998;110:397–404.

347. Cagle PT, Churg A. Differential diagnosis of benign and malignant mesothelial proliferations on pleural biopsies. *Arch Pathol Lab Med*. 2005;129:1421–27.

348. Shen J, Pinkus GS, Deshpande V, Cibas ES. Usefulness of EMA, GLUT-1, and XIAP for the cytologic diagnosis of malignant mesothelioma in body cavity fluids. *Am J Clin Pathol*. 2009;131:516–23.

349. Husain AN, Mirza MK, Gibbs A, Hiroshima K, Chi Y, Boumendjel R, et al. How useful is GLUT-1 in differentiating mesothelial hyperplasia and fibrosing pleuritis from epithelioid and sarcomatoid mesotheliomas? An international collaborative study. *Lung Cancer*. 2014;83:324–28.

350. Kato Y, Tsuta K, Seki K, Maeshima AM, Watanabe S, Suzuki K, et al. Immunohistochemical detection of GLUT-1 can discriminate between reactive mesothelium and malignant mesothelioma. *Mod Pathol*. 2007;20:215–20.

351. Hayes JP, Wiggins J, Ward K, Muldowney F, FitzGerald MX. Familial cryptogenic fibrosing pleuritis with Fanconi's syndrome (renal tubular acidosis). A new syndrome. *Chest*. 1995;107:576–78.

352. Baris YI, Sahin AA, Ozesmi M, Kerse I, Ozen E, Kolacan B, et al. An outbreak of pleural mesothelioma and chronic fibrosing pleurisy in the village of Karain/Urgup in Anatolia. *Thorax*. 1978;33:181–92.

353. Churg A, Cagle P, Colby TV, Corson JM, Gibbs AR, Hammar S, et al. The fake fat phenomenon in organizing pleuritis: a source of confusion with desmoplastic malignant mesotheliomas. *Am J Surg Pathol*. 2011;35:1823–29.

354. Lin XM, Chi C, Chen J, Liu Y, Li P, Yang Y. Primary pleural squamous cell carcinoma misdiagnosed as localized mesothelioma: a case report and review of the literature. *J Cardiothorac Surg*. 2013;8:50.

355. Pritchard SA, Howat AJ, Edwards JM. Immunohistochemical panel for distinction between squamous cell carcinoma, adenocarcinoma and mesothelioma. *Histopathology*. 2003;43:197–99.

356. Johnson JS, Edwards JM. Malignant mesothelioma mimicking squamous carcinoma in a pleural fluid aspirate. *Cytopathology*. 2001;12:54–56.

357. Ordonez NG. Value of cytokeratin 5/6 immunostaining in distinguishing epithelial mesothelioma of the pleura from lung adenocarcinoma. *Am J Surg Pathol*. 1998;22:1215–21.

358. Pelosi G, Fabbri A, Tamborini E, Perrone F, Testi AM, Settanni G, et al. Challenging lung carcinoma with coexistent DeltaNp63/p40 and thyroid transcription factor-1 labeling within the same individual tumor cells. *J Thorac Oncol*. 2015;10:1500–02.

359. Agackiran Y, Ozcan A, Akyurek N, Memis L, Findik G, Kaya S. Desmoglein-3 and napsin A double stain, a useful immunohistochemical marker for differentiation of lung squamous cell carcinoma and adenocarcinoma from other subtypes. *Appl Immunohistochem Mol Morphol*. 2012;20:350–55.

360. Kao SC, Griggs K, Lee K, Armstrong N, Clarke S, Vardy J, et al. Validation of a minimal panel of antibodies for the diagnosis of malignant pleural mesothelioma. *Pathology*. 2011;43:313–17.

361. Kannerstein M, Churg J, McCaughey WT, Hill DP. Papillary tumors of the peritoneum in women: mesothelioma or papillary carcinoma. *Am J Obstet Gynecol*. 1977;127:306–14.

362. Shukuya T, Serizawa M, Watanabe M, Akamatsu H, Abe M, Imai H, et al. Identification of actionable mutations in malignant pleural mesothelioma. *Lung Cancer*. 2014;86:35–40.

363. Kawai T, Hiroi S, Nakanishi K, Takagawa K, Haba R, Hayashi K, et al. Lymphohistiocytoid mesothelioma of the pleura. *Pathol Int*. 2010;60:566–74.

364. Galateau-Sallé F, Attanoos R, Gibbs AR, Burke L, Astoul P, Rolland P, et al. Lymphohistiocytoid variant of malignant mesothelioma of the pleura: a series of 22 cases. *Am J Surg Pathol.* 2007;31:711–16.

365. Yao DX, Shia J, Erlandson RA, Klimstra DS. Lymphohistiocytoid mesothelioma: a clinical, immunohistochemical and ultrastructural study of four cases and literature review. *Ultrastruct Pathol.* 2004;28:213–28.

366. Khalidi HS, Medeiros LJ, Battifora H. Lymphohistiocytoid mesothelioma. An often misdiagnosed variant of sarcomatoid malignant mesothelioma. *Am J Clin Pathol.* 2000;113:649–54.

367. Henderson DW, Attwood HD, Constance TJ, Shilkin KB, Steele RH. Lymphohistiocytoid mesothelioma: a rare lymphomatoid variant of predominantly sarcomatoid mesothelioma. *Ultrastruct Pathol.* 1988;12:367–84.

368. Clevenger J, Joseph C, Dawlett M, Guo M, Gong Y. Reliability of immunostaining using pan-melanoma cocktail, SOX10, and microphthalmia transcription factor in confirming a diagnosis of melanoma on fine-needle aspiration smears. *Cancer Cytopathol.* 2014;122:779–85.

369. Granter SR, Weilbaecher KN, Quigley C, Fisher DE. Role for microphthalmia transcription factor in the diagnosis of metastatic malignant melanoma. *Appl Immunohistochem Mol Morphol.* 2002;10:47–51.

370. Muramatsu Y, Isobe K, Sugino K, Kinoshita A, Wada T, Sakamoto S, et al. Malignant pleural mesothelioma mimicking the intrapulmonary growth pattern of epithelioid hemangioendothelioma. *Pathol Int.* 2014;64:358–60.

371. Bahrami A, Allen TC, Cagle PT. Pulmonary epithelioid hemangioendothelioma mimicking mesothelioma. *Pathol Int.* 2008;58:730–34.

372. Nind NR, Attanoos RL, Gibbs AR. Unusual intraparenchymal growth patterns of malignant pleural mesothelioma. *Histopathology.* 2003;42:150–55.

373. Attanoos RL, Dallimore NS, Gibbs AR. Primary epithelioid haemangioendothelioma of the peritoneum: an unusual mimic of diffuse malignant mesothelioma. *Histopathology.* 1997;30:375–77.

374. Lin BT, Colby T, Gown AM, Hammar SP, Mertens RB, Churg A, et al. Malignant vascular tumors of the serous membranes mimicking mesothelioma. A report of 14 cases. *Am J Surg Pathol.* 1996;20:1431–39.

375. Sullivan HC, Edgar MA, Cohen C, Kovach CK, HooKim K, Reid MD. The utility of ERG, CD31 and CD34 in the cytological diagnosis of angiosarcoma: an analysis of 25 cases. *J Clin Pathol.* 2015;68:44–50.

376. Fan C, Liu Y, Lin X, Han Y, He A, Wang E. Epithelioid angiosarcoma at chest wall which needs to be carefully distinguished from malignant mesothelioma: report of a rare case. *Int J Clin Exp Pathol.* 2014;7:9056–60.

377. Klabatsa A, Nicholson AG, Dulay K, Rudd RM, Sheaff MT. Diffuse pleural mesothelioma with epithelioid and angiosarcomatous components – a hitherto undescribed pattern of differentiation. *Histopathology.* 2012;60:1164–66.

378. Kao YC, Chow JM, Wang KM, Fang CL, Chu JS, Chen CL. Primary pleural angiosarcoma as a mimicker of mesothelioma: a case report. *Diagn Pathol.* 2011;6:130.

379. Ordonez NG. D2–40 and podoplanin are highly specific and sensitive immunohistochemical markers of epithelioid malignant mesothelioma. *Hum Pathol.* 2005;36:372–80.

380. Liu B, Liu L, Li Y. Giant solitary fibrous tumor of the pleura: a case report. *Thorac Cancer.* 2015;6:368–71.

381. Kamata T, Sakurai H, Nakagawa K, Watanabe SI, Tsuta K, Asamura H. Solitary fibrous tumor of the pleura: morphogenesis and progression. A report of 36 cases. *Surg Today.* 2016;46(3):335–40.

382. Creytens D, Libbrecht L, Ferdinande L. Nuclear expression of STAT6 in dedifferentiated liposarcomas with a solitary fibrous tumor-like morphology: a diagnostic pitfall. *Appl Immunohistochem Mol Morphol.* 2015;23:462–63.

383. Benabdejlil Y, Kouach J, Babahabib A, Elhassani ME, Rharrassi I, Boudhas A, et al. Intraperitoneal solitary fibrous tumor. *Case Rep Obstet Gynecol.* 2014;2014:906510.

384. Teo A, Hemmings C, Miller R. Sarcomatoid localised mesothelioma mimicking intrapulmonary synovial sarcoma: a case report and review of the literature. *Pathology.* 2010;42:182–84.

385. Cappello F, Barnes L. Synovial sarcoma and malignant mesothelioma of the pleura: review, differential diagnosis and possible role of apoptosis. *Pathology.* 2001;33:142–48.

386. Weinbreck N, Vignaud JM, Begueret H, Burke L, Benhattar J, Guillou L, et al. SYT–SSX fusion is absent in sarcomatoid mesothelioma allowing its distinction from synovial sarcoma of the pleura. *Mod Pathol.* 2007;20:617–21.

387. Somasundaram S, Khajanchi M, Vaja T, Jajoo B, Dey AK. Benign multicystic peritoneal mesothelioma: a rare tumour of the abdomen. *Case Rep Surg.* 2015;2015:613148.

388. Marien T, Zhou M, Brucker B. Benign multicystic mesothelioma masquerading as a urachal cyst. *Can J Urol.* 2014;21:7586–88.

389. Campbell B, Mehanna D, Stone J. Benign multicystic peritoneal mesothelioma: a rare cause of intra-abdominal cystic disease. *ANZ J Surg* 2017;87(6):e15–16.

390. Witek TD, Marchese JW, Farrell TJ. A recurrence of benign multicystic peritoneal mesothelioma treated through laparoscopic excision: a case report and review of the literature. *Surg Laparosc Endosc Percutan Tech.* 2014;24:e70–73.

391. Momeni M, Pereira E, Grigoryan G, Zakashansky K. Multicystic benign cystic mesothelioma presenting as a pelvic mass. *Case Rep Obstet Gynecol.* 2014;2014:852583.

392. Mino JS, Monteiro R, Pigalarga R, Varghese S, Guisto L, Rezac C. Diffuse malignant epithelioid mesothelioma in a background of benign multicystic peritoneal mesothelioma: a case report and review of the literature. *BMJ Case Rep.* 2014;2014:bcr2013200212.

393. Wang TB, Dai WG, Liu DW, Shi HP, Dong WG. Diagnosis and treatment of benign multicystic peritoneal mesothelioma. *World J Gastroenterol.* 2013;19:6689–92.

394. Tamhankar VA. Multicystic benign mesothelioma complicating pregnancy. *Case Rep Obstet Gynecol.* 2015;2015:687183.

395. Oks M, He T, Palkar A, Esposito MJ, Koenig SJ. Benign multicystic mesothelioma causing bilateral pneumothoraces. *Ann Am Thorac Soc.* 2015;12:1106–09.

396. Agarwal S, Mullick S, Gupta K, Prasad S. Pleural multicystic mesothelial proliferation: a mimicker of benign peritoneal mesothelioma. *Indian J Pathol Microbiol.* 2013;56:476–77.

397. Singh A, Chatterjee P, Pai MC, Chacko RT. Multicystic peritoneal mesothelioma: not always a benign disease. *Singapore Med J.* 2013;54:e76–78.

398. McCaughey WT, Colby TV, Battifora H, Churg A, Corson JM, Greenberg SD, et al. Diagnosis of diffuse malignant mesothelioma: experience of a US/Canadian Mesothelioma Panel. *Mod Pathol.* 1991;4:342–53.

399. Galateau-Sallé F, Vignaud JM, Burke L, Gibbs A, Brambilla E, Attanoos R, et al. Well-differentiated papillary mesothelioma of the pleura: a series of 24 cases. *Am J Surg Pathol.* 2004;28:534–40.

400. McCaughey WT, Al-Jabi M, Kannerstein M. A Canadian experience of the pathological diagnosis of diffuse mesothelioma. *IARC Sci Publ.* 1980;207–10.

401. Andrion A, Magnani C, Betta PG, Donna A, Mollo F, Scelsi M, et al. Malignant mesothelioma of the pleura: interobserver variability. *J Clin Pathol.* 1995;48:856–60.

402. Skov BG, Lauritzen AF, Hirsch FR, Skov T, Nielsen HW. Differentiation of adenocarcinoma of the lung and malignant mesothelioma: predictive value and reproducibility of immunoreactive antibodies. *Histopathology.* 1994;25:431–37.

403. Val-Bernal JF, Mayorga M, Val D, Garijo MF. Well-differentiated papillary mesothelioma manifesting in a hernia sac. *Pathol Res Pract.* 2014;210:609–12.

404. Nasit JG, Dhruva G. Well-differentiated papillary mesothelioma of the peritoneum: a diagnostic dilemma on fine-needle aspiration cytology. *Am J Clin Pathol.* 2014;142:233–42.

405. Irwin GW, Ervine A, Kennedy JA. Well-differentiated papillary mesothelioma: peritoneal implants are not always metastases in the presence of cancer. *Scott Med J.* 2014;59:e18–21.

406. Erdogan S, Acikalin A, Zeren H, Gonlusen G, Zorludemir S, Izol V. Well-differentiated papillary mesothelioma of the tunica vaginalis: a case study and review of the literature. *Korean J Pathol.* 2014;48:225–28.

407. Costanzo L, Scarlata S, Perrone G, Rossi L, Papa A, Di Matteo FM, et al. Malignant transformation of well-differentiated papillary mesothelioma 13 years after the diagnosis: a case report. *Clin Respir J.* 2014;8:124–29.

408. Washimi K, Yokose T, Amitani Y, Nakamura M, Osanai S, Noda H, et al. Well-differentiated papillary mesothelioma, possibly giving rise to diffuse malignant mesothelioma: a case report. *Pathol Int.* 2013;63:220–25.

409. Daya D, McCaughey WT. Well-differentiated papillary mesothelioma of the peritoneum. A clinicopathologic study of 22 cases. *Cancer.* 1990;65:292–96.

410. Burrig KF, Pfitzer P, Hort W. Well-differentiated papillary mesothelioma of the peritoneum: a borderline mesothelioma. Report of two cases and review of literature. *Virchows Arch A Pathol Anat Histopathol.* 1990;417:443–47.

411. Malpica A, Sant'Ambrogio S, Deavers MT, Silva EG. Well-differentiated papillary mesothelioma of the female peritoneum: a clinicopathologic study of 26 cases. *Am J Surg Pathol.* 2012;36:117–27.

412. Hoekstra AV, Riben MW, Frumovitz M, Liu J, Ramirez PT. Well-differentiated papillary mesothelioma of the peritoneum: a pathological analysis and review of the literature. *Gynecol Oncol.* 2005;98:161–67.

413. Churg A, Allen T, Borczuk AC, Cagle PT, Galateau-Sallé F, Hwang H, et al. Well-differentiated papillary mesothelioma with invasive foci. *Am J Surg Pathol.* 2014;38:990–98.

414. Trpkov K, Barr R, Kulaga A, Yilmaz A. Mesothelioma of tunica vaginalis of "uncertain malignant potential" – an evolving concept: case report and review of the literature. *Diagn Pathol.* 2011;6:78.

415. Zardawi SJ, Li BT, Zauderer MG, Wang JW, Atmore BB, Barnes TA, et al. Localized malignant pleural mesothelioma with renal metastasis.

Oxf Med Case Reports. 2015;2015: 170–72.

416. Giansanti M, Bellezza G, Guerriero A, Pireddu A, Sidoni A. Localized intrasplenic mesothelioma: a case report. *Int J Surg Pathol.* 2013;22:451–55.

417. Gelvez-Zapata SM, Gaffney D, Scarci M, Coonar AS. What is the survival after surgery for localized malignant pleural mesothelioma? *Interact Cardiovasc Thorac Surg.* 2013;16:533–37.

418. Andrews W, Paul S, Narula N, Altorki NK. Localized mesothelioma tumour arising synchronously with a primary contralateral lung cancer. *Interact Cardiovasc Thorac Surg.* 2013;17: 1061–62.

419. Nakano T, Hamanaka R, Oiwa K, Nakazato K, Masuda R, Iwazaki M. Localized malignant pleural mesothelioma. *Gen Thorac Cardiovasc Surg.* 2012;60:468–74.

420. Morimoto D, Fujimoto N, Nishi H, Asano M, Fuchimoto Y, Ono K, et al. Malignant pleural mesothelioma localized in the thoracic wall. *J Thorac Oncol.* 2012;7:e21–22.

421. Kim Y, Lee E, Jung W, Kim HK, Jung SH, Hong KD, et al. Localized malignant peritoneal mesothelioma arising in the mesentery of the ascending colon. *Am Surg.* 2012;78:E255–57.

422. Papalambros A, Sigala F, Vouza EG, Hepp W, Antonakis P. Sister Mary Joseph's nodule as primary localized malignant mesothelioma. Report of a case. *Zentralbl Chir.* 2011;136: 172–74.

423. Ouazzani A, Rondelet B, Sokolow Y, Ruiz Patino M, Remmelink M, Cappello M. Localized malignant lymphohistiocytoid pleural mesothelioma. *Acta Chir Belg.* 2011;111:38–43.

424. Hayashi H, Notohara K, Yoshioka H, Matsuoka T, Ikeda H, Kagawa K, et al. Localized malignant pleural mesothelioma showing a thoracic mass and metastasizing to the stomach. *Intern Med.* 2010;49:671–75.

425. Tanzi S, Tiseo M, Internullo E, Cacciani G, Capra R, Carbognani P, et al. Localized malignant pleural mesothelioma: report of two cases. *J Thorac Oncol.* 2009;4:1038–40.

426. Akamoto S, Ono Y, Ota K, Suzaki N, Sasaki A, Matsuo Y, et al. Localized malignant mesothelioma in the middle mediastinum: report of a case. *Surg Today*. 2008;38:635–38.

427. Takahashi H, Harada M, Maehara S, Kato H. Localized malignant mesothelioma of the pleura. *Ann Thorac Cardiovasc Surg*. 2007;13:262–66.

428. Allen TC, Cagle PT, Churg AM, Colby TV, Gibbs AR, Hammar SP, et al. Localized malignant mesothelioma. *Am J Surg Pathol*. 2005;29:866–73.

429. Robinson LA, Reilly RB. Localized pleural mesothelioma. The clinical spectrum. *Chest*. 1994;106:1611–15.

430. You Q, Zhao J, Shi G, Deng J, Teng X. Epithelioid malignant mesothelioma presenting with features of gastric tumor in a child. *Int J Clin Exp Pathol*. 2014;7:2636–40.

431. Kuroda K, Ishizawa S, Kudo T, Uotani H, Hosokawa A, Tanaka T, et al. Localized malignant mesenteric mesothelioma causing small bowel obstruction. *Pathol Int*. 2008;58:239–43.

432. Al-Qahtani M, Morris B, Dawood S, Onerheim R. Malignant mesothelioma of the tunica vaginalis. *Can J Urol*. 2007;14:3514–17.

433. Erdogan E, Demirkazik FB, Gulsun M, Ariyurek M, Emri S, Sak SD. Incidental localized (solitary) mediastinal malignant mesothelioma. *Br J Radiol*. 2005;78:858–61.

434. Hirano H, Takeda S, Sawabata Y, Okumura Y, Maeda H, Hanibuchi M, et al. Localized pleural malignant mesothelioma. *Pathol Int*. 2003; 53:616–21.

Chapter 12

Surgical Treatment of Pleural and Peritoneal Mesothelioma

Sean C. Wightman, Eugene A. Choi, and Wickii T. Vigneswaran

Background

Mesothelioma is a malignancy that originates from various serous mesothelial cell linings in the body. Malignant mesothelioma affects approximately 3000 people annually in the USA (1). In almost 85 per cent of patients this disease involves the pleura; peritoneal involvement is seen in about 14 per cent; and in less than 1 per cent mesothelioma can primarily involve the pericardium or tunica vaginalis (2,3).

In the majority of patients an environmental exposure to asbestos is noted. Although asbestos-related mesothelioma is most often attributed to occupational exposure, this is not always the case. Environmental exposure can happen in the home of workers exposed to asbestos that was carried on their clothes and people who live or lived near sites where the asbestos was mined or used (4). The most controversial link to mesothelioma is exposure to Simian virus 40 (SV40), a virus known to infect monkeys and apes which is highly carcinogenic. It was discovered that the polio vaccine used in the 1960s may have contained SV40 from some infected monkeys (5,6). SV40 was later demonstrated to cause mesothelioma in hamsters when the pleural space was infected with this virus. Erionite, a non-asbestos mineral fiber, has been identified as a cause of mesothelioma in Turkey where this is used as building material (7,8). Further investigation of the link between erionite exposure in Turkey and the high incidence of mesothelioma in certain families produced evidence that genetic predisposition might be also a factor. Higher incidence of mesothelioma among the family members has been explained by the presence of an inherited mutation in the *BRCA1*-associated protein 1 (*BAP1*) gene. Normally this gene inhibits tumor development; mutated *BAP1* is hypothesized to encourage the growth of tumor (9).

Exposure to ionizing radiation and chronic inflammation are also linked to development of mesothelioma (5,10). Increased incidence of pleural mesothelioma among patients who received radiation therapy for lymphoma and peritoneal mesothelioma and among patients with familial Mediterranean fever (FMF) with no exposure to asbestos supports these etiologies (11).

The three main histologic subtypes of malignant mesothelioma are epithelioid, sarcomatoid, and mixed or biphasic (12,13). The epithelioid type is further subtyped, which has been addressed elsewhere in this book. Patients with the diagnosis of malignant mesothelioma typically have local spread into surrounding structures and distant metastasis of the tumor is rare (14). Symptoms of mesothelioma do not typically arise until the disease has reached late stages. Often they are non-specific in nature, including weight loss, fatigue, and night sweats. In pleural mesothelioma, the presenting symptoms typically included fatigue and shortness of breath due to pleural effusions and the tumor restricting lung expansion causing restrictive lung disease. These symptoms often develop slowly, progressing for months before the time of diagnosis. Other noted symptoms may include chest pain, cough, and weight loss. Patients with primary abdominal mesothelioma present with increasing abdominal girth, abdominal pain, and weight loss (14,15). Often the disease affects males in the sixth or seventh decade of life.

Surgical Treatment of Malignant Pleural Mesothelioma

Surgery plays an important role in diagnosis, symptom control, and definitive treatment with "curative" intent. A precise diagnosis and differentiation of the histological subtype is required for treatment planning and prognostic prediction. This often can be obtained by open or video-assisted thoracoscopic (VATS) biopsy, although a CT- or ultrasound-guided core needle biopsy can be performed in patients with solid tumor; however, this method does not allow sampling from multiple sites, which is often recommended. Palliative treatment of the pleural effusion is best achieved by the placement of a cuffed tunneled pleural catheter, VATS talc pleurodesis, or partial pleurectomy. Patients with localized disease with good performance status and non-sarcomatoid histology are considered candidates for radical surgery. The aim of surgery is removal of all macroscopic tumor, termed maximal cytoreduction. It is estimated that 22 per cent of patients in the US are currently offered radical surgery and the estimate might be lower in European and developing countries (16). There still remains much controversy as to what maximal cytoreductive surgical procedure should be offered to individual patients (17).

Radical Cytoreductive Surgery

The two procedures that had been offered are extrapleural pneumonectomy and pleurectomy and decortication. Extrapleural pneumonectomy (EPP) involves en-bloc resection of parietal pleura, lung, ipsilateral pericardium, and ipsilateral

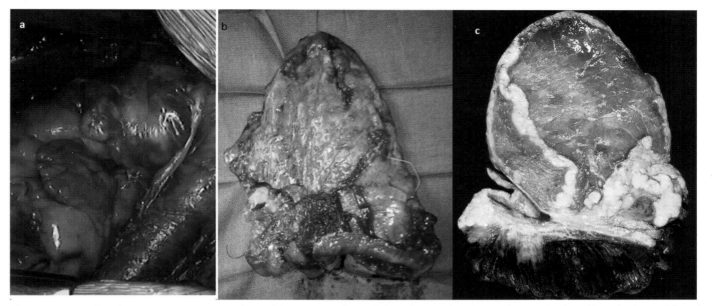

Figure 12.1 Extrapleural pneumonectomy (EPP) involves en-bloc resection of parietal pleura, lung, ipsilateral pericardium, and ipsilateral hemidiaphragm followed by prosthetic reconstruction of the diaphragm and often the pericardium. (a) Pleural cavity after extrapleural resection of lung. (b) The typical pathology specimen including en-bloc resection of lung with, pericardium and diaphragm, (c) with cross-section through the specimen.

hemidiaphragm followed by prosthetic reconstruction of the diaphragm and often the pericardium (Figure 12.1). The pleurectomy and decortication involves removal of the parietal and visceral pleura and in some instances the diaphragm (extended pleurectomy and decortication) and pericardium with prosthetic reconstruction (Figure 12.2). Although in EPP the surgical steps are well-defined, in pleurectomy decortication they are less so. Recently there has been a serious attempt to define the terminology and uniform definitions have been proposed by the International Association for the Study of Lung Cancer (IASLC) and the International Mesothelioma Interest Group (IMIG) (18). Lymph node dissection is performed in both procedures for adequate surgical staging.

Extrapleural Pneumonectomy (EPP)

Butchard et al. proposed the EPP for malignant pleural mesothelioma in 1976 (19). In their series the hospital mortality was 31 per cent and only 10 per cent of the patients survived beyond 2 years. This experience discouraged many thoracic surgeons offering EPP to patients until the report by Sugarbaker in 1996, where he reported a larger series of patients undergoing surgery with chemotherapy and adjuvant hemithoracic radiation therapy (20). He showed low hospital mortality and a 5-year survival of 46 per cent. In this series epithelioid histology, absent nodal disease, and resection with clear surgical margins had better outcomes. Many centers currently

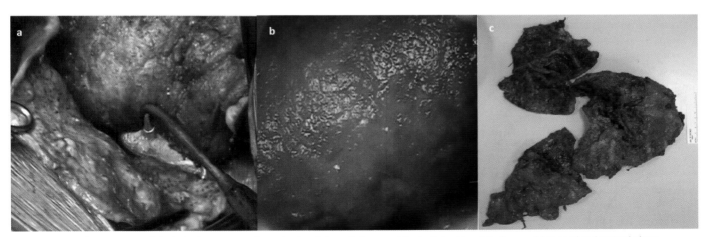

Figure 12.2 A pleurectomy and decortication removes the parietal and visceral pleura and the ipsilateral hemidiaphragm. (a) Visceral and parietal pleura dissected away from lung. (b) Lung without visceral pleura. (c) Specimen that was resected showing the pleura and diaphragm.

offer EPP in selected patients with neoadjuvant chemotherapy followed by adjuvant treatment of various types. However, evidence is still lacking from any randomized studies that demonstrate a clear advantage of EPP in patients with MPM. There are studies that support non-surgical treatment with equivalent survival among patients who can be considered for EPP, suggesting the outcome is based on case selection rather than the treatment itself. Recently reported low mortality for EPP and long survival in patients with early disease and epithelioid histology support the operation in selected patients. Intensity-modulated radiation therapy (IMRT) has been shown as promising following EPP for disease control, but long term data are still pending (21). Quality-of-life data are scarce following EPP and more studies are required to investigate this aspect of outcome following surgery.

Pleurectomy and Decortication (P/D)

McCormack et al. reported in 1976 a median survival of 21 months in patients with malignant pleural mesothelioma (MPM) following pleurectomy and decortication and adjuvant chemoradiation therapy (22). The main disadvantage of postoperative radiation therapy is that the lung is in the field of the radiation and may result in radiation pneumonitis. There is an increasing trend by several groups to advocate pleurectomy and decortication instead of EPP for MPM because of lower perioperative mortality and morbidity and better functional results (23–25). Recently, some groups have reported median survival over 24 months with high-dose lung-sparing adjuvant radiation therapy following P/D (26,27). Improved functional status and quality of life has been reported following P/D, which clearly provide a net benefit to this patient population (28,29).

Palliative Surgery

The patient presenting with pleural effusion requires drainage for relief of symptoms. If the patient is not a suitable candidate because of performance status or comorbidities for radical cytoreductive surgery, palliative treatment may be the only option available. Increasingly, an indwelling catheter is used to drain off recurrent pleural effusion, particularly if the lung is trapped. Video-assisted thoracoscopic talc pleurodesis provides good relief and improved quality of life if the lung is not trapped. In selected cases a limited pleurectomy will provide similar relief if the lung can be expanded with partial pleurectomy. However, the incidence of airleak and prolonged hospital stay has been reported among patients undergoing VATS partial pleurectomy (30).

Outcomes

Treatment options available to patients with pleural mesothelioma include supportive care, chemotherapy, surgery, and in some cases radiation or a combination of the above. With supportive care alone, life expectancy after diagnosis of MPM ranges from 6 to 9 months (9,30). With chemotherapy, median survival increases to around 12 months (9). Surgery increases survival up to 22 months in selected patients. Furthermore, surgery is an important component of mesothelioma treatment to relieve symptoms that can be debilitating and can have a vast impact on the patient's quality of life (1,10).

In the absence of randomized studies it is difficult to know which treatment or radical operation is better (31). The observed differences in median survival between reports may be due to selection bias. Quality of life is better after P/D than EPP. Perioperative complications and the operative mortality are lower in P/D and therefore this is considered a default operation for many (12–18). Two-year survival is reported to range from 40 per cent to 50 per cent (15,16). A review of the Society of Thoracic Surgeons Database demonstrated at least one major perioperative complication rate of 3.8 per cent among patients undergoing P/D compared to 24.2 per cent among patients undergoing EPP (11). EPP therefore should be considered only in few selected patients where "curative" resection is feasible without compromising quality of life (13–16,18).

Primary Peritoneal Mesothelioma

Diffuse malignant peritoneal mesothelioma (DMPM) is an exceedingly rare tumor (approximately 1–3 cases per million) and because of its rarity, may be associated with a delay before definitive diagnosis. Patients with DMPM often present with vague symptoms of abdominal pain, fatigue, as well as ascites (32). Less commonly, symptoms include weight loss, vomiting, fever, and diarrhea. Therefore, patients are usually diagnosed with advanced disease. Currently, there is no specific serum or histological marker available for mesothelioma and diagnosis is dependent on the presence and absence of multiple histological markers including calretinin, Wilms' tumor-1 antigen (WT-1), epithelial membrane antigen (EMA), and cytokeratin 5/6 (33,34).

DMPM has historically been thought to be a terminal diagnosis, resulting in approximately one-year survival after diagnosis. In general, peritoneal mesothelioma is a chemoresistant entity with very few effective drug treatments. Treatment with systemic chemotherapy, typically Pemetrexed and cisplatin, a regimen used to treat pleural disease, may extend median survival to 13 months (22). Other agents used against mesothelioma include gemcitabine, vinorelbine, as well as immunomodulatory drugs (35,36). Locoregional treatment of DMPM includes surgical resection alone, cytoreduction, and intraperitoneal peritoneal chemotherapy (HIPEC), and early postoperative intraperitoneal chemotherapy. Since its introduction, cytoreduction and HIPEC has been shown to be a therapeutic intervention for this disease and has drastically improved survival to around approximately at 50 per cent at 5 years (37). Curative resection can be achieved in a certain proportion of patients (5). The Milan Consensus Conference on Peritoneal Surface Malignancies (2006) outlined that the standard treatment of malignant peritoneal mesothelioma is integration of cytoreductive surgery and HIPEC (38). The invasive procedure

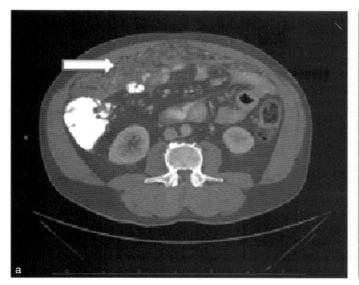 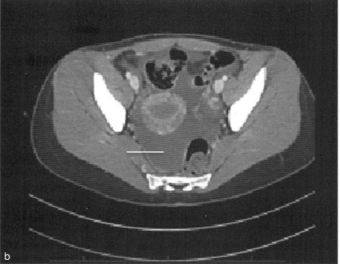

Figure 12.3 (a) A CT abdomen and pelvis showing peritoneal nodules and omental caking consistent with dry mesothelioma (indicated by the white arrow). (b) A CT abdomen and pelvis. Work-up found pelvic ascites (indicated by the white bar) and miliary nodules of the pelvic peritoneum consistent with wet mesothelioma.

involves resection of all visible tumor with a goal of removing to a level of no visible disease or disease remnants smaller than 0.25 cm (23). The major advantage of HIPEC is enhanced high concentrations of chemotherapy delivery without the major side effects associated with systemic chemotherapy delivery. Further, HIPEC alone has been shown to effectively treat refractory ascites and provides a method of palliation (39).

To assess whether cytoreductive and HIPEC is a viable option, patients must be evaluated to determine if they would indeed tolerate the procedure based on their other comorbidities, which may include cardiac risk stratification and pulmonary functions tests. They must also have disease which is amenable to optimal cytoreduction and possible curative resection. Patients undergo a complete history and physical examination and preoperative anesthesia evaluation, which may include further cardiac risk stratification and pulmonary function testing. To determine resectability and assist in surgical planning, cross-sectional imaging of the abdomen with either computed tomography (CT) or magnetic resonance imaging (MRI) of the abdomen and pelvis are necessary (40,41). Preoperative imaging can help determine if the disease is associated with ascites and distended bowel (wet mesothelioma) or if there is one large mass or multiple small peritoneal nodularity (dry mesothelioma); this can also help to visualize disease in critical, often unresectable locations (Figure 12.3). Additionally, a positron emission tomography (PET) scan combined with a CT scan may also help demonstrate the location of the disease (42). Several studies have reported higher sensitivity and specificity values for PET/CT compared to MRI (43). If the extent of peritoneal disease involvement cannot be determined CT, MRI, or PET alone, surgeons may consider a diagnostic laparoscopy to directly visualize the disease extent (44). However, laparoscopy may not assist in the assessment of the retroperitoneum or porta

hepatis, and the necessary trocar placement for laparoscopy may potentially seed disease. The systematic use of diagnostic laparoscopy requires further evaluation (45).

Procedure for Peritoneal Mesothelioma

The surgical procedure for primary peritoneal mesothelioma involves cytoreductive surgery to remove any visible tumor on the peritoneum combined with chemotherapy to remove microscopic disease intraoperatively. The patient is positioned in a modified lithotomy position in case a pelvis peritonectomy including sigmoidectomy and hysterectomy is required and to facilitate a rectal anastomosis as well as allow a flexible sigmoidoscopy or cystoscopy. A midline incision extending from the xiphoid to the pubis is made: the skin followed by the subcutaneous fat and the midline fascia is divided and the underlying anterior peritoneum is stripped with electrocautery and/or blunt dissection. A self-retaining retractor is used for consistent exposure of the abdomen.

The distribution and size of the disease is quantified according to the Peritoneal Cancer Index (PCI) score, proposed by Jacquet and Sugarbaker. The abdomen and pelvis are divided into nine regions and the small bowel is divided into four regions. In each region, a lesion size score is given: 0 for no implants seen, 1 for implants up to 0.5 cm, 2 for nodules 0.5–5 cm, and 3 for implants > 5 cm or confluent nodules (46). The goal of cytoreductive surgery is to resect all visible disease with visceral organ resection and peritonectomy. The peritonectomy procedure involves the greater omentectomy, right peritonectomy, left upper-quadrant peritonectomy, left parietal peritonectomy, right upper-quadrant peritonectomy, lesser omentectomy, stripping the omental bursa, and pelvis peritonectomy (47). In addition, a right colon

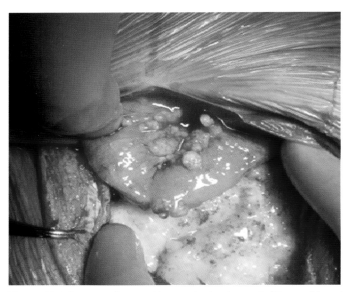

Figure 12.4 Recurrent disease with extensive involvement of the small bowel mesentery. Surgical small bowel resection and bypass were performed as well as a placement of a gastrostomy tube.

resection, splenectomy, Glissonian capsule resection, cholecystectomy, gastric resection, sigmoid colon resection, total abdominal hysterectomy, and bilateral salpingo-oophorectomy as well as other intestinal resection may be required (48).

The HIPEC portion involves intraoperative distribution of heated chemotherapy within the abdominal cavity. Inflow and outflow catheters are placed into the abdomen and connected to a pump with a heater element. Perfusion can be performed in an open or closed technique (49). Peritoneal fluid is circulated until a temperature of 42–43°C is reached and chemotherapy is then added to the heated peritoneal fluid. The abdomen is continuously agitated to promote heat and drug dispersion. Hyperthermia is used to increase cytotoxicity of the chemotherapy agent and chemotherapy penetrance of tissue; additionally, preclinical models suggest that heat can directly destroy tumor cells (50). The selection of the chemotherapy agent for perfusion is varied, but in general, cisplatin is the most active single agent and drug combinations with cisplatin have been demonstrated to be effective in terms of treatment response. Oxaliplatin has recently been used as chemotherapy agent in HIPEC for peritoneal mesothelioma. The estimated one- and three-year survival rates were 100 per cent and 91 per cent, respectively (51). After 90 minutes of circulation, the abdomen is then irrigated and the temperature probes and drains removed. Bowel anastomoses are performed after the perfusion to return the bowel to continuity. Drains are placed prior to abdominal closure with an optional small feeding tube. Patients are monitored postoperatively typically in a monitored unit setting. The patients should be monitored to sustain an elevated urine output for chemotherapy clearance.

Outcomes

Most single and multi-institutional studies of cytoreductive surgery and HIPEC for the treatment of DMPM have demonstrated a benefit in median overall and progression-free survival, ranging from 19 to 90 months and from 7 to 28 months, respectively (52). PCI scores and completeness of cytoreduction (CC) scores are predictors of survival. In a multi-institutional study of cytoreductive surgery and HIPEC for peritoneal mesothelioma, the two strongest predictors of survival were PCI score ($p = 0.002$) and CC score ($p = 0.001$) (53). The completeness of cytoreduction is defined by a scaling score: CC0 is defined as no visible residual tumor, CC1 is residual tumor nodules < 2.5 mm, CC2 is residual tumor nodules between 2.5 mm and 2.5 cm, and CC3 is residual tumor > 2.5 cm. A recent Italian study has demonstrated better survival of patients who had complete peritonectomy (including peritoneum appearing to be free of gross disease) versus selective peritonectomy (including peritoneum with visible disease). The 5-year overall survival of the selective parietal peritonectomy and the complete parietal peritonectomy was 40 per cent and 63.9 per cent, respectively ($p = 0.02$). Similar to patients with pleural mesothelioma, patients with DMPM with an epithelial subtype have better outcome after cytoreductive surgery and HIPEC. Other significant prognostic factors include absence of nodal metastases and administration of HIPEC. The procedure is well tolerated and associated with an acceptable morbidity and mortality rate. The main complications from this procedure include 0–7 per cent mortality, need for re-operation, chemotherapy side effects, and risk of fistula formation (5,25). Recurrence of peritoneal disease is about 50 per cent at 3 years (5) and the small bowel has been reported as the common site of recurrence (Figure 12.4) (54).

Summary

Surgery is an integral component of treatment of patients with isolated pleural or peritoneal mesothelioma, who are in good performance status with epithelioid or biphasic histology. This uncommon disease is best treated in specialized centers with expertise in all aspect of multidisciplinary care including diagnosis, treatment, and follow-up.

References

1. Henley SJ, Larson TC, Wu M, Antao VC, Lewis M, Pinheiro GA, et al. Mesothelioma incidence in 50 states and the District of Columbia, United States, 2003–2008. *Int J Occup Environ Health.* 2013;19(1):1–10.

2. Moolgavkar SH, Meza R, Turim J. Pleural and peritoneal mesotheliomas in SEER: age effects and temporal trends, 1973–2005. *Cancer Causes Control.* 2009;20(6):935–44.

3. Vigneswaran WT, Stefanacci PR. Pericardial mesothelioma. *Curr Treat Options Oncol.* 2000;1(4):299–302.

4. Miller A. Mesothelioma in household members of asbestos-exposed workers: 32 United States cases since 1990. *Am J Ind Med*. 2005;47(5):458–62.

5. Carbone M, Rizzo P, Pass H. Simian virus 40: the link with human malignant mesothelioma is well established. *Anticancer Res*. 2000;20(2A):875–77.

6. Rizzo P, Bocchetta M, Powers A, Foddis R, Stekala E, Pass HI, Carbone M. SV40 and the pathogenesis of mesothelioma. *Semin Cancer Biol*. 2001;11(1):63–71.

7. Baris YI, Grandjean P. Prospective study of mesothelioma mortality in Turkish villages with exposure to fibrous zeolite. *J Natl Cancer Inst*. 2006;98(6):414–17.

8. Carbone M, Emri S, Dogan AU, Steele I, Tuncer M, Pass HI, et al. A mesothelioma epidemic in Cappadocia: scientific developments and unexpected social outcomes. *Nat Rev Cancer*. 2007;7(2):147–54.

9. Zauderer MG, Bott M, McMillan R, Sima CS, Rusch V, Krug LM, et al. Clinical characteristics of patients with malignant pleural mesothelioma harboring somatic *BAP1* mutations. *J Thorac Oncol*. 2013;8(11):1430–33.

10. Farioli A, Violante FS, Mattioli S, Curti S, Kriebel D. Risk of mesothelioma following external beam radiotherapy for prostate cancer: a cohort analysis of SEER database. *Cancer Causes Control*. 2013;24(8):1535–45.

11. Gentiloni N, Febbraro S, Barone C, Lemmo G, Neri G, Zannoni G, Capelli A, Gasbarrini G. Peritoneal mesothelioma in recurrent familial peritonitis. *J Clin Gastroenterol*. 1997;24(4):276–79.

12. Law MR, Hodson ME, Heard BE. Malignant mesothelioma of the pleura: relation between histological type and clinical behaviour. *Thorax*. 1982;37(11):810–15.

13. Antman K, Shemin R, Ryan L, Klegar K, Osteen R, Herman T, et al. Malignant mesothelioma: prognostic variables in a registry of 180 patients, the Dana-Farber Cancer Institute and Brigham and Women's Hospital experience over two decades, 1965–1985. *J Clin Oncol*. 1988;6(1):147–53.

14. Camacho LH, Mora-Bowen A, Munden R, Smythe WR, Ordoñez NG. Malignant mesothelioma: natural history, pathologic features and future therapies. *Am J Med*. 2007;120(7): e7–9.

15. Sridhar KS, Doria R, Raub WA, Thurer RJ, Saldana M. New strategies are needed in diffuse malignant mesothelioma. *Cancer* 1992;70(12):2969–79.

16. Flores RM, Riedel E, Donington JS, Alago W, Ihekweazu U, Krug L, et al. Frequency of use and predictors of cancer-directed surgery in the management of malignant pleural mesothelioma in a community-based (Surveillance, Epidemiology, and End Results [SEER]) population. *J Thorac Oncol*. 2010;5(10):1649–54.

17. Flores RM, Pass HI, Seshan VE, Dycoco J, Zakowski M, Carbone M, et al. Extrapleural pneumonectomy versus pleurectomy/decortication in the surgical management of malignant pleural mesothelioma: results in 663 patients. *J Thorac Cardiovasc Surg*. 2008;135(3):620–26.

18. Rice D. Standardizing surgical treatment in malignant pleural mesothelioma. *Ann Cardiothorac Surg*. 2012;1(4):497–501.

19. Butchart EG, Ashcroft T, Barnsley WC, Holden MP. Pleuropneumonectomy in the management of diffuse malignant mesothelioma of the pleura. Experience with 29 patients. *Thorax*. 1976;31: 15–24.

20. Sugarbaker DJ, Garcia JP, Richards WG, Harpole DH Jr, Healy-Baldini E, DeCamp MM Jr, et al. Extrapleural pneumonectomy in the multimodality therapy of malignant pleural mesothelioma. Results in 120 consecutive patients. *Ann Surg*. 1996;224(3):288–94; discussion 294–96.

21. Cho BC, Feld R, Leighl N, Opitz I, Anraku M, Tsao MS, et al. A feasibility study evaluating Surgery for Mesothelioma After Radiation Therapy: the "SMART" approach for resectable malignant pleural mesothelioma. *J Thorac Oncol*. 2014;9(3):397–402.

22. McCormack PM, Nagasaki F, Hilaris BS, Martini N. Surgical treatment of pleural mesothelioma. *J Thorac Cardiovasc Surg*. 1982;84:834–42.

23. Burt BM, Cameron RB, Mollberg NM, Kosinski AS, Schipper PH, Shrager JB, et al. Malignant pleural mesothelioma and the Society of Thoracic Surgeons Database: an analysis of surgical morbidity and mortality. *J Thorac Cardiovasc Surg*. 2014;148(1):30–35.

24. Lang-Lazdunski L, Bille A, Lal R, Cane P, McLean E, Landau D, et al. Pleurectomy/decortication is superior to extrapleural pneumonectomy in the multimodality management of patients with malignant pleural mesothelioma. *J Thorac Oncol*. 2012;7(4):737–43.

25. Mollberg NM, Vigneswaran Y, Kindler HL, Warnes C, Salgia R, Husain AN, et al. Quality of life after radical pleurectomy decortication for malignant pleural mesothelioma. *Ann Thorac Surg*. 2012;94(4):1086–92.

26. Minatel E, Trovo M, Polesel J, Baresic T, Bearz A, Franchin G, et al. Radical pleurectomy/decortication followed by high dose of radiation therapy for malignant pleural mesothelioma. Final results with long-term follow-up. *Lung Cancer*. 2014;83(1):78–82.

27. Rosenzweig KE, Zauderer MG, Laser B, Krug LM, Yorke E, Sima CS, et al. Pleural intensity-modulated radiotherapy for malignant pleural mesothelioma. *Int J Radiat Oncol Biol Phys*. 2012;83(4):1278–83.

28. Bölükbas S, Eberlein M, Schirren J. Prospective study on functional results after lung-sparing radical pleurectomy in the management of malignant pleural mesothelioma. *J Thorac Oncol*. 2012;7(5):900–05.

29. Burkholder D, Hadi D, Kunnavakkam R, Kindler H, Todd K, Celauro AD, et al. Effects of Extended Pleurectomy and Decortication on Quality of Life and Pulmonary Function in Patients With Malignant Pleural Mesothelioma. *Ann Thorac Surg*. 2015;99(5):1775–80.

30. Merritt N, Blewett CJ, Miller JD, Bennett WF, Young JE, Urschel JD. Survival after conservative (palliative) management of pleural malignant mesothelioma. *J Surg Oncol*. 2001;78(3):171–74.

31. Taioli E, Wolf AS, Flores RM. Meta-analysis of survival after pleurectomy decortication versus extrapleural pneumonectomy in mesothelioma. *Ann Thorac Surg*. 2015;99(2):472–80.

32. Jin S, Cao S, Cao J, Shen J, Hu J, Che D, et al. Predictive factors analysis for malignant peritoneal mesothelioma. *J Gastrointest Surg*. 2015;19(2):319–26.

33. Lee M, Alexander HR, Burke A. Diffuse mesothelioma of the peritoneum: a

pathological study of 64 tumors treated with cytoreductive therapy. *Pathology*. 2013; 45(3):464–73.

34. Husain AN, Colby T, Ordonez N, Krausz T, Attanoos R, Beasley MB, et al. Guidelines for pathologic diagnosis of malignant mesothelioma: 2012 update for the consensus statement from the International Mesothelioma Interest Group. *Arch Pathol Lab Med*. 2013;137(5): 647–67.

35. Nakashima K, Inatsu H, Kitamura K, Hikosaka T, Hoshiko S, Ashiduka S. Advanced diffuse malignant peritoneal mesothelioma responding to palliative chemotherapy. *Clin J Gastroenterol*. 2012;5(6):373–76.

36. Karpathiou G, Argiana E, Koutsopoulos A, Froudarakis ME. Response of a patient with pleural and peritoneal mesothelioma after second-line chemotherapy with lipoplatin and gemcitabine. *Oncology*. 2007;73(5–6):426–29.

37. Alexander HR, Hanna N, Pingpank JF. Clinical results of cytoreduction and HIPEC for malignant peritoneal mesothelioma. *Cancer Treat Res*. 2007;134:343–55.

38. Deraco M, Bartlett D, Kusamura S, Baratti D. Consensus statement on peritoneal mesothelioma. *J Surg Oncol*. 2008;98(4):268–72.

39. Turner KM, Varghese S, Alexander HR Jr. Surgery for peritoneal mesothelioma. *Curr Treat Options Oncol*. 2011;12(2):189–200.

40. Yan TD, Haveric N, Carmignani CP, Chang D, Sugarbaker PH. Abdominal computed tomography scans in the selection of patients with malignant peritoneal mesothelioma for comprehensive treatment with cytoreductive surgery and perioperative intraperitoneal chemotherapy. *Cancer*. 2005;103(4):839–49.

41. Low RN, Barone RM. Combined diffusion-weighted and gadolinium-enhanced MRI can accurately predict the peritoneal cancer index preoperatively in patients being considered for cytoreductive surgical procedures. *Ann Surg Oncol*. 2012;19(5):1394–1401.

42. Vilardell AD, Rasiej MJ, Taub RN, Ichise M. Clinical utility of 18F-Fdg positron emission tomography in malignant peritoneal mesothelioma. *Q J Nucl Med Mol Imaging*. 2016;60(1):54–61.

43. Klumpp BD, Schwenzer N, Aschoff P, Miller S, Kramer U, Claussen CD, et al. Preoperative assessment of peritoneal carcinomatosis: intraindividual comparison of 18F-FDG PET/CT and MRI. *Abdom Imaging*. 2013;38(1):64–71.

44. Tabrizian P, Jayakrishnan TT, Zacharias A, Aycart S, Johnston FM, Sarpel U, et al. Incorporation of diagnostic laparoscopy in the management algorithm for patients with peritoneal metastases: a multi-institutional analysis. *J Surg Oncol*. 2015;111(8):1035–40.

45. Iversen LH, Rasmussen PC, Laurberg S. Value of laparoscopy before cytoreductive surgery and hyperthermic intraperitoneal chemotherapy for peritoneal carcinomatosis. *Br J Surg*. 2013;100(2):285–92.

46. Cotte E, Passot G, Gilly FN, Glehen O. Selection of patients and staging of peritoneal surface malignancies. *World J Gastrointest Oncol*. 2010;2(1): 31–35.

47. Sugarbaker PH. Parietal peritonectomy. *Ann Surg Oncol*. 2012;19(4):1250.

48. Sugarbaker PH. Peritonectomy procedures. *Cancer Treat Res*. 2007;134:247–64.

49. Halkia E, Tsochrinis A, Vassiliadou DT, Pavlakou A, Vaxevanidou A, Datsis A, et al. Peritoneal carcinomatosis: intraoperative parameters in open (coliseum) versus closed abdomen HIPEC. *Int J Surg Oncol*. 2015;2015:610597.

50. Qi D, Hu Y, Li J, Peng T, Su J, He Y, et al. Hyperthermia induces apoptosis of 786-O cells through suppressing Ku80 expression. *PLoS ONE*. 2015;10(4):e0122977.

51. Hubert J, Thiboutot E, Dubé P, Cloutier AS, Drolet P, Sideris L. Cytoreductive surgery and hyperthermic intraperitoneal chemotherapy with oxaliplatin for peritoneal mesothelioma: preliminary results and survival analysis. *Surg Oncol*. 2015;24(1):41–46.

52. Helm JH, Miura JT, Glenn JA, Marcus RK, Larrieux G, Jayakrishnan TT, et al. Cytoreductive surgery and hyperthermic intraperitoneal chemotherapy for malignant peritoneal mesothelioma: a systematic review and meta-analysis. *Ann Surg Oncol*. 2015;22(5):1686–93.

53. Yan TD, Deraco M, Baratti D, Kusamura S, Elias D, Glehen O, et al. Cytoreductive surgery and hyperthermic intraperitoneal chemotherapy for malignant peritoneal mesothelioma: multi-institutional experience. *J Clin Oncol*. 2009;27(36):6237–42.

54. Baratti D, Kusamura S, Cabras AD, Dileo P, Laterza B, Deraco M. Diffuse malignant peritoneal mesothelioma: failure analysis following cytoreduction and hyperthermic intraperitoneal chemotherapy (HIPEC). *Ann Surg Oncol*. 2009;16(2):463–72.

Chapter 13

Non-surgical Treatment of Malignant Mesothelioma

Manuel Fernández-Bruno, Silvia Fernández, Macarena González, Jordi Remon, and Pilar Lianes

Introduction

Malignant mesothelioma is a rare malignancy that arises most commonly from the mesothelial surfaces of the pleural cavity. Frequently most of the patients have advanced disease at diagnosis and are not eligible for multimodality treatment.

Today, we know that malignant pleural mesothelioma (MPM) has an extremely poor prognosis with a median overall survival (OS) of locally advanced or metastatic disease without treatment of 6–9 months and 9–18 months for treated patients, with fewer than 5 percent of patients surviving 5 years, regardless of the therapeutic approach (1). We will focus this chapter on reviewing the different treatment options that we have when this rare and aggressive malignancy begins or progresses to an advanced and non-surgical stage.

Historically, the development of systemic treatment for MPM has been difficult because of the small numbers of patients, problems in determining whether an individual patient is benefiting from treatment, and the poor prognosis associated with advanced disease (2,3). Also, we know that MPM has always been a difficult neoplasm to stage clinically and to evaluate by classical RECIST response evaluation criteria in terms of determining its response to treatments in clinical trials (4).

Nowadays, emerging therapies may offer hope for improved palliation, prolonging survival, and even potentially curing some patients, but the systemic management of MPM in patients who are not suitable for surgical approaches is still an issue and topic for discussion.

We will discuss the chemotherapy combination antifolate/platinum doublet that has demonstrated a significant efficacy benefit (I,A) compared with other chemotherapy schemes in the systemic approach; we will comment about first- and second-line treatment, the role of the maintenance treatment and the new target agents that we have for this neoplasm.

Front-line Therapy

The combination doublet chemotherapy of cisplatin with an antifolate drug, either pemetrexed (a multitarget antifolate drug) or raltitrexed (a thymidylate synthase (TS) inhibitor) has demonstrated statistical superiority in survival time, time to disease progression (TTP), and response rates (RR) compared with cisplatin alone in two phase III trials (5,6), as we see in Table 13.1. There is evidence that three-drug chemotherapy

combinations did not improve efficacy over two-drug combinations (2).

Vogenzal et al. showed in the EMPHACIS trial that the combination schedule with cisplatin plus pemetrexed increased OS to 12.1 months from 9.3 months in comparison with the control arm with cisplatin alone ($p = 0.02$). TTP was 5.7 months vs. 3.9 months, respectively ($p = 0.001$), and RR was 41.3 percent vs. 16.7 percent, respectively ($p < 0.0001$) (6). This trial included 456 patients with MPM. A multivariate regression analysis of prognostic factors in this trial was subsequently provided showing that factors predictive of overall survival were therapy group, vitamin supplementation group, Karnofsky index (IK) (90–100 versus 70–80), disease stage, histologic subtype, and white blood cell count ($\geq 8200/\mu l$ versus lower values) (7). Hence, prognostic factors like non-epithelial histology subtypes, a poor performance status (PS), and the presence of anemia, high white blood cells, and thrombocytosis should be carefully considered before deciding on the treatment option (8). In addition to the demonstrated survival benefit, combination therapy was associated with improvements in symptoms and quality of life. All parameters favored the combination therapy group, including global quality of life, pain, dyspnea, fatigue, anorexia, and cough (9).

A similar survival benefit was observed in the second phase III trial of van Meerbeeck et al. with 250 patients conducted by the European Organisation for Research and Treatment of Cancer (EORTC) Lung Cancer Group. The addition of raltitrexed (another antifolate drug) to cisplatin in this trial demonstrated an increased OS to 11.4 months, compared with 8.8 months with cisplatin as the single agent ($p = 0.048$). However, TTP (5.3 months vs. 4.0 months, respectively; $p = 0.058$) and RR (23.6 percent vs. 13.6 percent, respectively; $p = 0.056$) were not statistically significantly different between the treatment arms (6).

Following the study of Vogelzang et al., the combination of pemetrexed and cisplatin, with prophylactic folic acid and vitamin B12, has been approved by the United States Food and Drug Administration (FDA) for the treatment of patients with malignant pleural mesothelioma whose disease is either unresectable or who are not otherwise candidates for curative surgery. Thereafter, within several years, platinum and antifolate, especially pemetrexed, has been established as a standard of care in front-line chemotherapy for mesothelioma worldwide.

Finally, there are also aspects to be considered by the physician when using these drugs in front-line therapy: the duration

Table 13.1 Main efficacy results of the pivotal phase III trials in the first-line setting in patients with advanced MPM

	EMPHACIS Trial (5)		EORTC Trial (6)	
	Cisplatin plus pemetrexed	Cisplatin	Cisplatin plus raltitrexed	Cisplatin
N	226	222	126	124
RR, %	41.3	16.7	23.6	13.6
P value	<0.0001		0.56	
OS, months	12.1	9.3	11.4	8.8
HR	0.77		0.76	
P value	0.02		0.048	
TTP, months	5.7	3.9	5.3	4
HR	0.68		0.78	
P value	0.001		0.058	

HR: hazard ratio; OS: overall survival; RR: response rate; TTP: time to progression.

of the treatment, the main differences between both antifolate drugs, the effectiveness of the combination of other drugs for unfit patients and patients diagnosed with the sarcomatoid subtype.

In both pivotal trials the treatment continued until disease progression, but the median number of cycles was six in the pemetrexed trial and five in the raltitrexed one, and was reduced to four in the clinical practice by analogy with non small-cell lung cancer (NSCLC). In advanced NSCLC, the administration of more than four cycles will confer more toxicity than clinical benefit in survival terms.

On the other hand, pemetrexed is a multitarget antifolate drug compared with raltitrexed, which only inhibits thymidylate synthase (TS), and a supplementation of folic acid and vitamin B12 is needed to reduce the hematological toxicity. This fact explains the differences in the toxicity profiles in both studies. A recent analysis of the efficacy and cost-effectiveness of first-line chemotherapy in MPM shows that the schedules cisplatin-pemetrexed and cisplatin-raltitrexed are not different in terms of RR, TTP, and OS. Both combinations are cost-effective, but the analysis found that the schedule cisplatin–raltitrexed offers marginally higher quality-adjusted life years (QALY) and life years at a substantially lower total cost than cisplatin–pemetrexed (10). No large non-inferiority trial in patients with MPM to evaluate the substitution of pemetrexed by raltitrexed has been performed yet, probably due to the large number of patients needed.

However, from the results of both phase III trials, we still don't have data to extrapolate the benefit to the subgroups of patients with a moderate or poor PS, the elderly (those > 75 years of age), and patients with sarcomatous histologic subtype. Unfit and elderly patients represent a considerable number of newly diagnosed patients that usually have comorbidities that prevent the use of a standard regimen with cisplatin. In an effort to decrease toxicity, carboplatin was substituted for cisplatin in conjunction with pemetrexed in another trial. There are two phase II trials that have shown indirectly similar results

and efficacy for the carboplatin plus pemetrexed combination in young and elderly patients, with a slightly worse hematological toxicity in the older age group (11). Another phase II trial confirmed the efficacy of the carboplatin–pemetrexed combination as first-line treatment with an overall RR of 29 percent (12). This RR is lower than that reported for the combination of cisplatin plus pemetrexed; however, as we know, radiologic RR is difficult to assess in patients with MPM, and assessment has varied widely between studies. An analysis of the data obtained from 1700 patients with MPM who received pemetrexed plus cisplatin or pemetrexed plus carboplatin under an international expanded access program found that the time to disease progression and the one-year survival were similar (63.1 percent vs. 64.0 percent) in both groups (13). As we know, palliative chemotherapy in unfit patients with ECOG scale of performance status (PS) 2 should not be delayed and should be considered before the appearance of functional clinical signs (14). These results support the combination of pemetrexed plus carboplatin being a possible alternative regimen in this population if cisplatin toxicity is a particular concern.

Other treatment options could be the substitution of a non-platinum partner with an antifolate in patients with MPM. A phase II trial that evaluated the combination of pemetrexed plus gemcitabine in 108 chemotherapy-naïve patients with MPM showed moderate clinical activity, with a RR of 26 percent and a median OS inferior to the outcome observed with cisplatin plus an antifolate (10 months) and significant hematological toxicity, with severe neutropenia occurring in more than 50 percent of patients (15).

Finally, the last question is whether pemetrexed combinations are effective in patients with sarcomatoid histology, which represent almost 10 percent of MPM and provides patients with a prior resistance to chemotherapy treatments, having the worst survival, ranging from 3.5 to 8 months (16).

In a retrospective analysis, 29 of 672 patients analyzed were diagnosed with sarcomatoid MPM and treated with a platinum plus pemetrexed combination. The results showed that standard chemotherapy had only a negligible impact on the prognosis of these patients, with stable disease observed in 21 percent of patients, and a median progression-free survival (PFS) and OS of 3.3 and 7.6 months, respectively (17). In a recent systematic review of response rates of this histology in clinical trials, only the 13.9 percent (95 percent CI: 8.6, 21.6) of RR were achieved for patients with sarcomatoid tumors (18).

Other combination regimens have been tested in the front line without presenting the same success. Cisplatin and gemcitabine were incorporated into clinical practice following results from two phase II trials (19,20). Although the activity of gemcitabine was limited in single-agent studies, response rates for these combinations have ranged from 15 percent to 48 percent, with acceptable levels of toxicity. Median durations of response and overall survival have been similar to those for other regimens. However, given the lack of phase III evidence, the use of gemcitabine as first-line therapy is not supported.

The combination of cisplatin and doxorubicin has been studied in other trials achieving objective response rates varying from 14 per cent to 42 percent, and median survival ranged from 7 to 12 months. The trial with the highest reported response rate (42 percent) and longest median survival (12 months) also had the most prominent gastrointestinal toxicity (21,22).

Maintenance Treatments

The use of continuation or switch maintenance therapy strategy with a single agent, especially with pemetrexed (23), even after an induction treatment with a platinum plus pemetrexed schedule has been effective in NSCLC but has not been evaluated properly in the mesothelioma setting and has not yet been analyzed through a large randomized trial.

The role of pemetrexed as maintenance therapy after an induction with four courses of platinum plus pemetrexed is still being evaluated by a phase II trial led by the Cancer and Leukemia Group B (CALGB) and switch maintenance strategies with a focal adhesion kinase inhibitor, defactinib (VS6063), and gemcitabine are currently under way.

In conclusion, the more convenient administration of maintenance therapy in patients with MPM is still an open question, and the only randomized phase III trial that has evaluated this issue has yielded disappointing results.

Second-line Therapy

Although data are limited, second-line chemotherapy may be effective in patients with malignant pleural mesothelioma, but currently there is still no second-line standard of care.

Phase III randomized evaluation of pemetrexed compared with best supportive care (BSC) as second-line treatment in premetexed-naïve patients was negative for the primary endpoint, OS (8.4 months in the chemotherapy arm vs. 9.7 months for BSC group; $p = 0.74$), possibly because of the significant imbalance in post-discontinuation chemotherapy between arms (51.7 percent in the BSC arm vs. 28.5 percent in the

chemotherapy arm; $p < 0.0002$). Notwithstanding the second-line was associated with an increase in RR (18.7 percent vs. 1.7 percent; $p < 0.0001$) and delayed disease progression (3.7 months vs. 1.5 months; $p = 0.0002$), although it failed to show a benefit in quality of life (QoL) (24). Nevertheless, it is reasonable to use second-line pemetrexed if it has not been used before. Other agents like vinorelbine and gemcitabine have shown appreciable activity in phase II trials as single agents in the second-line setting (25).

Second-line treatment in patients with MPM remains an ideal field to test new chemotherapy agents as well as new therapeutic strategies, so in the absence of a standard treatment, including patients in clinical trials should be a strategy to be considered.

Novel Target Therapies

The lack of responses and the resistance of MPM to conventional treatment have prompted research to identify possible new molecular targets.

Today we know that angiogenesis is an important factor in MPM. Mesothelioma cells secrete and express several angiogenic factors such as VEGF, VEGFR, platelet-derived growth factor (PDGF), and platelet-derived growth factor receptor (PDGFR). Consequently, several anti-angiogenic drugs have been tested in this setting. Bevacizumab, a VEGF-blocking monoclonal antibody, did not show any efficacy advantage in OS ($p = 0.91$) or PFS ($p = 0.88$) when it was combined with cisplatin/gemcitabine over chemotherapy alone in a phase II randomized trial with chemotherapy-naïve patients with MPM. The trial showed a median OS of 15.7 months in the bevacizumab arm, which is better than most other multicenter studies in MPM. If it had been a single-arm trial, the authors could have erroneously concluded that this combination was an active regimen. This study confirms previous data regarding activity of gemcitabine/cisplatin in patients with MPM. However, some cytotoxic agents, but not gemcitabine, stimulate angiogenesis and tumor regrowth by mobilizing circulating endothelial progenitors from bone marrow. This could explain the negative results of this trial. Pretreatment VEGF levels correlated with PFS and OS, suggesting the potential utility of VEGF as a prognostic factor. Bevacizumab-treated patients with lower pretreatment VEGF levels had a longer PFS and OS (26).

Another phase II trial evaluated the addition of bevacizumab to cisplatin and pemetrexed as first-line treatment in advanced MPM. The PFS at 6 months was 56 percent with a median PFS of 6.9 months and a median OS of 14.8 months, but the study failed to meet the primary endpoint of 33 percent improvement in PFS at 6 months compared with historical controls treated with chemotherapy alone (27). These data have been confirmed this year with the preliminary results of Zalcman's phase III MAPS trial, which shows that the addition of bevacizumab to the cisplatin–pemetrexed doublet provides a significantly longer survival in patients with MPM, making this triplet a new treatment paradigm (28).

Table 13.2 Results of main clinical trials carried out with novel drugs in patients with advanced or unresectable MPM as first- or second-line treatment

	Drug	*N*	PR, %	SD, %	PFS, months	OS, months
As second-line treatment						
Jahan et al. (29)	Vatalanib	47	6	72	4.1	10
Garland et al. (30)	Cediranib	54	9	34	2.6	9.5
Campbell et al. (31)	Cediranib	50	10	34	1.9	4.4
Rossoni et al. (33)	NGR-hTNF	57	2	44	9.1*	24.8*
Stevenson et al. (37)	GC-1008	13	NR	23	1.4	13
Garland et al. (39)	Erlotinib	63	NR	42	2	10
Laurie et al. (41)	Sunitinib	35	NR	NR	2.8	8.3
Dubey et al. (42)	Sorafenib	51	6	54	3.6	9.7
Garland et al. (45)	Everolimus	61	NR	NR	3	5
As first-line treatment						
Hassan et al. (36)	Amatuximab	89	39	51	6.1	14.5
O'Brien et al. (46)	Bortezomib	82	NR	NR	5.1	13.5

NR: not reported; OS: overall survival; PFS: progression-free survival; PR: partial response; SD: stable disease.
* In patients with disease control and weekly NGR-hTNF administration.

Other VEGF targeting strategies, such as blocking the tyrosine kinase (TK) domain of the VEGFR with vatalanib, have not shown substantial evidence of efficacy (29). Cediranib is another VEGFR and PDGFR TK inhibitor. Cediranib at 45 mg daily as monotherapy has shown modest activity in MPM after platinum-based therapy (RR: 9 percent, PFS: 2.6 months and OS: 9.5 months). However, some patient tumors were highly sensitive to cediranib (34 percent of patients with stable disease and one-year survival rate of 36 percent) (30,31). These results highlight the need to identify a predictive biomarker for this drug.

The immunotherapy strategy has shown significant preclinical activity of the human tumor necrosis factor α (TNF-α) mediated through apoptosis of tumor endothelial cells via caspase activation, but has proven to be too toxic for use in clinical trials. To help favorably shift the dose–response curve, TNF-α was fused to a cyclic tumor-homing peptide, NGR (asparagine–glycine–arginine), which selectively binds to CD13 overexpressed on the epithelial cells of solid tumors (32).

In a phase II trial in 57 previously treated patients evaluating NGR-hTNF every three weeks or weekly, 46 percent of patients achieved disease control and median PFS was 2.8 months. For 14 patients with disease control on weekly NGR-hTNF, the median PFS and OS were 9.1 and 24.8 months, respectively, compared with 4.4 and 13.3 months, respectively, in the 3-weekly schedule. PS of 0 and a low baseline neutrophil to lymphocyte ratio ($p = 0.04$) were two variables associated with improved OS (33). The results of a second-line randomized phase III trial with MPM (NCT01098266) comparing the best investigator choice (BIC) plus weekly NGR-hTNF with BIC plus placebo reported OS and PFS benefit with NGR-hTNF plus chemotherapy in patients with a short prior treatment-free interval. A confirmatory first-line phase III trial is deserved (34).

SS1P is an immunotoxin-linked antibody against mesothelin. Front-line treatment in 19 patients with cisplatin plus pemetrexed and SS1P (45 μg/kg) was well tolerated, and achieved partial responses of 50 percent. Additionally, serum mesothelin response in 63–83 percent of patients correlated with radiological responses in all patients who obtained a partial response (35).

Amatuximab (MORAb-009) is a high-affinity chimeric monoclonal antibody against mesothelin. A phase II trial combined MORAb-009 and cisplatin plus pemetrexed for 6 cycles and then MORAb-009 was given as maintenance therapy in 89 patients. After six cycles of chemotherapy, 63 percent of patients received amatuximab as single agent. By independent radiological review, 39 percent of patients had partial responses and 51 percent had stable disease, with a median PFS of 6.1 months and a median OS of 14.5 months (36). It is possible that patients who received maintenance therapy had longer PFS and it is important to know which biomarker could be associated with the efficacy of this new drug. Another monoclonal antibody against TGF-β, GC-1008 – a pleiotropic cytokine overexpressed by MPM – achieved a median OS of 14 months in 13 patients (37).

PDGF is a growth factor inducing mesothelial cell proliferation. The PDGF-α receptor is overexpressed in mesothelioma cells and high serum PDGF in patients with MPM seems to be an independent prognostic marker of poor survival (38). Imatinib is a TK inhibitor of c-kit and PDGFR, but as a single agent is not an effective treatment of MPM disease. Two phase II trials are testing imatinib in combination with cisplatin and pemetrexed as first-line treatment of patients with MPM

(NCT 00402766). In another trial, the combination of gemcitabine plus imatinib is being tested after failure on cisplatin plus pemetrexed (NCT 00551252).

Despite the 50 percent expression of epidermal growth factor receptor (EGFR) in mesothelioma tissue, activation mutations are not usually present and the results of trials using erlotinib (39) and gefitinib (40) have been disappointing. Other drugs such as sunitinib (41) and sorafenib (42) have shown limited activity as single agents in the treatment of patients with MPM, and results with all these agents are difficult to interpret because of patient selection.

Insulin growth factor receptor (IGFR) is also expressed in MPM. Cixutumumab, a humanized monoclonal antibody against IGFR, is active against MPM cells and a phase II clinical trial to confirm this efficacy is currently ongoing.

Dasatinib, an inhibitor of the Src family of non-receptor TK and PDGFR, has also been tested in MPM, but as a second-line single agent has no activity and is associated with pulmonary toxicities, such as pleural effusion observed in 9 percent of patients. Colony-stimulating factor-1 (CSF-1) could be used as a dasatinib biomarker of outcome (43). Ranpirnase is a ribonuclease. In a phase III trial, single-agent doxorubicin was compared with doxorubicin plus ranpirnase, but the combination did not improve OS (44). Other drugs such as everolimus, an oral mTOR inhibitor, did not achieve positive results in a recent phase II trial (45). Bortezomib, a proteasome inhibitor (46), and pazopanib, an oral angiogenesis inhibitor, are currently being evaluated in phase II trials.

Table 13.2 summarizes and compares the results obtained from the most important clinical trials carried out with new drugs in patients with MPM.

References

1. Aisner J. Current approach to malignant mesothelioma of the pleura. *Chest.* 1995;107:332S.

2. Berghmans T, Paesmans M, Lalami Y, Louviaux I, Luce S, Mascaux C, et al. Activity of chemotherapy and immunotherapy on malignant mesothelioma: a systematic review of the literature with meta-analysis. *Lung Cancer.* 2002;38:111.

3. Tomek S, Emri S, Krejcy K, Manegold C. Chemotherapy for malignant pleural mesothelioma: past results and recent developments. *Br J Cancer.* 2003;88:167.

4. Byrne MJ, Nowak AK. Modified RECIST criteria for assessment of response in malignant pleural mesothelioma. *Ann Oncol.* 2004;15:257–60.

5. Vogelzang NJ, Rusthoven JJ, Symanowski J, Denham C, Kaukel E, Ruffie P, et al. Phase III study of pemetrexed in combination with cisplatin versus cisplatin alone in patients with malignant pleural mesothelioma. *J Clin Oncol.* 2003;21:2636–44.

6. van Meerbeeck JP, Gaafar R, Manegold C, Van Klaveren RJ, Van Marck EA, Vincent M, et al. Randomized phase III study of cisplatin with or without raltitrexed in patients with malignant pleural mesothelioma: an intergroup study of the European Organisation for Research and Treatment of Cancer Lung Cancer Group and the National Cancer Institute of Canada. *J Clin Oncol.* 2005;23:6881–89.

7. Symanowski JT, Rusthoven J, Nguyen B, et al. Multiple regression analysis of prognostic variables for survival from the phase III study of pemetrexed plus cisplatin vs. cisplatin in malignant pleural mesothelioma (abstract). *Proc Am Soc Clin Oncol* 2003;22:647a.

8. Curran D, Sahmoud T, Therasse P, van Meerbeeck J, Postmus PE, Giaccone G. Prognostic factors in patients with pleural mesothelioma: the European Organization for Research and Treatment of Cancer experience. *J Clin Oncol.* 1998;16:145–52.

9. Gralla RJ, Hollen PJ, Liepa AM, et al. Improving quality of life in patients with malignant pleural mesothelioma: results of the randomized pemetrexed + cisplatin vs cisplatin trial using the LCSS-meso instrument (abstract). *Proc Am Soc Clin Oncol.* 2003;22:621a.

10. Woods B, Paracha N, Scott DA, Thatcher N. Raltitrexed plus cisplatin is cost-effective compared with pemetrexed plus cisplatin in patients with malignant pleural mesothelioma. *Lung Cancer.* 2012;75:261–67.

11. Ceresoli GL, Castagneto B, Zucali PA, Favoretto A, Mencoboni M, Grossi F, et al. Pemetrexed plus carboplatin in elderly patients with malignant pleural mesothelioma: combined analysis of two phase II trials. *Br J Cancer.* 2008;99:51–56.

12. Katirtzoglou N, Gkiozos I, Makrilia N, Tsaroucha E, Rapti A, Stratakos G, et al. Carboplatin plus pemetrexed as first-line treatment of patients with malignant pleural mesothelioma: a phase II study. *Clin Lung Cancer.* 2010;11:30–35.

13. Santoro A, O'Brien ME, Stahel RA, Nackaerts K, Baas P, Karthaus M, et al. Pemetrexed plus cisplatin or pemetrexed plus carboplatin for chemonaive patients with malignant pleural mesothelioma: results of the International Expanded Access Program. *J Thorac Oncol.* 2008;3:756–63.

14. O'Brien ME, Watkins D, Ryan C, Priest K, Corbishley C, Norton A, et al. A randomized trial in malignant mesothelioma of early versus delayed chemotherapy in symptomatically stable patients: the MED trial. *Ann Oncol.* 2006;17:270–75.

15. Janne PA, Simon GR, Langer CJ, Taub RN, Dowlati A, Fidias P, et al. Phase II trial of pemetrexed and gemcitabine in chemotherapy-naive malignant pleural mesothelioma. *J Clin Oncol.* 2008;26:1465–71.

16. Galetta D, Catino A, Misino A, Logroscino A, Fico M. Sarcomatoid mesothelioma: future advances in diagnosis, biomolecular assessment, and therapeutic options in a poor-outcome disease. *Tumori.* 2016;102(2):127–30.

17. Gattoni E, Grosso F, Roveta A, Libener R, Degiovanni D, Mancuso M, et al. Outcomes of sarcomatoid malignant pleural mesothelioma, a distinct clinical entity. *ASCO Meeting Abstracts.* 2012;30:7084.

18. Mansfield AS, Symanowski JT, Peikert T. Systematic review of response rates

of sarcomatoid malignant pleural mesotheliomas in clinical trials. *Lung Cancer*. 2014;86(2):133–36.

19. Byrne MJ, Davidson JA, Musk AW, Dewar J, van Hazel G, Buck M, et al. Cisplatin and gemcitabine treatment for malignant mesothelioma: a phase II study. *J Clin Oncol*. 1999;17:25–30.

20. Nowak AK, Byrne MJ, Williamson R, Ryan G, Segal A, Fielding D, et al. A multicentre phase II study of cisplatin and gemcitabine for malignant mesothelioma. *Br J Cancer*. 2002;87:491–96.

21. Chahinian AP, Antman K, Goutsou M, Corson JM, Suzuki Y, Modeas C, et al. Randomized phase II trial of cisplatin with mitomycin or doxorubicin for malignant mesothelioma by the Cancer and Leukemia Group B. *J Clin Oncol*. 1993;11:1559.

22. Henss H, Fiebig HH, Schildge J, Arnold H, Hasse J. Phase-II study with the combination of cisplatin and doxorubicin in advanced malignant mesothelioma of the pleura. *Onkologie*. 1988;11:118.

23. Ciuleanu T, Brodowicz T, Zielinski C, Kim JH, Krzakowski M, Laack E, et al. Maintenance pemetrexed plus best supportive care versus placebo plus best supportive care for non-small-cell lung cancer: a randomised, double-blind, phase 3 study. *Lancet*. 2009;374: 1432–40.

24. Jassem J, Ramlau R, Santoro A, Schuette W, Chemaissani A, Hong S, et al. Phase III trial of pemetrexed plus best supportive care compared with best supportive care in previously treated patients with advanced malignant pleural mesothelioma. *J Clin Oncol*. 2008;26:1698–704.

25. Zauderer MG, Kass SL, Woo K, Sima CS, Ginsberg MS, Krug LM, et al. Vinorelbine and gemcitabine as second-line or third-line therapy for malignant pleural mesothelioma. *Lung Cancer*. 2014;84:271–74.

26. Kindler HL, Karrison TG, Gandara DR, Lu C, Krug LM, Stevenson JP, et al. Multicenter, double-blind, placebo-controlled, randomized phase II trial of gemcitabine/cisplatin plus bevacizumab or placebo in patients with malignant mesothelioma. *J Clin Oncol*. 2012;30:2509–15.

27. Dowell JE, Dunphy FR, Taub RN, Gerber DE, Ngov L, Yan J, et al. A multicenter phase II study of cisplatin, pemetrexed, and bevacizumab in patients with advanced malignant mesothelioma. *Lung Cancer*. 2012;77(3):567–71.

28. Zalcman G, et al. Bevacizumab 25mg/kg plus cisplatin-pemetrexed (CP) triplet versus CP doublet in Malignant Pleural Mesothelioma (MPM): Results of the IFCTGFPC-0701 MAPS randomizes phase 3 trial. *ASCO Meeting Abstracts*. 2015;400s:7500.

29. Jahan T, Gu L, Kratzke R, Dudek A, Otterson GA, Wang X, et al. Vatalanib in malignant mesothelioma: a phase II trial by the Cancer and Leukemia Group B (CALGB 30107). *Lung Cancer*. 2012;76:393–96.

30. Garland LL, Chansky K, Wozniak AJ, Tsao AS, Gadgel SM, Veerschraegen CF, et al. Phase II study of cediranib in patients with malignant pleural mesothelioma: SWOG S0509. *J Thorac Oncol*. 2011;6:1938–45.

31. Campbell NP, Kunnavakkam R, Leighl NB, et al. Cediranib (C) in patients (pts) with malignant mesothelioma (MM): A phase II trial of The University of Chicago Phase II Consortium. *ASCO Meeting Abstracts*. 2011;29:7027.

32. Curnis F, Arrigoni G, Sacchi A, Fischetti L, Arap W, Pasqualini R, et al. Differential binding of drugs containing the NGR motif to CD13 isoforms in tumor vessels, epithelia, and myeloid cells. *Cancer Res*. 2002;62:867–74.

33. Rossoni G, Gregorc V, Vigano MG, Butta A, Ghio D, Lambiase A, et al. NGR-hTNF as second-line treatment in malignant pleural mesothelioma (MPM). *ASCO Meeting Abstracts*. 2012;30:7076.

34. Gaafar RM, Favoretto A, Gregorc V, Grossi F, Jassem J, Polychronis A, et al. Phase III trial (NGR015) with NGR-hTNF plus best investigator choice (BIC) versus placebo plus BIC in previously treated patients with advanced malignant pleural mesothelioma (MPM). *ASCO Meeting Abstracts*. 2015;400s:7501.

35. Hassan R, Sharon E, Thomas A, Zhang J, Ling A, Miettinen M, et al. Phase 1 study of the antimesothelin immunotoxin SS1P in combination with pemetrexed and cisplatin for front-line therapy of pleural mesothelioma and correlation of tumor response with serum mesothelin, megakaryocyte potentiating factor and cancer antigen 125. *Cancer*. 2014;120(21):3311–19.

36. Hassan R, Jahan TM, Kindler HL, Bazhenova L, Reck M, Thomas A, et al. Phase II clinical trial of amatuximab, a chimeric antimesothelin antibody with pemetrexed and cisplatin in advanced unresectable pleural mesothelioma. *Clin Cancer Res*. 2014;20(23):5927–36.

37. Stevenson J, Kindler HL, Schwed D, et al. Phase II trial of anti-transforming growth factor-beta (TGFβ) monoclonal antibody GC1008 in relapsed malignant pleural mesothelioma (MPM). *ASCO Meeting Abstracts*. 2012;30:7077.

38. Filiberti R, Marroni P, Neri M, Ardizzoni A, Betta PG, Cafferata MA, et al. Serum PDGF-AB in pleural mesothelioma. *Tumour Biol*. 2005;26:221–26.

39. Garland LL, Rankin C, Gandara DR, Rivkin SE, Scott KM, Nagle RB, et al. Phase II study of erlotinib in patients with malignant pleural mesothelioma: a Southwest Oncology Group Study. *J Clin Oncol*. 2007;25:2406–13.

40. Govindan R, Kratzke RA, Herndon JE, 2nd, Niehans GA, Vollmer R, Watson D, et al. Gefitinib in patients with malignant mesothelioma: a phase II study by the Cancer and Leukemia Group B. *Clin Cancer Res*. 2005;11:2300–04.

41. Laurie SA, Gupta A, Chu Q, Lee CW, Morzycki W, Feld R, et al. Brief report: a phase II study of sunitinib in malignant pleural mesothelioma. the NCIC Clinical Trials Group. *J Thorac Oncol*. 2011;6:1950–54.

42. Dubey S, Janne PA, Krug L, Pang H, Wang X, Heinze R, et al. A phase II study of sorafenib in malignant mesothelioma: results of Cancer and Leukemia Group B 30307. *J Thorac Oncol*. 2010;5:1655–61.

43. Dudek AZ, Pang H, Kratzke RA, Otterson GA, Hodgson L, Vokes EE, et al. Phase II study of dasatinib in patients with previously treated malignant mesothelioma (cancer and leukemia group B 30601): a brief report. *J Thorac Oncol*. 2012;7:755–59.

44. Reck M, Krzakowski M, Jassem J, et al. Randomized, multicenter phase III study of ranpirnase plus doxorubicin (DOX) versus DOX in patients with unresectable malignant mesothelioma (MM). *ASCO Meeting Abstracts*. 2009;27:7507.

45. Garland LL, Ou S-H, Moon J, Mack PC, Testa J, Tsao AS, et al. SWOG 0722: a phase II study of mTOR inhibitor everolimus (RAD001) in malignant pleural mesothelioma (MPM). *J Thorac Oncol.* 2015;10(2):387–91.

46. O'Brien M, Gaafar RM, Popat S, Grossi F, Price A, Talbot DC, et al. Phase II study of first-line bortezomib and cisplatin in malignant pleural mesothelioma and prospective validation of progression free survival rate as a primary end-point for mesothelioma clinical trials (European Organisation for Research and Treatment of Cancer 08052). *Eur J Cancer.* 2013;49(13):2815–22.

Primary Carcinoma of the Pleura and Peritoneum

Bonnie Balzer

So-called "Primary Pleural Carcinoma"

The literature contains a small number of case reports of patients with putative primary pleural carcinoma. However, in 1956, Babolini et al. suggested that this entity was questionable, and described their findings as the "pleural form of primary lung cancer" (1). Indeed, the diagnosis of primary pleural carcinoma in cases reported in the literature has seldom been based on comprehensive histopathologic examination and has relied heavily upon clinicoradiologic parameters such as anatomic location and size of the tumor, radiologic appearance, and clinical history (2,3). Historically, in the setting of a large pleural tumor with no involvement of the lung parenchyma and no known history of malignancy, a theoretical case could have been made for at least considering the possibility that the pleura was the primary site. As pathology practice has evolved to its current standard with the advent of immunohistochemistry combined with advanced imaging, once extrapulmonary carcinomas are excluded, carcinomas with extensive pleurotropic growth are all now classified and subtyped as primary lung carcinomas. More importantly, these tumors are treated as lung primaries to the benefit of the patient whose access to therapies, clinical expertise, study participation and prognostication are well-established for lung carcinoma and non-existent for so-called "primary pleural carcinomas."

Pathologic Features

Rigorous criteria for accepting a carcinoma as pleural-based have never been formally established, and of particular importance is whether or not *any* lung parenchymal involvement disqualifies a case from consideration (2,4,5). In each of the types of carcinoma reported in the literature as primary pleural carcinoma, lung involvement has been permitted, albeit to a limited extent, and pleural infiltration was considered the overriding feature. Primary lung carcinomas, particularly those at the periphery of the lobes, and malignancies originating in the mediastinum (e.g., thymic) often show direct pleural spread and may grow through the pleura, forming large tumor beds. These patterns of involvement have the capacity to mimic a primary tumor of the pleura, histologically, clinically, and radiologically. Prior odds would indicate that by far the most common carcinoma to show pleurotropic growth by local invasion is of pulmonary origin. In current practice, carcinomas involving the pleura are classified as secondary spread from primary lung carcinomas which may occur by direct seeding or invasion or by metastasis. Although any subtype of lung carcinoma can show this pattern of spread, in practice the vast majority of carcinomas displaying this pleural predominant infiltration are adenocarcinomas. This is not surprising because adenocarcinoma comprises ~ 40 percent of non-small cell lung carcinomas, making it the most common histologic subtype of lung carcinoma (5,6). Adding to the diagnostic difficulty is the fact that the most common histologic subtype of metastatic carcinomas to the pleura from extrapulmonary primary sites are also adenocarcinomas, e.g., breast or gynecologic carcinomas in women which can show extensive pleurotropic growth and significant histologic heterogeneity (7).

Other histologic subtypes of carcinoma reported as pleural primaries include two cases of mucoepidermoid carcinoma (8), and one case of squamous cell carcinoma (9).

Pseudomesotheliomatous Carcinoma of the Pleura

Approximately 80 cases of "pseudomesotheliomatous carcinoma," a term first utilized by Harwood et al. in 1976 (10), have been reported. Unlike squamous cell carcinoma and mucoepidermoid carcinoma, which show classic microscopic features as would be present in any organ, pseudomesotheliomatous carcinoma has a distinctive appearance and is the closest approximation to the original but dubious concept of primary pleural carcinoma.

Radiologic Features

Most cases diagnosed as pseudomesotheliomatous carcinoma cases demonstrate predominantly pleural involvement with pleural thickening and nodularity similar to that seen in malignant mesothelioma. Pleural effusions are common (11).

Clinical Features

Pseudomesotheliomatous carcinoma, like malignant mesothelioma, has a distinctive male predominance (7:1) (11). Age ranges from 23 to 96 with a mean of ~ 63 years. The clinical presentation of pseudomesotheliomatous carcinoma and malignant mesothelioma are essentially identical. In a retrospective review (2), dyspnea on exertion was the most common complaint and most patients exhibited more than one symptom including chest pain/discomfort, cough, fatigue, and weight loss

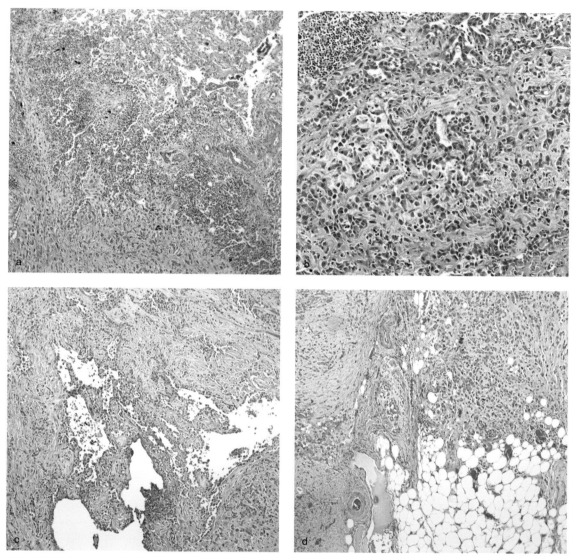

Figure 14.1 Pseudomesotheliomatous carcinoma in a 72-year-old female who underwent extrapleural pneumonectomy. (a) Interface between lung and pleura. (b) High-power view of epithelioid cells forming irregular nests. (c) Tubulopapillary architecture. (d) Infiltration of the tumor into the pleura and fat and vascular invasion.

(11). As with mesothelioma, pseudomesotheliomatous carcinoma shows a definite association with asbestos exposure in selected cases (11). Environmental risk factors also include smoking (2,11).

Pathology

Pseudomesotheliomatous carcinoma is a clinicopathologic entity loosely defined as a poorly differentiated epithelioid malignancy which shares a microscopic and immunohistochemical phenotype indistinguishable from poorly differentiated pulmonary adenocarcinoma. It exhibits pleural predominant (although not exclusive) growth and partially or fully encases the lung, sometimes with involvement of the chest wall and/or diaphragm. Grossly, cases described under this heading demonstrate atelectatic lung nearly completely encased by a thickened pleura often with fusion of the visceral and parietal pleura (10). Microscopically, the most characteristic feature is the diffuse and unrelenting infiltration of pleura by cords, glands, and acinar and stratified papillary arrays of malignant epithelioid, cuboidal, hobnail, or rhabdoid cells. Cytologically, the cells show nuclear hyperchromasia, nucleomegaly, and prominent eosinophilic cytoplasm. Despite the high-grade appearance there is a striking uniformity to the cells with only random pleomorphism and limited anaplasia, resembling some features of epithelioid mesothelioma. At the junction of the pleura and lung only minimal pulmonary parenchymal involvement is present (Figures 14.1–14.4). The managerial consolidation of pleural and pulmonary carcinoma reduces the clinically significant differential diagnosis to metastatic carcinoma of extrapulmonary type and malignant

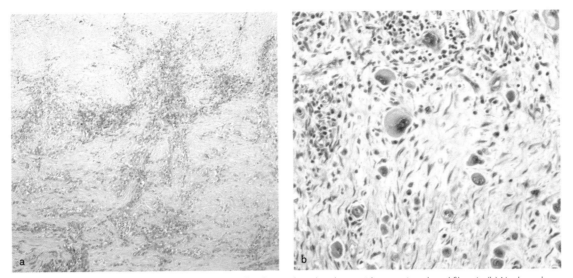

Figure 14.2 (a) Pseudoepitheliomatous carcinoma diffusely invading the pleura with extensive pleural fibrosis. (b) Nuclear pleomorphism and cytologic enlargement with some cells showing multinucleation.

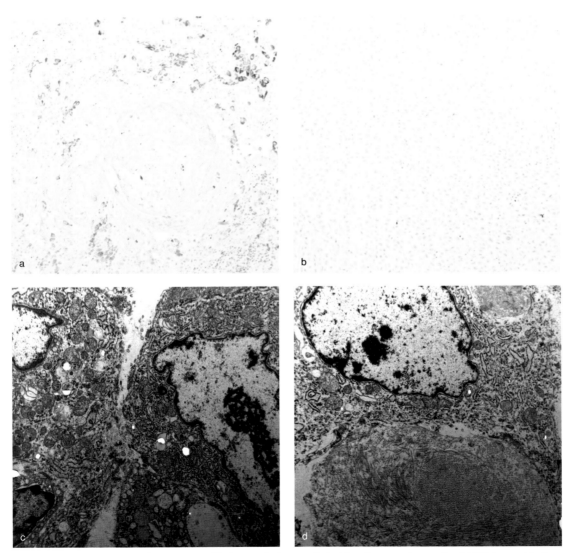

Figure 14.3 (a) Immunostain demonstrating CK5/6 positivity in some foci while others remain negative. (b) TTF-1 negativity in pseudomesotheliomatous carcinoma. (c) Ultrastructure of pseudomesotheliomatous carcinoma showing numerous mitochondria. (d) Intermediate filaments on electron microscopy. (Electron microscopy performed and photographed by Danial Leal.)

Table 14.1 Immunohistochemical selectivities (in %) in pleuropulmonary adenocarcinomas of pulmonary vs. non-pulmonary origin (33–40)

DX	LUNG	BRST	Cholan	Endom	PANC	GALL	GYNM	GASTR	URO
CK7	>85	~90	95	95	~95	~95	100	70	90
CK20	<10	<5	~45	5	~45	~30	0	~45	40
TTF-1	70+	0	90+*	~5	0	0	5–10	1	0
Mamma	<1	85	0	0	0	0	0	0	0
CDX2	~12	0	0	0	0	0	10–15	>90	0
GATA-3	12	>90	10	<10	37	<5	<10	<10	90
ER/PR	<5	~70	0	70	0	0	90	0	0
PAX-8	0	0	0	98	<1	<1	~70	<1	23
GCDFP	<5	~55	0	~40	<1	NA	<1	0	0
WT-1	3	10	0	0	0	0	>80	NA	>90

Notations: Mucinous adenocarcinoma is not included (>90 percent CK20+); BRST: breast; Cholan: cholangiocarcinoma; Endom: endometrium; GALL: gallbladder; GASTR: gastric cancer; GYNM: ovarian, serous, pelvic, fallopian tube carcinoma; Mamma: mammaglobin; PANC: pancreas; URO: urothelial.

mesothelioma which would have different therapeutic modalities. In the absence of a documented history or radiologic studies indicating an extrapulmonary mass, ancillary studies are frequently required to make a definitive diagnosis between these two entities.

Immunohistochemistry

Although morphologic features do play a significant role in differentiating among types of carcinoma, successful lineage assignment of adenocarcinomas is more challenging and often requires evaluation with at least a limited panel of immunostains. Even with the expanding arrays of antibodies available, distinguishing pulmonary carcinomas from their metastatic mimics and from mesothelioma can still be elusive, especially when applied to small specimens and biopsies, which are increasingly common.

Pulmonary vs. Non-pulmonary Adenocarcinoma with Extensive Pleural Spread

Although lung-specific markers are not available, it is possible to separate primary from metastatic carcinomas to the lungs, or at least to categorize them into clinically useful categories for treatment (12). The majority of lung adenocarcinomas demonstrate a CK7+/CK20– immunoprofile. Table 14.1 lists the most common sites of metastasis to the lung and immunostains which can be employed for narrowing the differential diagnosis and establishing a definitive diagnosis. Selection of any one immunostain is largely dependent on the morphology and clinical information available.

Pulmonary Adenocarcinoma with Extensive Pleural Spread vs. Malignant Mesothelioma

Application of immunohistochemistry has demonstrated varying sensitivities and specificities (14). In this particular setting,

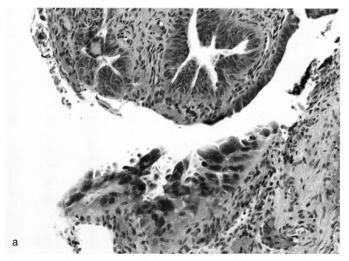
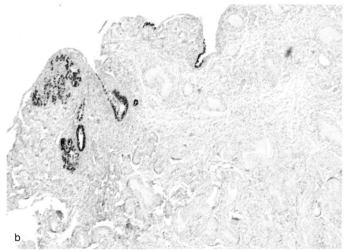

Figure 14.4 (a) Fallopian tubal fimbria with serous tubal intraepithelial carcinoma demonstrating high-grade cytology replacing the surface epithelium. (b) Strong p53 nuclear reactivity supporting the diagnosis of STIC.

a limited panel can consist of two mesothelioma-associated markers (e.g., calretinin, WT-1, and podoplanin; ±CK5/6, mesothelin), and two to three adenocarcinoma-associated markers (e.g., CK7, MOC-31, CEA, Ber-EP4, ±B72.3, claudin 4). Addition of pulmonary organ-selective markers (e.g., TTF-1, napsin A, Surfactant A), supplemented if necessary by non-pulmonary organ-selective markers, will usually succeed in distinguishing pulmonary carcinomas from mesothelioma. Some ultrastructural studies of pseudoepitheliomatous carcinoma revealed the presence of sparse and short microvilli in tumor cells, suggesting origin from Type II pneumocytes, but electron microscopy has limited utility in the differential diagnosis (11,13).

Recently, differences in DNA methylation profiles have shown promise in separating adenocarcinoma from malignant mesothelioma (15), but most practice settings do not have routine access to such techniques. Another study has demonstrated a P16/CDKN2A deletion in malignant mesothelioma (16,17). Molecular profiling has detected additional abnormalities in malignant mesothelioma which differ from adenocarcinoma, but these are not yet translated into routine testing in standard pathology practice (18,19).

Treatment and Prognosis

Prognosis is poor, ranging from 8 to 13 months, despite aggressive, usually multimodal (chemotherapy, radiation, surgery), treatment (2).

"Primary Peritoneal" Carcinoma

Primary peritoneal carcinoma (PPC), was accepted in the past as carcinoma arising from the extended Müllerian system. However, our understanding of this type of carcinoma has undergone a significant shift in recent decades as a result of several factors, including meticulous morphologic examination of fully resected specimens and investigative studies utilizing molecular techniques and genetic testing uncovering new information (20). Although this journey to the currently held theory of the origins of PPC is intriguing, it is beyond the scope of this chapter, and interested readers are referred to several reviews on the topic (20,21).

Radiology

Radiologic characteristics of peritoneal carcinoma are relatively non-specific and correlate with the extent and location of disease, whether limited to the pelvis or involving the entire intra-abdominal cavity. Generally, findings include ascites, omental enlargement, peritoneal nodularity, and ovarian enlargement which is usually bilateral.

Clinical

Sporadic high-grade papillary serous carcinoma (HGPSC) is more common than papillary serous carcinoma (PSC) associated with the BRCA1 and BRCA2 hereditary breast–ovarian cancer syndrome (22). Mutations in the tumor suppressor genes BRCA1 and BRCA2 are inherited in an autosomal dominant pattern and PSC associated with germline BRCA mutations accounts for 10–15 percent of ovarian carcinoma, most of which is of the high-grade serous subtype. The lifetime risk (to age 70) in a patient with a BRCA1 mutation for developing ovarian cancer is 35–70 percent and in BRCA2 mutation carriers this lifetime risk is 10–30 percent, compared with the general population for which the risk is less than 2 percent. Although outcomes data are limited, the prognoses of HGPSC controlled for stage is comparable for BRCA mutation carriers as for patients lacking the mutations. Prophylactic bilateral salpingo-oophorectomy has been shown to significantly reduce the risk of developing carcinoma in BRCA mutation carriers, although it does not eliminate it entirely (23).

Peritoneal tumors of Müllerian cell origin are considered to occur exclusively in women, although rare cases have been reported in men (24,25). The symptoms of peritoneal progression from extra-ovarian carcinomas are often non-specific and frequently caused by advanced disease. Symptoms present are pelvic or abdominal pain, bloating, indigestion, abdominal distention, early satiety, and pain with intercourse.

Pathology

Classification of ovarian and extra-ovarian peritoneal carcinomas has changed significantly over the past decade, with the most recent iteration broadly categorizing tumors into type I and type II neoplasms based upon their histologic, clinical, and molecular features (26,27). The type I tumors include low-grade serous, low-grade endometrioid, and grade-independent mucinous, clear cell, and transitional cell carcinomas. These tumors are hypothesized to originate from atypical proliferative borderline tumors, endometriosis, or within benign cystic proliferations, and adenofibromas, rather than from the peritoneal serous membranes. Molecular alterations which drive the type I pathway involve the KRAS, BRAF, or ERBB2 genes, and TP53 mutations are lacking (27). This group of tumors exhibits an indolent clinical course and a slow tempo for progression to invasive carcinoma. Type II carcinomas – the main focus of this section – account for the majority of extra-ovarian carcinomas involving the peritoneum (21). This category includes high-grade serous and high-grade endometrioid carcinomas, undifferentiated carcinomas, and carcinosarcomas. Until recently, identification of an *in situ* or precursor lesion has eluded investigators, but studies now indicate that the majority of Type II carcinomas appear to originate from intraepithelial carcinoma in the fallopian tube that rapidly progress to extensively involve the peritoneum. Type II carcinomas are marked by TP53 mutations and they lack mutations of KRAS, BRAF, or ERBB2. Rarely do cases of Type I carcinoma evolve or progress to Type II carcinomas (28).

Type II cancers are generally detected at an advanced clinical stage and patients often present with peritoneal carcinomatosis with the ovaries harboring a large burden of disease involving

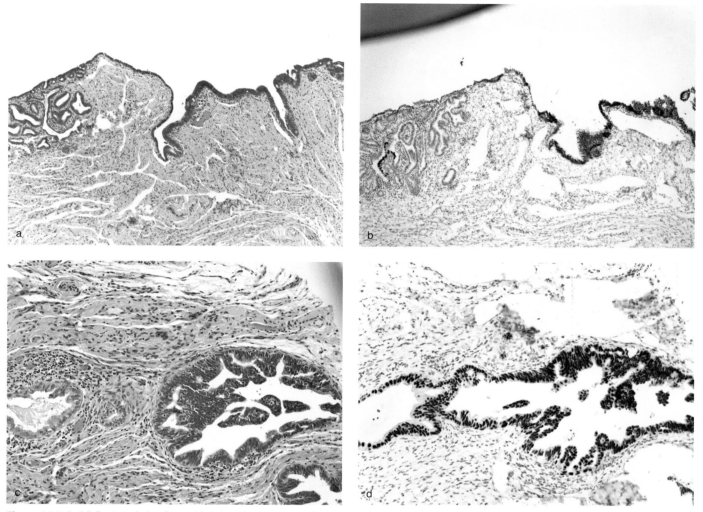

Figure 14.5 (a,c) Fallopian tubal surface epithelial involvement in non-fimbriated areas showing characteristic high-grade serous type cytology. (b,d) Strong p53 nuclear immunoreactivity which characterizes this lesion.

all the pelvic organs obscuring an obvious precursor and/or primary site of origin. In the past, the assumption that the bulk of the tumor burden was the primary site of disease in serous carcinomas has led to assignment of these carcinomas as ovarian in the majority of cases. However, a small but persistent subset of cases demonstrated extensive peritoneal carcinomatosis with little ovarian involvement. In 1993 the Gynecologic Oncology Group established guidelines for classifying tumors as primary peritoneal carcinoma (29). These were (1) ovaries that are of normal size or enlarged only as a result of a benign process; (2) extent of extra-ovarian involvement greater than surface ovarian involvement; (3) ovaries that do not show evidence of cortical invasion or are confined to the ovarian surface epithelium and invasion into cortical stroma is less than 5×5 mm; (4) histologically, carcinoma is primarily of serous type. Regardless of the specific site of origin, HGPSC predominantly involving the peritoneum is currently and has always been managed as high-stage ovarian serous carcinoma (30).

Within the last decade of studies, evidence has been uncovered implicating a fallopian tube precursor to Type II cancers, and the current prevailing theory is that the majority of ovarian surface epithelial carcinomas are invariably derived from a fallopian tube precursor (20,21). Evidence supporting this hypothesis has centered on the fact that in the majority of HGPSC cases, serous tubal intraepithelial carcinoma (STIC) lesions are found, most commonly in the fimbriated ends of the fallopian tubes (Figure 14.4). Microscopically, STIC lesions resemble HGPSC but are confined to the epithelium (Figure 14.5). In some cases, invasion can be found in the fallopian tube (Figure 14.6). Furthermore, in ~20 percent of the fallopian tubes submitted from patients who undergo prophylactic salpingo-oophorectomy for germ-line mutations of *BRCA1* and *BRCA2*, STIC lesions are identified, sometimes as the only pathologic abnormality (27). This finding also discredits the alternative theory of so-called "primary peritoneal carcinoma" with intraepithelial backspread to the fallopian tube.

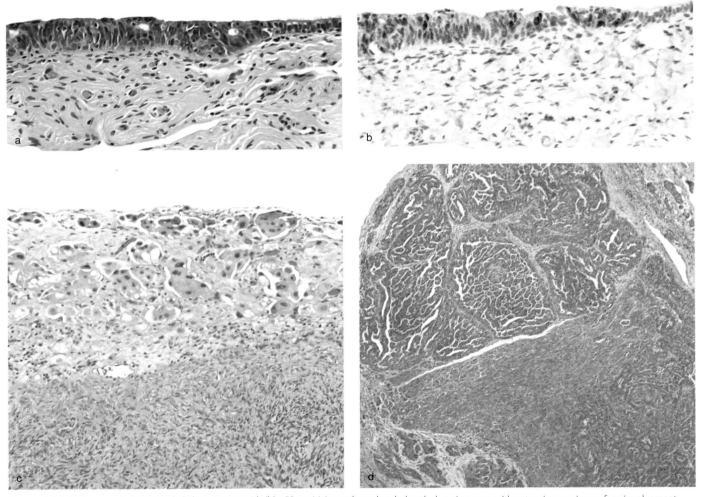

Figure 14.6 (a) Serous tubal intraepithelial carcinoma with (b) p53 positivity as the only tubal pathology in a case with extensive ovarian surface involvement (c) and peritoneal spread (d).

Additional support for the fallopian tubes as the origin of HGSPC derives from molecular studies demonstrating *TP53* mutations in >95 percent of HGPSC that are essentially identical to those detected in >90 percent of STICs. In a minority of cases where fallopian tubal involvement is not detected, HGPSC are postulated to arise from ovarian cortical inclusion cysts, in part because they exhibit a ciliated epithelial cell lining similar to that found in the fallopian tube. The emerging morphologic, immunohistochemical, and molecular information may permit future strategies for assigning a primary site to Type II serous carcinomas (30); however, currently, they may be collectively referred to as pelvic serous carcinoma and managed as high-stage ovarian serous carcinoma.

Histopathologic Changes

The classic morphology of HGPSC consists of the papillary architecture interspersed with slit-like spaces (Figure 14.7). High-grade epithelial cells with elongated nuclei and a columnar appearance line the fibrovascular cores in stratified arrays. Cytologically, the cells display marked nuclear hyperchromasia and nucleomegaly with "random anaplasia," occasional

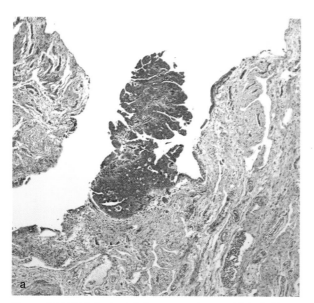
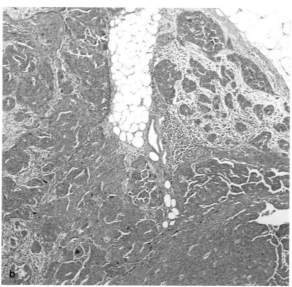

Figure 14.7 (a) Fallopian tubal serous carcinoma with foci of invasion, and (b) extensive peritoneal carcinomatosis both demonstrating the high-grade focally anaplastic nuclear features and slit-like spaces.

multinucleation, and easily found mitotic figures. Psammomatous calcifications (psammoma bodies) are found in a significant number of cases and necrosis is often found. In general with extensive sampling and complete submission of the fallopian tubes, STICs, precursor lesions, are identified (Figure 14.8). A subset of HGPSC are associated with *BRCA* dysfunction whether in germline or somatic mutations or promotor hypermethylation. Solid and transitional growth patterns, severe nuclear anaplasia and nucleomegaly with bizarre forms, the presence of tumor infiltrating lymphocytes and an increased mitotic index embody a constellation of histologic findings which are distinctive in *BRCA*-related tumors (31).

Immunohistochemistry

Pelvic serous carcinoma, whether of ovarian, fallopian tube, or peritoneal origin, all show a similar immunohistochemical profile. The majority of serous tumors exhibit a CK7+ CK20– profile. Most also exhibit nuclear reactivity with WT-1 and PAX-8 (a nephric lineage transcription factor). Variable nuclear immunoreactivity is displayed with PAX-2 (a nuclear

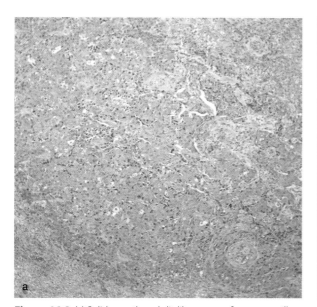
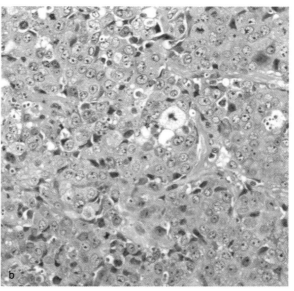

Figure 14.8 (a) Solid growth and slit-like spaces of serous papillary carcinoma of the peritoneum. (b) High-power view of marked anaplastic epithelioid cells, grayish nuclei with numerous mitotic figures, and nucleolar prominence.

Table 14.2 Immunohistochemical stains as applied to pelvic serous carcinoma and its metastatic mimics. Immunohistochemical selectivities (in %) in adenocarcinomas (12,33–35,37–41)

Stain	PSC	CRC	GEJ	BRST	LUNG	Pan/bil	Endom	Uro	Pap RCC	Cerv
CK7	+	−	+	+	+	+	+	+	+	+
CK20	−	+	−	−	−	−	−	+	−	−
CDX-2	−	+	+/−	−	−	+	−	−	−	−
GATA-3	−	−	−	+	−	+ 10%	−	+	−	−
ER/PR	+	−	−	+	−	−	+ or −	−	−	+
p16	+	−	−	−	−	−	+	+	−	+
p53	+	−	−	+ or −	−	−	+	+ or −	−	−
p63	−	−	−	+ or −	−	−	−	+	−	−
TTF-1	−	−	10+	10	+	−	−	−	−	−
PAX-8	+	−	−	−	−	−	−	−	+	+
WT-1	+	−	−	−	−	−	+ or −	−	−	−
DPC4	+	NA	NA	NA	NA	−	NA	NA	NA	NA

Notation: BRST: breast carcinoma; Cerv: cervix; CRC: colorectal carcinoma; Endom: endometrial serous carcinoma; GEJ: gastroesophageal junction carcinoma; Pan/bil: pancreatobiliary; Pap RCC: papillary renal cell carcinoma; PSC: pelvic serous carcinoma; Uro: urothelial carcinoma.

transcription factor similar to PAX-8), estrogen and progesterone receptors. The immunophenotype appears to be preserved in the majority of tumors tested following neoadjuvant therapy and in the majority of recurrences following remission.

Treatment and Prognosis

The majority of patients with high-grade serous carcinoma are treated with chemotherapy, either after or before surgery. Peritoneal involvement regardless of the site of origin (ovary, fallopian tube, etc.) is considered stage III disease. Poor prognostic indicators are high-grade morphology and high-stage disease.

Selected Differential Diagnostic Scenarios

Pelvic serous carcinoma often presents at high stage with peritoneal carcinomatosis and malignant ascites with the potential to obscure an obvious primary site of origin. Sampling of large surgical specimens, for example in cases of debulking, with complete sectioning of the fallopian tubes often reveals small foci of serous tubal intraepithelial or invasive serous carcinoma of the fallopian tube. In such cases the diagnosis is straightforward. In cases with limited specimen sampling available and/or with a history of a primary carcinoma from elsewhere, notably breast or lung, metastases from non-pelvic peritoneal sites enter the differential. Adding to the challenge is that, increasingly, small biopsies are employed as the first step in establishing a diagnosis and precursor or STIC lesion will not be sampled. Judicious use of immunohistochemical studies may be necessary to identify lineage in these cases. Common extra-pelvic sites of peritoneal carcinomatosis include gastroesophageal, gastric, colorectal, appendiceal, pancreatic, gallbladder, urothelial, breast, and lung (Table 14.2). Expression

of WT-1 and PAX-8 and/or PAX-2 supports a Müllerian immunophenotype and most gastrointestinal, lung, and breast primaries are negative for WT-1 and PAX-8.

Breast carcinoma, the most common non-Müllerian-derived carcinoma to produce peritoneal carcinomatosis in women (Figure 14.9), is almost always immunoreactive with

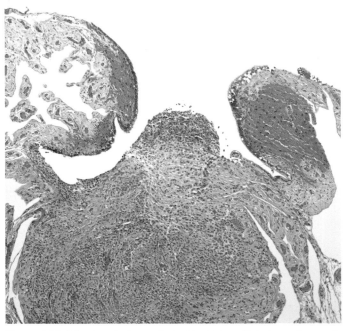

Figure 14.9 Fallopian tube in a patient with a history of lobular carcinoma of the breast demonstrating metastasis to the surface epithelium and stroma characterized by cords and sheets of epithelioid cuboidal epithelial cells but with little cytologic resemblance to serous carcinoma.

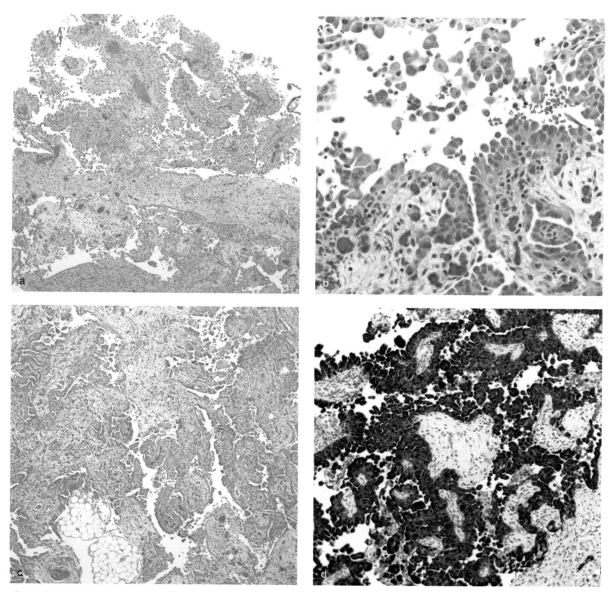

Figure 14.10 (a) Malignant mesothelioma epithelioid pattern demonstrating papillae and fibrovascular cores lined by uniformly atypical cells. (b) Higher-power view of peritoneal mesothelioma showing the cuboidal cytology and marked nuclear atypia, but discohesion in contrast to high-grade serous carcinoma. (c) Surface growth pattern of epithelioid malignant mesothelioma similar to peritoneal serous carcinomatosis. (d) Strong calretinin positivity supporting mesothelial differentiation.

GATA-3. Mammaglobin and GCDFP-15 are less sensitive but equally selective for mammary origin. Each of these three markers is generally negative in ovarian carcinomas. Comparison with ER and PR expression from the primary breast carcinoma, if available, is useful; however, in the setting of treatment, recurrence, and/or tumor progression receptor status may be altered.

Peritoneal carcinomatosis from metastatic lung adenocarcinoma can be a diagnostic challenge because pulmonary adenocarcinomas may show many different subtypes, including papillary. Despite the potential for histologic overlap, immunohistochemistry is useful in separating lung from Müllerian carcinoma, because the majority of lung adenocarcinomas are thyroid transcription factor 1 (TTF-1) positive, while negative for WT-1 and PAX-8, and the opposite is true of Müllerian carcinoma (Figure 14.10).

In younger patients germ cell tumors may give rise to peritoneal carcinomatosis, and although serous adenocarcinoma is less common, it does occur in younger age groups. Morphologically, embryonal carcinoma is the most similar to serous adenocarcinoma, but these tumors can be separated using OCT4, which shows nuclear positivity in embryonal carcinoma but is negative in serous adenocarcinomas. The site of origin in peritoneal carcinomatosis with less than classic Müllerian histopathology and no known primary requires a panel of

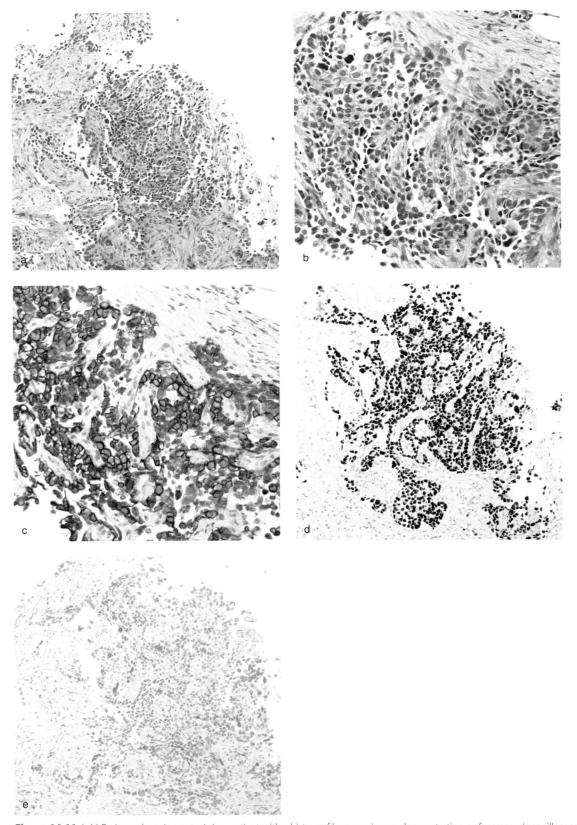

Figure 14.11 (a,b) Peritoneal carcinomatosis in a patient with a history of lung carcinoma demonstrating surface pseudopapillary growth resembling serous carcinoma. Notably, despite the widespread disease, ascites was lacking, in contrast to serous carcinoma. (c) Cytokeratin-positive tumor cells could be seen in both lung and serous carcinoma. (d) TTF-1 is strongly positive in tumor cells that lack WT-1 expression (e), supporting metastatic lung carcinoma.

immunostains which could initially include CK7, CK20, WT-1, GATA-3, PAX-8, TTF-1, and CDX2 (Table 14.2).

In some cases malignant mesothelioma enters the differential diagnosis of pelvic serous carcinoma, especially in cases of diffuse peritoneal spread without significant organ-based disease (Figure 14.11). Because WT-1 will react with tumor cells of both mesothelioma and Müllerian carcinoma, calretinin, thrombomodulin, CK5/6, and D2–40 (podoplanin) are recommended as mesothelioma-selective markers, whereas PAX-8, MOC-31, B72.3, and Ber-EP4 will be positive in serous adenocarcinoma. Recently, a fusion of EWSR1 with YY1 has been detected in a subset of peritoneal mesotheliomas by RNA sequencing (32), which in theory could be used to separate it from serous adenocarcinoma in diagnostically challenging cases. Approximately a third of peritoneal mesotheliomas show germline and somatic inactivation of BRCA-associated protein 1 (BAP1). The loss of BAP1 is a very rare event in gynecologic serous adenocarcinoma and this test may be important to distinguish mesothelioma from these tumors (42).

In summary, both pleural and peritoneal predominant carcinomas are considered secondary spread or metastasis. Treatment differs, in some carcinomas significantly, for management of carcinomas originating from different organs. Furthermore, the advent of targeted therapy increases the importance of distinguishing the site of origin in these cases. Attention to microscopic examination of specific areas such as the pleuropulmonary junction and fimbriated ends of completely submitted fallopian tubes in combination with judiciously selected immunohistochemical stains will aid in making the distinction among the differential diagnostic considerations discussed above.

References

1. Babolini, B. The pleural form of primary cancer of the lung. *Dis Chest*. 1956;29(3):314–23.

2. Attanoos RL, Gibbs AR. Pseudomesotheliomatous carcinomas of the pleura: a 10-year analysis of cases from the Environmental Lung Disease Research Group, *Cardiff Histopathol*. 2003;43(5):444–52.

3. Koss MN, Travis WD, Moran CA, Hochholzer L. Pseudomesotheliomatous adenocarcinoma: a reappraisal. *Semin Diagn Pathol*. 1992;9:117–23.

4. Saito R, Kasajima A, Taniuchi S, Fujishima F, Ishida K, Nakamura Y, et al. Case reports of primary pulmonary adenocarcinoma with pleural spread: so-called pseudomesotheliomatous adenocarcinoma *Pathol Int*. 2012;62(10):709–15.

5. Travis WD, Travis LB, Devesa SS. Lung cancer. *Cancer*. 1995;5:191–202.

6. Devesa SS, Shaw GL, Blot WJ. Changing patterns of lung carcinoma. *Cancer Epidemiol Biomarkers Prev*. 1991;1:29–34.

7. Roberts ME, Neville E, Berrisford RG, Antunes F, Ali NJ, BTS Pleural Disease Guideline Groups. Management of a malignant pleural effusion: British Thoracic Society Pleural Disease Guideline 2010. *Thorax*. 2010;65(Suppl 2):ii32–40.

8. Moran CA, Suster S. Primary mucoepidermoid carcinoma of the pleura. A clinicopathologic study of two cases. *Am J Clin Pathol*. 2003;120:381–85.

9. Lin X, Chi C, Chen J, Liu Y, Li P, Yang Y. Primary pleural squamous cell carcinoma misdiagnosed as localized mesothelioma: a case report and review of the literature. *J Cardiothorac Surg*. 2013;8:50.

10. Harwood TR, Gracey DR, Yokoo H. Pseudomesotheliomatous carcinoma of the lung: a variant of peripheral lung cancer. *Am J Clin Pathol*. 1976;65(2):159–67.

11. Dodson RF, Hammar SP. Analysis of asbestos concentration in 20 cases of pseudomesotheliomatous lung cancer. *Ultrastruct Pathol*. 2015;39(1):13–22.

12. Jagirdar J. Application of immunohistochemistry to the diagnosis of primary and metastatic carcinoma to the lung. *Arch Pathol Lab Med*. 2008;132:384–96.

13. Pardo J, Torres W, Martinez-Peñuela A, Panizo A, de Alava E, García JL. Pseudomesotheliomatous carcinoma of the lung with a distinct morphology, immunohistochemistry, and comparative genomic hybridization profile. *Ann Diagn Pathol*. 2007;11(4):241–51.

14. Ordonez NG. What are the current best immunohistochemical markers for the diagnosis of epithelioid mesothelioma? A review and update. *Hum Pathol*. 2007;38:1–16.

15. Christensen BC, Marsit CJ, Houseman EA, Godleski JJ, Longacker JL, Zheng S, et al. Differentiation of lung adenocarcinoma, pleural mesothelioma, and nonmalignant pulmonary tissues using DNA methylation profiles. *Cancer Res*. 2009;69:6315–21.

16. Ladanyi M. Implications of P16/CDKN2A deletion in pleural mesotheliomas. *Lung Cancer*. 2005;49(Suppl 1):S95–98.

17. Lopez-Rios F, Chuai S, Flores R, Shimizu S, Ohno T, Wakahara K, et al. Global gene expression profiling of pleural mesotheliomas: overexpression of aurora kinases and P16/CDKN2A deletion as prognostic factors and critical evaluation of microarray-based prognostic prediction. *Cancer Res*. 2006;66:2970–79.

18. Lee AY, Raz DJ, He B, Jablons DM. Update on the molecular biology of malignant mesothelioma. *Cancer*. 2007;109:1454–61.

19. Lee Y, Miron A, Drapkin R, Nucci MR, Medeiros F, Saleemuddin A, et al. A candidate precursor to serous carcinoma that originates in the distal fallopian tube. *J Pathol*. 2007;211(1):26–35.

20. Dubeau L. The cell of origin of ovarian epithelial tumours. *Lancet Oncol*. 2008;9(12):1191–97.

21. Nik NN, Vang R, Shih IeM, Kurman RJ. Origin and pathogenesis of pelvic (ovarian, tubal, and primary peritoneal) serous carcinoma. *Ann Rev Pathol*. 2014;9:27–45.

22. King M-C, Marks J, Mandell J, New York Breast Cancer Study Group. Breast and Ovarian cancer risks due to inherited mutations in *BRCA1* and *BRCA2*. *Science*. 2003;302(5645):643–46.

23. Kauff ND, Satagopan JM, Robson ME, Scheuer L, Hensley M, Hudis CA, et al. Risk-reducing salpingo-oophorectomy in women with a *BRCA1* or *BRCA2* mutation. *N Engl J Med.* 2002:346:1609–15.

24. Jermann M, Vogt P, Pestalozzi BC. Peritoneal carcinoma in a male patient. *Oncology.* 2003;64(4):468–74.

25. Shmueli E, Leider-Tredjo L, Schwartz I, Aderka D, Inbar M. Primary papillary serous carcinoma in the peritoneum in a man. *Ann Oncol.* 2001;12(4)563–67.

26. Ayhan A, Kurman RJ, Yemelyanova A, Vang R, Logani S, Seidman JD, et al. Defining the cut point between low-grade and high-grade ovarian serous carcinomas: a clinicopathologic and molecular genetic analysis. *Am J Surg Pathol.* 2009;33(8):1220–24.

27. Vang R, Shih IeM, Kurman R. Ovarian low-grade and high grade serous carcinoma: pathogenesis, clinicopathologic and molecular biologic features, and diagnostic problems. *Adv Anat Pathol.* 2009; 16(5):267–82.

28. Dehari R, Kurman RJ, Logani S, Shih IeM. The development of high-grade serous carcinoma from atypical proliferative (borderline) serous tumors and low-grade micropapillary serous carcinoma: a morphologic and molecular genetic analysis. *Am J Surg Pathol.* 2007;31(7):1007–12.

29. Bloss JD, Liao S, Buller RE, Manetta A, Berman ML, McMeekin S, et al. Extra ovarian peritoneal serous papillary carcinoma: a case-control retrospective comparison to papillary adenocarcinoma of the ovary. *Gynecol Oncol.* 1993;50:347–51.

30. Singh N, Gilks CB, Hirshowitz L, Wilkinson N, McCluggage WG. Adopting a uniform approach to site assignment in tubo-ovarian high-grade serous carcinoma: the time has come. *Int J Gynecol Pathol.* 2016;35(3):230–37.

31. Soslow RJ, Han G, Park KJ, Garg K, Olvera N, Spriggs DR, et al. Morphologic patterns associated with *BRCA1* and *BRCA2* genotype in ovarian carcinoma. *Mod Pathol.* 2012;25:625–36.

32. Panagopoulos I, Thorsen J, Gorunova L, Micci F, Haugom L, Davidson B, et al. RNA sequencing identifies fusion of the *EWSR1* and *YY1* genes in mesothelioma with t(14;22)(q32;q12). *Genes Chromosomes Cancer.* 2013;52(8):733–40.

33. Bhargava R, Beriwal S, Dabbs D. An immunohistologic validation survey for sensitivity and specificity. *Am J Clin Pathol.* 2007;127:103–13.

34. Comin CE, Novelli L, Cavazza A, Rotellini M, Cianchi F, Messenrini L. Expression of thrombomodulin, calretinin, cytokeratin 5/6, D2–40 and WT-1 in a series of primary carcinomas of the lung: an immunohistochemical study in comparison with epithelioid pleural mesothelioma. *Tumori.* 2014;100(5):559–67.

35. Espinosa I, Gallardo A, D'Angelo E, Mozos A, Lerma E, Prat J. Simultaneous carcinomas of the breast and ovary: utility of Pax-8, WT-1, and GATA3 for distinguishing independent primary tumors from metastases. *Int J Gynecol Pathol.* 2015;34(3):257–65.

36. Lau SK, Chu PF, Weiss LM. Immunohistochemical expression of estrogen receptor in pulmonary adenocarcinoma. *Appl Immunohistochem Mol Morphol.* 2006;14:83–87.

37. Laury AR, Perets R, Piao H, Krane JF, Barletta JA, French C, et al. A comprehensive analysis of PAX8 expression in human epithelial tumors. *Am J Surg Pathol.* 2011;35(6):816–26.

38. Mazziotta RM, Borczuk AC, Powerll CA, Mansukhani M. CDX2 immunostaining as a gastrointestinal marker: expression in lung carcinomas is a potential pitfall. *Appl Immunohistochem Mol Morphol.* 2005;13:55–60.

39. Miettinen M, McCue PA, Sarlomo-Rikala M, Rys J, Czapiewski P, Wazny K, et al. Gata3: a multispecific but potentially useful marker in surgical pathology: a systematic anlysis of 2500 epithelial and nonepithelial tumors. *Am J Surg Pathol.* 2014;38(1):13–22.

40. Tong GX, Yu WM, Beaubier NT, Weeden EM, Hamele B, Mansukhai MM, et al. Expression of PAX8 in normal and neoplastic renal tissues: an immunohistochemical study. *Mod Pathol.* 2009;22:1218–27.

41. Nofech-Mozes S, Khalifa M, Ismiil N, Reda S, Saad W, Hanna WM, et al. Immunophenotyping of serous carcinoma of the female genital tract. *Mod Pathol.* 2008;21:1147–55.

42. Andrici J, Jung J, Sheen A, D'Urso L, Sioson L, Pickett J, et al. Loss of BAP1 expression is very rare in peritoneal and gynecologic serous adenocarcinomas and can be useful in the differential diagnosis with abdominal mesothelioma. *Hum Pathol.* 2016;51:9–15.

Chapter 15

Lymphoid Malignancies of the Pleura and Peritoneum

Richard Attanoos

Introduction

All forms of hematologic malignancy may involve the various serosal sites usually as secondary involvement from known lymph nodal, marrow-based, or extra-nodal disease. Primary serosal pericardial, pleural, and peritoneal lymphomas are rare. During the development of their disease process about 16 percent of patients with non-Hodgkin's lymphoma (NHL) subsequently develop serosal (usually pleural) disease (1). Serous effusions are seen in 20–30 percent of NHL and Hodgkin's lymphoma. In contrast, primary serosal lymphomas are extremely rare. Most represent rare topographic manifestations of diffuse large B-cell lymphoma that have emerged as defined entities in the recent WHO classification of lymphoid malignancies, typically with a phenotype resembling terminally differentiated B cells or plasma cell lineage, most are associated with immunodeficiency, viral infection and poor prognosis (2). The pathogenesis of these primary pleural lymphomas is not completely understood, but likely involves a complex interrelationship between chronic serosal inflammatory disease, immunosenescence/acquired immunodeficiency, host genetic factors, and viral infection serving as a catalyst for uncontrolled B-cell proliferation and eventual lymphoma. Clinically non-aggressive (formally termed "low-grade") primary serosal lymphomas are also extremely uncommon and most represent marginal zone lymphoma (3).

Primary Pleural Lymphomas

Two distinct types of primary pleural lymphomas are defined as recognized entities in the 2008 WHO classification (2) – the primary effusion lymphoma formerly termed *body cavity based lymphoma* in patients with human immunodeficiency virus (HIV), and the diffuse large B-cell lymphoma associated with chronic inflammation formerly termed *pyothorax-associated pleural lymphoma*. Primary pleural NHL arising in an immunocompetent subject without a history of chronic pyothorax are exceptional.

Primary Effusion Lymphoma

This neoplasm typically presents without solid tumor masses and as multicavitary effusions (Figures 15.1 and 15.2). The pleural cavity is the most common site followed by peritoneal and pericardial cavities. Patients typically have either acquired HIV

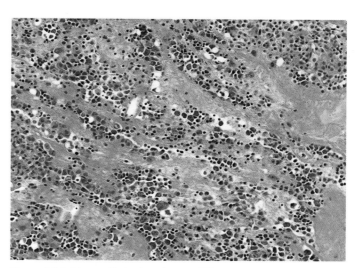

Figure 15.1 Primary effusion lymphoma, ×100.

infection, severe immunodeficiency of another source, or senile immunosenescence in elderly patients (4,5).

By light microscopic examination the tumor cells are typically immunoblastic in nature with large nuclei and prominent nucleoli, although plasmablastic, anaplastic, and Reed–Sternberg-like cell forms are seen. It is not uncommon for there to be cellular autolysis, degeneration, and apoptosis present.

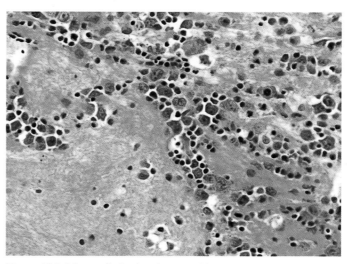

Figure 15.2 Primary effusion lymphoma, ×400.

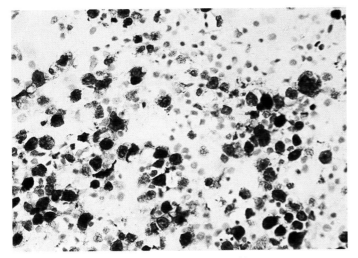

Figure 15.3 Primary effusion lymphoma MUM1, ×400.

The tumor immunophenotype demonstrates that these lymphoma cells usually express leukocyte common antigen (CD45), plasma cell-related markers (CD138, VS38c), as well as MUM1 (Figure 15.3) and activation-associated markers (CD30, CD38) (Figure 15.4). The pan B-cell markers (CD19, CD20, CD79a, PAX-5) are typically negative (Figures 15.5 and 15.6). Surface immunoglobulin is also negative and cytoplasmic immunoglobulins are detectable in only about 20 percent of cases. Molecular genetic studies show clonal rearrangements of immunoglobulin genes, confirming that these primary effusion lymphomas are monoclonal B-cell neoplasms. It is important to appreciate that aberrant expression of pan T-cell antigens (CD2, CD3, CD5, CD7) may be observed. An awareness of this should prevent misdiagnosis. The lymphoma cells are positive for human herpes virus 8 (HHV-8)/Kaposi's sarcoma herpes virus (KSHV) and most cases are co-infected with Epstein–Barr virus (EBV) (Figure 15.7). The EBV antibody LMP-1 is almost always negative.

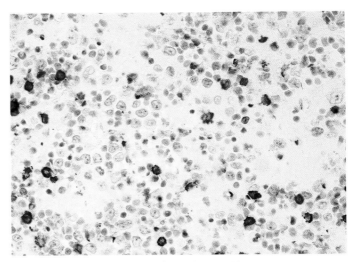

Figure 15.5 Primary effusion lymphoma CD20, ×400.

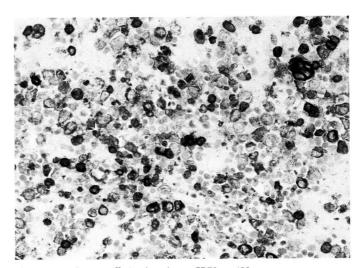

Figure 15.6 Primary effusion lymphoma CD79a, ×400.

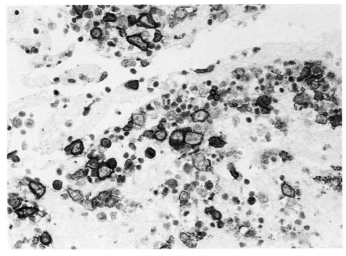

Figure 15.4 Primary effusion lymphoma CD30, ×400.

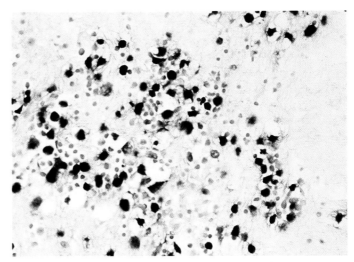

Figure 15.7 Primary effusion lymphoma Epstein–Barr encoding region (EBER), ×400.

The disease course is extremely poor irrespective of treatment, with median survival at less than 6 months.

Diffuse Large B-cell Lymphoma Associated with Chronic Inflammation

This is an EBV-associated B-cell neoplasm that occurs in the context of long-standing chronic inflammation. This tumor entity was first reported in the pleura in 1987 by Iuchi and colleagues in three Japanese subjects (6). Since that time, the tumor entity has emerged in other sites. Most cases arise in anatomical sites with limited vascularization (immunoprivileged regions). However, the most common site remains the pleural cavity, where the lymphoma develops in persons with a history of pyothorax resulting from artificial pneumothorax for the treatment of tuberculosis, or arises de novo following chronic tuberculous pleuritis (7). Similar cases have been reported in the peritoneum, pericardium, and in association with fibrin thrombi (8). Age at diagnosis ranged between the fifth and eighth decades. The interval between the initial inflammatory event and the presentation of lymphoma exceeds 10 years and there is a strong male preponderance of at least 10:1 (9,10). Subjects with this disease typically present with chest wall pain and swelling together with fever. A minority (25 percent) of patients develop respiratory symptoms.

On macroscopic inspection, the tumor shows marked serosal thickening with firm consistency and tan discoloration. Necrosis is common. These lymphomas usually show invasion into adjacent structures such as lung, mediastinum, pericardium, diaphragm, and liver. Widespread dissemination of diffuse large B-cell lymphoma associated with chronic inflammation is uncommon.

On microscopic examination the tumor shows features consistent with other forms of diffuse large B-cell lymphoma comprising rich mixtures of centroblastic or immunoblastic morphology. Apoptosis may be a prominent feature, particularly in areas of extensive necrosis. There may be a prominent inflammatory component present mostly small lymphocytes and plasma cells. Angiocentric destruction observed in some forms of EBV-related T-cell-rich B-cell lymphoma is not a common feature in this lymphoma.

The tumor cells express common leukocyte antigen (CD45) and pan B-cell antigens (CD19, CD20, and CD79a). Most cases have been known to show a post-germinal center B-cell phenotype (CD10−, Bcl-6−, MUM1+, BLIMP-1+, CD138+). CD30 is often expressed (CD15 is negative). Aberrant expression of T-cell antigens (CD2, CD3, CD4, CD7) is again not uncommon. Molecular genetic studies show immunoglobulin heavy chain variable region rearrangements consistent with clonal B-cell neoplasm.

The tumor cells in this entity express latent infection genes Epstein–Barr virus 2 and latent membrane protein (LMP-1) together with the EBV genome in the tumor cells. It is important to recall that HHV-8 (KSHV) viral genomes are not present in diffuse large B-cell lymphoma associated with chronic inflam-

mation, and this represents a distinct feature in contrast with primary effusion lymphoma. Most subjects with diffuse large B-cell lymphoma associated with chronic inflammation have elevated serum anti-EBV antibodies.

Diffuse large B-cell lymphoma associated with chronic inflammation is an aggressive lymphoma with median survival of 9 months. The 5-year overall survival is approximately 30 percent. Chemo-radiotherapy and surgical resection have provided variable results (11).

Primary Marginal Zone B-cell Lymphoma

This is a rare tumor in the serosa similar to its more common nodal and extranodal counterparts (12). It is an indolent B-cell NHL comprising morphologically varied small lymphocytic, monocytoid, or centrocytoid cells often associated with plasma cell differentiation. The immunophenotypic features are as those defined elsewhere: CD20+, CD79a+, Bcl-2+, CD5−, CD10−, CD23−, CD43+. CD21 and CD35 are often positive in tumor cells and also highlight any associated follicular dendritic cell networks in lymphoid follicles.

Clinical assessment is essential to determine if this is a primary or secondary manifestation of disease.

Secondary Lymphoid Malignancies Involving the Serosa

Lymphomatous or leukemic infiltrates involving the pleura are relatively common, observed in approximately 15 percent of patients with NHL during the course of their illness (13). The morphologic, immunophenotypic, and molecular genetic features of the disease reflect that observed in counterpart nodal or marrow-based disease. Diffuse large B-cell lymphoma, follicular lymphoma, and small lymphocytic lymphoma/chronic lymphocytic leukemia are the most commonly reported lymphomas involving the pleura (14). Plasma cell tumors are well described at serosal sites. For classical Hodgkin lymphoma to involve the pleura is a rare event.

It is not uncommon to identify dense lymphoid and plasma cell infiltrates in serosal biopsies and these may, on occasion, raise concern for neoplasia, both from the perspective of plasma cell tumors (solitary plasmacytoma/multiple myeloma) and lymphoid malignancy (B-cell NHL with variable plasma cell differentiation).

In reactive inflammatory serosal infiltrates, the lymphocytic component may be mild to severe, associated with secondary germinal centers and plasma cells. The reactive lymphoid follicles when present typically form at the interface between the deep connective tissue of the serosa and the fat. These secondary lymphoid follicles express the B-cell markers (CD20 and CD79a), germinal centers express CD10, Bcl-6, and there are well-maintained follicular dendritic cell networks (defined by CD21 and CD23). The reactive germinal centers are Bcl-2 negative, and the proliferation marker Ki-67 shows prominent expression with accentuated polarity. Reactive lymphoid

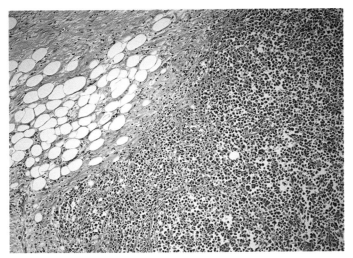

Figure 15.8 Plasmablastic lymphoma peritoneum, ×100.

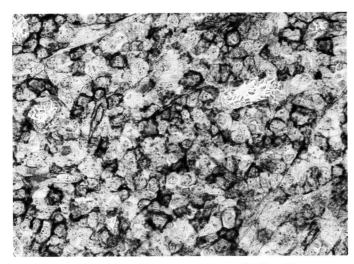

Figure 15.10 Plasmablastic lymphoma peritoneum CD138, ×400.

infiltrates are predominantly of T-cell phenotype expressing CD3 with mixed T helper (CD4) and T cytotoxic (CD8) cells. B cells (CD20, CD79a) are typically less marked, although the reactive infiltrate is mixed in nature.

In contrast, non-blastic lymphomatous infiltrates tend to be more florid and monomorphic than reactive infiltrates. In most cases, small lymphocytic lymphoma/chronic lymphocytic leukemia is the most common manifestation of secondary lymphoma in the serosa. Small lymphocyte-like cells are sometimes seen with occasional larger blasts (paraimmunoblasts). Neoplastic infiltrates should be suspected when the predominant cell is of the B-cell phenotype (CD20 > CD3 and there is extensive Bcl-2 expression with low Ki-67). Neoplastic follicles appear more ill-defined with indistinct mantle zones, devoid of tangible body macrophages and lacking polarity. Follicular

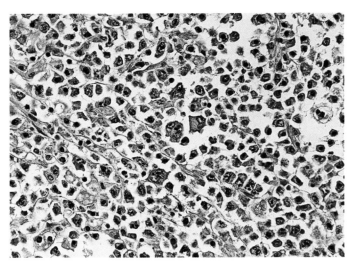

Figure 15.9 Plasmablastic lymphoma peritoneum, ×400

dendritic cell networks (CD21, CD23, CD35) appear "moth-eaten," reflecting colonization by lymphoma cells. Light chain monotypia may be demonstrable in some lymphoma with florid plasmacellular differentiation. The lymphoma cell population will show a distinct immunophenotype dependent on the lymphoma (Table 15.1).

Plasma cell tumors may be composed of sheets of plasma cells with varied morphologic features ranging from mature plasma cells (with the "clock face" nuclear chromatin pattern, eccentric nucleus, perinuclear "hof," and basophilic cytoplasm), to areas with multinucleation, cytological atypia, and intranuclear (Dutcher bodies) and intracytoplasmic (Russell bodies) inclusions of immunoglobulins (Figures 15.8 and 15.9) (15).

A variety of malignant lymphomas may show plasmacellular differentiation. This may be most commonly seen in the non-blastic B-cell lymphomas (SLL/CLL, marginal zone lymphoma, follicular lymphoma, and mantle cell lymphoma).

Immunohistochemical markers used to separate reactive from neoplastic plasma cell infiltrates focus on demonstrating lineage and monotypia. Plasma cell markers CD138 and CD38, together with CD79a, immunoglobulin heavy chains and light chains are expressed (Figure 15.10). CD20 and PAX-5 are negative. A point of potential confusion is that the epithelial marker EMA labels plasma cells and CD45 may be equivocal/negative. Some cases are positive for CAM 5.2, others for S100. Conversely, VS38c (a plasma cell marker) often labels carcinoma. CD56 (neural cell adhesion molecule) is sometimes useful, being positive in plasma cell tumors and negative in reactive plasma cells. Plasma cell tumor-mimicking malignant mesothelioma has been reported and associated with massive pleural effusion (16). In the peritoneum, solitary plasmacytoma has been associated with nodular amyloid and myeloma with disseminated disease (15) (Figure 15.11).

Table 15.1 Immunomarkers used to identify the non-blastic B-cell lymphomas

	Follicular lymphoma	SLL/CLL	Mantle cell lymphoma	Lymphoplasmacytic lymphoma	Marginal zone lymphoma
CD5	−	+	+	−	−
CD10	+	−	−	−	−
CD23	−	+	−	−	−
Cyclin D1	−	−	+	−	−
Bcl-2	+	+	+	+	+

Lymphoid Malignancies of the Pleura and Peritoneum and Asbestos

The incidence rates of lymphoid malignancy are increasing with around a five- to eightfold variation worldwide (17), being highest in North America and Western Europe and lower in Eastern Europe and Asia, and this has been attributed to various factors (subject to the individual lymphoma entity type). The knowledge that there are observed geographic variations and temporal trends in incidence rates of various lymphomas has suggested that there may be environmental factors which account for some cases of the disease. Indeed, many lymphomas are associated with various latent viral infections (as seen in the primary pleural lymphomas with EBV+, HIV+/−, HHV-8+/−), bacterial infection (*Helicobacter pylori* with marginal zone lymphoma MALT type), immunosuppression, autoimmune conditions, ultraviolet light, ionizing radiation, and in some cases chemicals (herbicides) (18).

A small number of case reports have identified the coincidental presence of lymphomas in persons with presumed asbestos-induced mesothelioma, and this has prompted the suggestion that there may be a causal association (19,20). Malignant mesothelioma and most clinically non-aggressive lymphomas arise in elderly persons, so a chance occurrence is not proof of causation. In one large national survey of 17,800 asbestos insulators no increase in the incidence of lymphoma or leukemia was identified (21).

There is no established causal association between the various lymphoid malignancies of the pleura and peritoneum and asbestos.

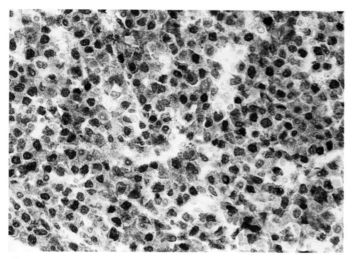

Figure 15.11 Plasmablastic lymphoma peritoneum MUM1, ×400.

References

1. Das DK, Gupta SK, Ayyagarai S, Bambery DK, Datta BN, Datta U. Pleural effusions in non-Hodgkin's lymphoma: a cytomorphologic, cytochemical and immunologic study. *Acta Cytol*. 1987;31:119.

2. Swerdlow SH, Campo E, Harris NL, et al. WHO classification of tumours of haematopoietic and lymphoid tissues. In: Bosman FT, Jaffe ES, Lakhani SR, Ohgaki H, editors. *World Health Organization classification of tumours*. Lyon: IARC; 2008.

3. Ahmad H, Pawardi J, Falk S, Morgan JA, Balacumaraswami L. Primary pleural lymphomas. *Thorax*. 2003;58:908–09.

4. Nador RG, Cesarman E, Chadburn A, Dawson DB, Ansari MQ, Sald J, et al. Primary effusion lymphoma: a distinct clinicopathologic entity associated with the Kaposi's sarcoma-associated herpes virus. *Blood*. 1996;88(2):645–56.

5. Cesarman E, Chang Y, Moore PS, Said JW, Knowles DM. Kaposi's sarcoma-associated herpesvirus-like DNA sequences in AIDS-related body-cavity-based lymphomas. *N Engl J Med*. 1995;332(18):1186–91.

6. Iuchi K, Ichimiya A, Akashi A, Mizuta T, Lee YE, Tada H, et al. Non-Hodgkin's lymphoma of the pleural cavity developing from long standing pyothorax. *Cancer*. 1987;60:1771–75.

7. Takakuwa T, Tresnasari K, Rahadiani N, Miwa H, Daibata M, Aozasa K. Cell origin of pyothorax-associated lymphoma: a lymphoma strongly associated with Epstein–Barr virus infection. *Leukemia*. 2008;22(3):620–27.

8. Loong F, Chan AC, Ho BC, Chau YP, Lee HY, Cheuk W, et al. Diffuse large B-cell lymphoma associated with chronic inflammation as an incidental finding and new clinical scenarios. *Mod Pathol*. 2010;23(4):493–501.

9. Keung YIK, Cobos E, Morgan D, McConnell TS. Non pyothorax associated primary pleural lymphoma with complex karyotypic abnormalities.

Leukaemia Lymphoma. 1996;23: 621–24.

10. Hirai S, Hamanaka Y, Mitsui N, Morifuji K, Sutoh M. Primary malignant lymphoma arising in the pleura without preceding long-standing pyothorax. *Ann Thorac Cardiovasc Surg.* 2004;10:297–300.

11. Nakatsuka S, Yao M, Hoshida Y, Yamamoto S, Iuchi K, Aozasa K. Pyothorax associated lymphoma: a review of 106 cases. *J Clin Oncol.* 2002;20(20):4255–60.

12. Mitchell A, Meunier C, Ouellette D, Colby T. Extranodal marginal zone lymphoma of mucosa-associated lymphoid tissue with initial presentation in the pleura. *Chest.* 2006;129(3):791–94.

13. Vega F, Padula A, Valbuena JR, Stancu M, Jones D, Medeiros LJ. Lymphomas involving the pleura. A clinicopathologic study of 34 cases diagnosed by pleural biopsy. *Arch Pathol Lab Med.* 2006;130:1497–502.

14. Steiropoulos P, Kouliatsis G, Karpathiou G, Popidou M, Froudarakis ME. Rare cases of primary pleural Hodgkin and non-Hodgkin lymphomas. *Respiration.* 2009;77:459–63.

15. Gemechu T, Ali A. Solitary plasmacytoma of the mesentery with nodular amyloid deposits: a case report with immunohistochemical evaluation. *Ethiop Med J.* 2001;39(1):53.

16. Colonna A, Gualco G, Bacchi CE, Bacchi CE, Leite MA, Rocco M, et al. Plasma cell myeloma presenting with diffuse pleural involvement: a hitherto unreported pattern of a new mesothelioma mimicker. *Ann Diagn Pathol.* 2010;14(1):30–35.

17. Parkin DM, Muir, CS, Whelan SL, et al. *Cancer Incidence in Five Continents.* Lyon: IARC; 1992.

18. Newton R, Hjalgrim, Law G, et al. A review of the epidemiology of non-Hodgkin lymphomas. In: Cummingham D, Morgan G, Miles A, editors. *The effective management of non-Hodgkin's lymphoma* (2nd edition). London: Aesculapalius Medical Press; 2004.

19. Kagan E, Jacobson RJ. Lymphoid and plasma cell malignancies: asbestos related disorders of long latency. *Am J Clin Pathol.* 1983;80:14–20.

20. Hara N, Fujimoto, N, Miyamoto Y, Yamagishi T, Asano M, Fuchimoto Y, et al. Lymphoproliferative disorder in pleural effusion in a subject with past asbestos exposure. *Respir Med Case Rep.* 2015;16:169–71.

21. Selikoff IJ, Hammond EC, Seidman H. Mortality experience of insulation workers in the United States and Canada 1943–1976. *Ann N Y Acad Sci.* 1979:330:91–116.

Chapter 16

Mesenchymal and Other Unusual Tumors of the Pleura and Peritoneum

Nicole A. Cipriani and Peter Pytel

Introduction

Mesenchymal tumors of the pleura, pericardium, and peritoneum are relatively rare compared to metastases, mesotheliomas, and carcinomas. The most common serosal mesenchymal neoplasm is solitary fibrous tumor; however, other benign or malignant tumors of soft tissue can also rarely occur on the serous membranes. Serosal sites are not the primary or typical location for most of these soft-tissue tumors, and many of the data are therefore presented as case reports or case series published in the radiology or pathology literature (1–4). The main reason to include soft-tissue tumors in this book on the pathology of serous membranes is the fact that they may be mistaken for those tumors more typically encountered in these locations. This chapter focuses on soft-tissue tumors that are relatively common or represent a particular diagnostic pitfall.

Several aspects of the presentation may provide helpful clues to the diagnosis of serosal tumors. The distribution of disease as either a localized mass or a diffuse process is important. Details of the history including age, prior radiation exposure, prior asbestos exposure, and immunocompromised state have to be considered (5–8). In the chest region, sarcomas primarily based in the chest wall include Ewing sarcoma family tumors (EFT), chondrosarcoma, osteosarcoma, and malignant peripheral nerve sheath tumor (MPNST). Intrathoracic sarcomas more often include angiosarcoma or leiomyosarcoma (2). In some settings, these sarcomas may mimic mesothelioma and carcinoma, which are more common malignancies encountered in this location. Many soft-tissue lesions beyond the scope of this chapter can arise in the tissues surrounding the abdominal cavity including the abdominal wall and the retroperitoneum. Soft-tissue lesions that are primary intraperitoneal include desmoplastic small round cell tumor, fibromatosis, and peritoneal sarcomatosis, which is most commonly observed in the context of gastrointestinal stromal tumors. On rare occasions, some sarcomas have been described as potential mimics of serosal disease processes, including clear cell sarcoma, alveolar soft part sarcoma, low-grade fibromyxoid sarcoma, and extraskeletal osteosarcoma (5–8).

Solitary Fibrous Tumor (SFT)

Overview

SFT is the second most common primary pleural neoplasm following diffuse malignant mesothelioma, and accounts for approximately 5 percent of all pleural tumors (9,10). It is the most common mesenchymal neoplasm and is thought to originate from submesothelial mesenchymal cells. SFT was originally dubbed "localized mesothelioma" due to its suspected mesothelial origin, and has also been known as "localized fibrous tumor of the pleura," more closely approximating its mesenchymal phenotype (11).

Clinical Features

SFT occurs equally in males and females and in a wide age distribution; however, onset in the fifth and sixth decades is most frequent (11). Visceral pleural origin is more frequent than parietal, and intrapulmonary cases account for a small percentage (12). Neither genetic predisposition nor environmental exposures have been associated with development of SFT. Clinical presentation ranges from asymptomatic to thoracic symptoms (cough, dyspnea, or chest pain). Paraneoplastic syndromes are not infrequent: hypertrophic pulmonary osteoarthropathy has been described in up to 20 percent of SFT patients and hypoglycemia (Doege–Potter syndrome) in up to 6 percent, due to tumor secretion of hyaluronic acid or insulin-like growth factor II, respectively (11). Chest x-ray demonstrates a well-circumscribed, usually peripheral opacity. CT confirms soft-tissue attenuation and more clearly delineates the size and location of the mass, which is occasionally lobulated and frequently displaces nearby structures (Figure 16.1a). Contrast-enhancement may occur due to rich vascularity. Occasional hemorrhage or necrosis is present. A vascular pedicle can be identified in many SFTs (up to 80 percent) (11,12). Core-needle biopsy may provide sufficient diagnostic tissue; however, fine-needle aspiration generally does not yield adequate cells due to the fibrous background.

Pathologic Features

Gross features of SFT include a smooth outer surface with occasional prominent vasculature and/or a fibrovascular pedicle. Lobulations may be evident (Figure 16.1b). Size ranges from a few centimeters to > 20 cm. The cut surface can be fleshy to firm and tan–pink to white, depending on the relative predominance of cells versus stroma (Figure 16.1c). Areas of necrosis or hemorrhage may be present in large or high-grade cases (11,13,14).

Microscopically, SFT is well-circumscribed with pushing borders and an occasional pseudocapsule. The classic descriptor "patternless pattern" implies a sheet-like growth pattern of spindle cells without discrete architectural arrangement. A vague

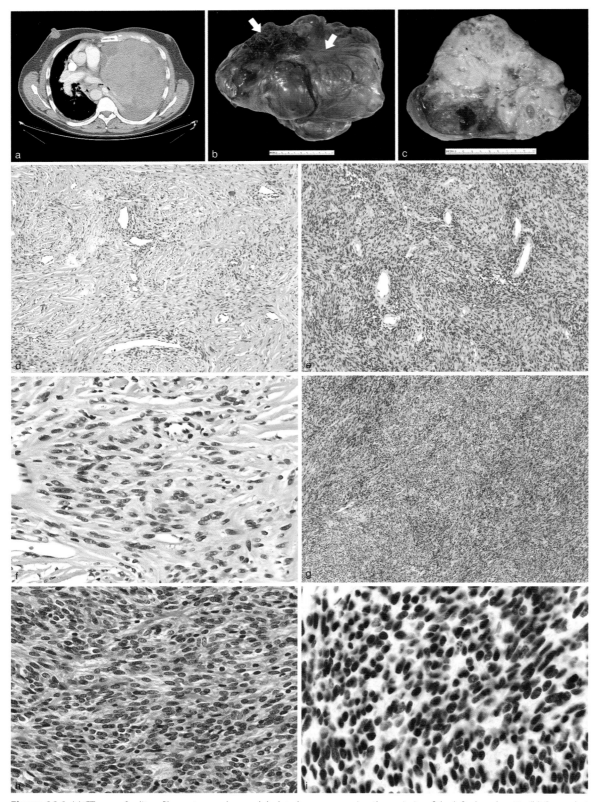

Figure 16.1 (a) CT scan of solitary fibrous tumor shows a lobulated mass occupying the majority of the left pleural cavity. (b) Gross photograph, outer surface, confirms lobulated architecture. The mass is covered by a glistening membrane and demonstrates a vascular pedicle (arrows). (c) Gross photograph, cut surface, shows fleshy tan–pink tumor with focal hemorrhage and cystic degeneration. (d) Example of a relatively hypocellular SFT rich in collagenous stroma and thin-walled, dilated blood vessels. (e) SFT can show moderate cellularity and a "patternless pattern" of spindle cells. (f) Higher power demonstrates relatively bland spindle cells with oval to elongate nuclei embedded in a collagenous stroma. (g) High-grade SFT showing hypercellularity and fasciculated growth pattern. (h) Increased nuclear density and decreased stroma should suggest high-grade SFT. (i) Nuclear immunoreactivity for STAT6.

Table 16.1 Tapias score for predicting recurrence in pleural SFT (18)

Tumor characteristic	Points
Pleural origin: visceral/intrapulmonary	0
Pleural origin: parietal	1
Morphology: pedunculated	0
Morphology: sessile	1
Greatest dimension: < 10 cm	0
Greatest dimension: ≥ 10 cm	1
Hypercellularity	1
Necrosis or hemorrhage	1
Mitoses: < 4 per 10 high-power fields	0
Mitoses: ≥ 4 per 10 high-power fields	1
Minimum score = 0; maximum score = 6.	

fascicular growth pattern can be present in some cases. Cellularity can range from hypocellular with abundant stromal collagen to moderately cellular with sparse collagen (Figure 16.1d,e). Cells range from plump with oval nuclei and minimal amounts of cytoplasm to spindled with elongate nuclei and tapering cytoplasm. Chromatin is usually fine with occasional small nucleoli (Figure 16.1f). Stroma demonstrates variable amounts of collagen, which may separate cells into chords or nests. Thin-wall, dilated, branching (so-called hemangiopericytoma-like) blood vessels are frequent. Mitoses should number no more than four per 10 high-power fields (13,14).

High-grade or so-called "malignant SFT" is characterized by hypercellularity, necrosis, nuclear atypia, or greater than four mitoses per 10 high-power fields (Figure 16.1g,h) (9,11,15). Attempts to use these histologic features to predict recurrence or metastasis have been somewhat unsuccessful, as the features of benign-behaving and aggressive SFTs can be overlapping. Multiple scoring systems to predict recurrence of pleural SFT have been published (England's criteria, de Perrot classification, and Tapias score) (16–18). The Tapias score has performed the best, as ROC curve demonstrated an area under curve of 0.7730, compared to 0.697 and 0.524 for England and de Perrot, respectively (see Table 16.1) (18). Low-risk patients (score < 3) had 4 percent recurrence and 89 percent survival at 15 years. High-risk patients (score ≥ 3) had 28 percent recurrence and 66 percent survival at 15 years. Proliferation index (Ki67 or MIB index > 5 percent) has been shown by some to be predictive of decreased disease-free survival (19).

Dedifferentiation in SFT has been proposed as histologic evidence of increasingly aggressive behavior, aside from the malignant SFT described above (20). Dedifferentiation is defined as the presence of a discrete high-grade sarcoma component that demonstrates epithelioid, round cell, or spindle cell morphology with increased mitosis and necrosis.

Ancillary Testing

Immunostain for CD34 is strongly positive in the majority of cases. CD99 and Bcl-2 can be positive in 70–90 percent of cases

(13,21). EMA, SMA, and S100 are generally negative (14). Beta-catenin can show nuclear expression in up to 40 percent (22). Dedifferentiated SFT shows loss of CD34 and gain of p53 and p16 by IHC (20). Recently, NAB2–STAT6 fusion has been identified in the majority of SFTs, and is accompanied by nuclear expression of STAT6 by IHC (Figure 16.1i). Both located on chromosome 12q13, STAT6 is a transcriptional activator and NAB2 is a transcriptional repressor that becomes an activator when fused to STAT6. STAT6 can be positive in a minority of dedifferentiated liposarcomas and deep benign fibrous histiocytomas, but otherwise is a highly sensitive and specific marker of SFT (21).

Treatment and Prognosis

Complete surgical resection is the treatment of choice for most SFTs. Pedunculated tumors can be resected at the base of the vascular pedicle whereas sessile tumors require some dissection. Adjuvant radiotherapy is reserved for rare cases with positive margins, chest wall invasion, recurrent pleural effusions, or sessile tumors with malignant features (11). Concurrent chemoradiotherapy (with ifosfamide and doxorubicin) has been used in inoperable cases (10).

Overall 5-year survival ranges from 80 to 100 percent. Recurrence is highest in malignant sessile SFTs (63 percent versus 2 percent in benign pedunculated) (11,17). Metastases are rare but can occur with highest frequency in the liver and central nervous system. Spleen, retroperitoneum, adrenal gland, GI tract, kidney, and bone have also been involved. CT scan every 6 months for 2 years after resection is recommended, followed by yearly scans (11).

Schwannoma
Overview

Different peripheral nerve sheath tumors can arise in peritoneum, pleura, and mediastinum. Most common are schwannomas (discussed in detail below), but neurofibromas, perineuriomas, and malignant peripheral nerve sheath tumors are also encountered (23,24).

Clinical Features

Schwannomas are typically adult-age tumors without clear gender predilection. Most cases are sporadic, but familial cases often with multiple lesions are seen in association with neurofibromatosis type 2 linked to *NF2* gene mutations and schwannomatosis linked to *SMARCB1/INI1* gene mutations (both on chromosome 22). Schwannomas may present with neurologic symptoms related to compression of central or peripheral nervous system structures, or they may come to attention as a mass lesion. In most cases these slow-growing tumors cause slowly evolving deficits, but in rare cases, schwannomas may present acutely because of intratumoral hemorrhage. In the chest, the most common location for schwannomas is the posterior mediastinum, but they are also rarely encountered in other mediastinal compartments. In the lungs, they can be found as endobronchial or as pleural/subpleural lesions (25).

Pathologic Features

In soft tissues, schwannomas are encapsulated by a layer of perineurial cells and, therefore, appear as well-demarcated lesions that usually measure less than 5 cm in size but can sometimes reach larger dimensions in deep locations like the retroperitoneum (25–27). In some cases, the tumor arises from a peripheral nerve that can be identified on imaging studies or intraoperatively. In those cases, the tumor is located as a lesion abutting the nerve without diffuse infiltration of the nerve fascicles. Complete nerve-sparing surgical resection is therefore often feasible. On cross-sections, the tumor reveals a firm tan surface. Frequently associated secondary degenerative changes may disrupt this appearance by resulting in cystic areas or areas of organizing hemorrhage. In general, schwannomas represent a relatively uniform proliferation of Schwann cells with typical morphologic features including buckled or wavy tapered and spindled nuclei. The prototypical histologic features of schwannoma are alternating dense and loose areas referred to as Antoni A and Antoni B, respectively (Figure 16.2a). In the dense areas, cells are often arranged in fascicles and may show palisading, resulting in the appearance of Verocay bodies. The Antoni B areas are rich in loose extracellular matrix and often lack such distinctive architectural arrangements of the cells. Other helpful features are the presence of hyalinized and sometimes prominently clustered blood vessels. Focal infiltration by macrophages, focal hemosiderin deposition, and randomly admixed cells with cytologic atypia are frequently encountered. Named morphologic variants (Figure 16.2b–f) include cellular schwannomas, plexiform schwannomas, and microcystic/reticular schwannomas (25–27).

Ancillary Testing

The lesional cells in schwannomas stain strongly and uniformly for S100 (Figure 16.2d) and Sox10 (25–27). The capsular perineurial cells can be highlighted by EMA. Some schwannomas express calretinin and GFAP (Figure 16.2f). The latter can be a reason for non-specific cross-reactivity to cytokeratin AE1/3 (Figure 16.2e). Collagen IV and laminin can be utilized to highlight the presence of pericellular basement membrane, which is one of the ultrastructural hallmarks of Schwann cells. Recent studies have suggested that the long-held belief of axons being excluded from schwannomas is not entirely accurate (28). Staining for neurofilament, therefore, has to be interpreted with caution. The most common cytogenetic aberration in schwannomas is complete or partial loss of chromosome 22. Many sporadic tumors also harbor inactivating NF2 mutations. Cases with SMARCB1 mutations are reported to exhibit partial loss of SMARCB1/INI1 staining by immunohistochemistry (25–27).

Typical schwannomas do not pose much of a diagnostic challenge. Cellular variants may mimic other spindle cell neoplasms including sarcomas. Positive staining for cytokeratin AE1/3 on the basis of cross-reactivity with GFAP can be misleading, raising the question of a spindle cell carcinoma or a thymic tumor if in the mediastinum (Figure 16.2e). Cases with extensive secondary degenerative and ancient changes can be difficult to classify. In some cases, the distinction from neurofibroma or perineurioma can be a challenge. Hybrid forms are described.

Treatment and Prognosis

Schwannomas are benign. The recurrence risk is low in completely resected schwannomas but higher in cellular and plexiform ones that may be less amenable to complete resection. True malignant transformation of Schwannoma to malignant peripheral nerve sheath tumor is an exceptionally rare event only documented in case reports. If present, this malignant transformation is typically associated with epithelioid change (25).

Inflammatory Myofibroblastic Tumor (IMT)
Overview

IMT, as its name suggests, is a tumor comprising cells with a myofibroblastic phenotype characteristically admixed with inflammatory cells. It has also been called "inflammatory pseudotumor" or "plasma cell granuloma" prior to the discovery that many lesions harbor recurrent genetic anomalies involving the ALK (anaplastic lymphoma kinase) gene and subsequent classification of this subset as a true neoplasm. Although relatively frequent in the lung (compared to extrathoracic sites), it represents only up to 1 percent of lung tumors (29).

Clinical Features

IMT occurs equally in both genders and can occur in patients of all ages but does tend to occur in children and young adults. It is the most frequently diagnosed primary lung lesion in children (29). It can occur both in soft tissue and visceral sites, with the thorax (including pleura, lung, and mediastinum), abdomen, pelvis, and retroperitoneum representing the most common sites (30). No specific etiologic factors have been attributed to the development of IMT, although a relationship to underlying lung disease or infection has been seen in some cases, possibly representing inflammatory pseudotumors. Clinical presentation ranges from asymptomatic to non-specific pulmonary symptoms, including cough, hemoptysis, and dyspnea (31). Systemic symptoms include fever, weight loss, anemia, and growth failure in children (32). On CT, IMT appears as a slow-growing, solitary mass with a predilection for the peripheral or subpleural lower lobes. IMT is usually oval and well-circumscribed, but can have irregular, ill-defined borders

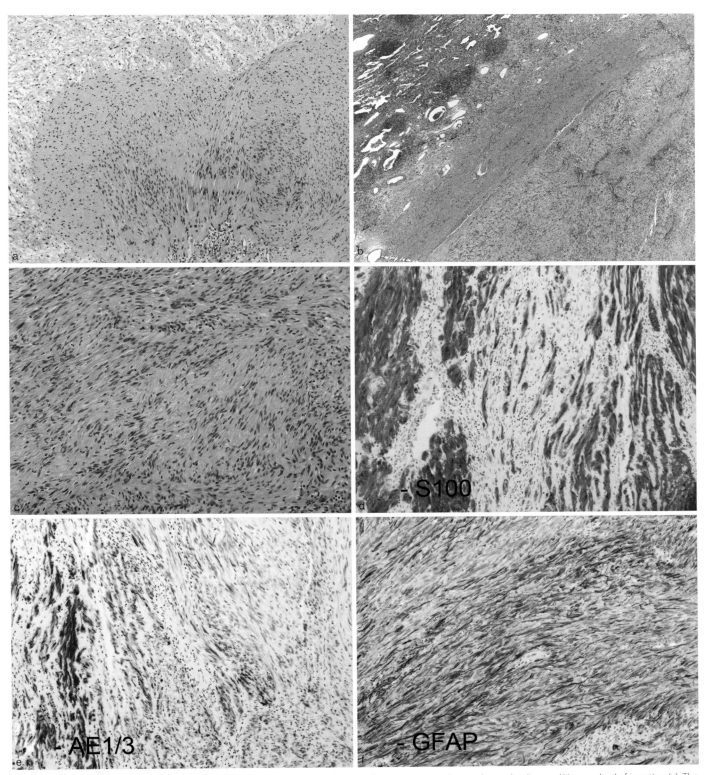

Figure 16.2 Typical features of Schwannoma include alteration between dense and loose areas as well as nuclear palisading and Verocay body formation (a). The case illustrated in images (b)–(f) presented as large mediastinal mass compressing adjacent lung parenchyma (b, left upper corner). The tumor uniformly comprises cellular dense areas with some fasciculate arrangement of cells but no nuclear palisading (c). Clusters of lymphocytes are admixed. The tumor cells show strong uniform staining for S100 (d). Labeling for cytokeratin AE1/3 (e) attributable to cross-reactivity of AE1 with GFAP (f) can be a diagnostic pitfall in cellular schwannomas like this case.

(Figure 16.3a). Size ranges from 1 to 15 cm. Calcification, cystic degeneration, and necrosis are rare but can occur, with calcification occurring more frequently in children than adults (33). Contrast-enhancement can be moderate, high, or delayed (29). Core-needle biopsy could raise the possibility of IMT; however, definitive diagnosis is generally made on surgical excision specimens.

Pathologic Features

Grossly, IMT is well-circumscribed and solid or multinodular with a uniform, white–tan, fleshy cut surface (Figure 16.3b). Degenerative change or hemorrhage is rarely present. Size ranges from less than 1 to greater than 20 cm (34).

Microscopically, IMT is characterized by variably elongated, stellate, or plump spindle cells with a prominent associated inflammatory infiltrate comprising predominantly lymphocytes and plasma cells with occasional eosinophils and rare neutrophils (Figure 16.3c–e) (30). Mitoses are variably present, but should not be atypical.

Three typical histologic patterns have been described. The first pattern is hypocellular with a myxoid to edematous stroma and a capillary network resembling nodular fasciitis. Lesional cells have vesicular nuclei and eosinophilic cytoplasm. Eosinophils can be prominent but plasma cells are lacking. The second pattern is variably hypercellular with a fascicular to storiform growth pattern and occasional dense stromal collagen. Nuclei are elongated. Plasma cells often predominate. The third pattern is characterized by abundant scar-like collagen and even calcification or, rarely, ossification (35).

Atypical features include hypercellularity, fascicular or herringbone growth pattern, multinucleated or ganglion-like giant cells, round cells, necrosis, and atypical mitoses (30). Malignant transformation should be considered in the presence of large cells with vesicular nuclei, prominent nucleoli, and atypical mitoses (34).

Ancillary Testing

The lesional spindle cells demonstrate immunohistochemical evidence of myofibroblastic differentiation, including positivity for smooth muscle actin ($>$ 90 percent of cases), muscle-specific actin (90 percent), vimentin ($>$ 90 percent), and desmin (70 percent). Cytokeratin is occasionally present (30 percent), but only focally (32,35).

Rearrangements of the *ALK* gene on chromosome 2p23 have been demonstrated in 50–75 percent (30). Pediatric cases appear to harbor *ALK* rearrangements more frequently than adults (36). Rearrangements in *ROS1* or *PDGFR*β have recently been described in ALK-negative cases (37).

Immunohistochemical staining for ALK is present in 50–60 percent of cases morphologically consistent with IMT (Figure 16.3f), and correlates to *ALK* overexpression by reverse transcriptase polymerase chain reaction (RT-PCR) (30,32,33,38).

Staining patterns include diffuse cytoplasmic, granular cytoplasmic, and nuclear membranous (38). Immunostaining for *ROS1* has also been shown in *ROS1*-rearranged cases in a cytoplasmic distribution, with or without nuclear staining (39).

Treatment and Prognosis

IMT is generally considered a neoplasm of intermediate biologic potential with a potential to locally recur but infrequently metastasize (30,32,34). Metastastatic sites include lung, brain, liver, and bone (30,32). Occasional spontaneous regression has been documented (40). Significant prognostic differences have not been demonstrated between ALK-negative and ALK-positive cases. Morphologic predictors of behavior have also been inadequate, and even atypical histologic features do not necessarily correlated to outcome (30).

The treatment of choice is complete surgical resection when possible. Chemotherapy (including ALK-inhibitor crizotinib) and/or radiation therapy is reserved for unresectable cases or incomplete resections (31,41). Recurrence can occur in up to 25 percent of cases, but is considerably less ($<$ 10 percent) if completely resected (40).

Desmoid Tumor

Overview

Deep, aggressive, or desmoid-type fibromatosis (DF) is considered a neoplasm of intermediate biologic potential, with the capacity to locally infiltrate but not metastasize. In contrast to superficial fibromatosis (also known as Dupuytren's contracture when located in the palm), deep fibromatosis is a clonal neoplasm occurring either sporadically or in the setting of familial adenomatous polyposis (42).

Clinical Features

Most cases of DF occur sporadically with only 5–10 percent arising in familial adenomatous polyposis (FAP) patients; however, the incidence in the FAP population alone can be up to 30 percent. Multifocality is present in up to 10 percent, and should initiate workup for FAP (42). A history of trauma or prior operation is often elicited. Age range is variable, but peaks between 10 and 40 years. During reproductive age, the incidence of DF is higher in females, but shows equal gender distribution in the pediatric and older age groups (43). DF is generally divided into (1) intra-abdominal (associated with small bowel mesentery and representing most cases of FAP-associated DF), (2) abdominal wall (most cases of pregnancy-related DF), and (3) extra-abdominal (intramuscular or deep fascial, including pelvic and shoulder girdle and head and neck) (42). The clinical presentation of DF is usually that of a slow-growing, painless mass occasionally with rapid enlargement (44). CT often identifies the mass (Figure 16.4a); however, MRI is the main imaging modality, which demonstrates a single or multiple

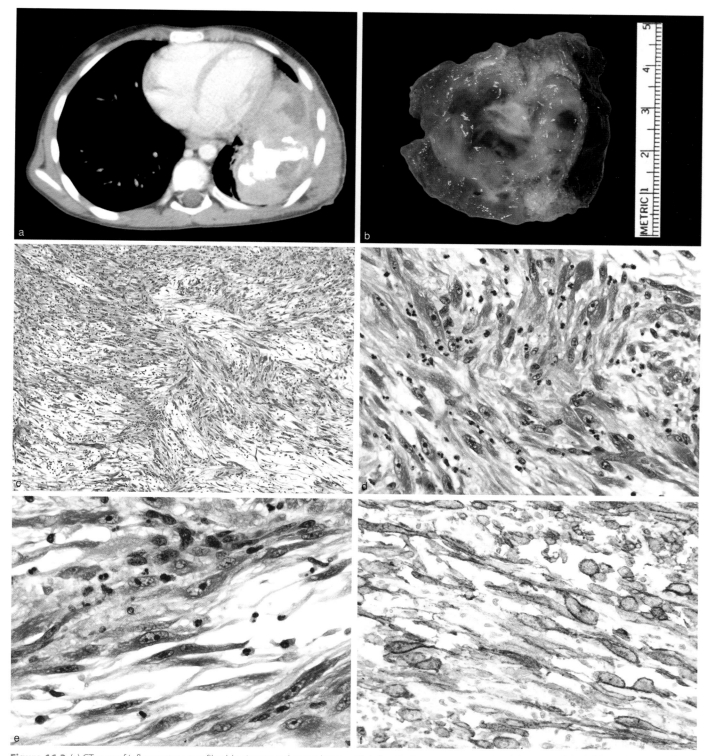

Figure 16.3 (a) CT scan of inflammatory myofibroblastic tumor shows a large, well-defined heterogeneous mass involving most of the left hemithorax. Confluent areas of high density and low density likely represent calcification and necrosis, respectively. (b) Gross photograph, cut surface, demonstrates tan glistening tissue consistent with myxoid stromal change. Central hemorrhage and fibrosis are evident. (c) Moderately cellular neoplasm with variably collagenous to myxoid stroma. (d) Spindle cells have oval nuclei and tapering cytoplasm. Numerous admixed inflammatory cells are present. (e) Variably prominent nucleoli are present. Scattered eosinophils are appreciated. (f) Cytoplasmic and membranous immunoreactivity for ALK.

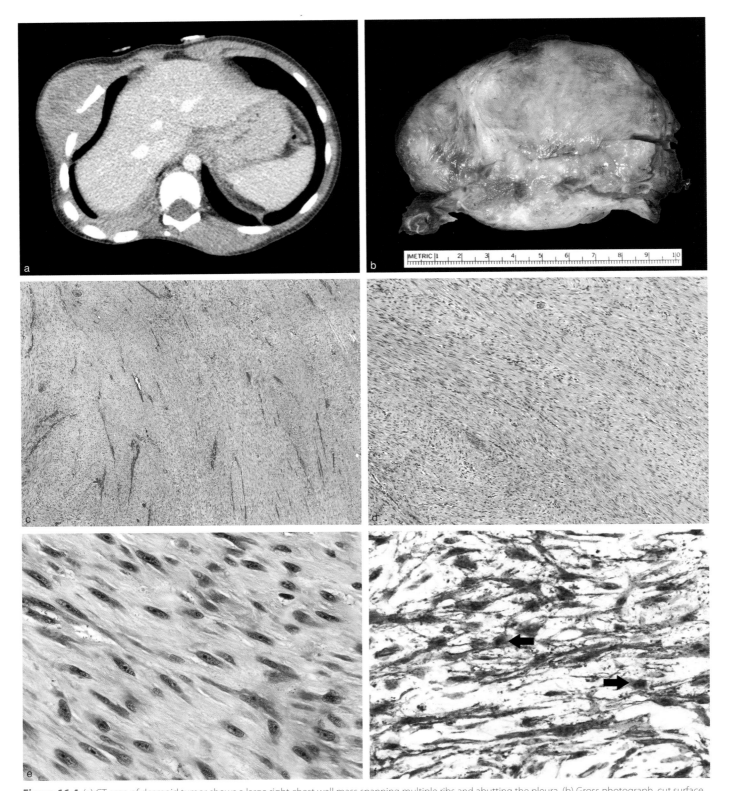

Figure 16.4 (a) CT scan of desmoid tumor shows a large right chest wall mass spanning multiple ribs and abutting the pleura. (b) Gross photograph, cut surface, shows a firm, white, fasciculated tumor. (c) Sweeping eosinophilic fascicles of spindle cells with scattered compressed blood vessels. (d) Parallel arrangement of cells and abundant collagenous stroma is appreciated. (e) Nuclei are elongated with small, single nucleoli. Cytoplasm is scant and tapering. (f) Nuclear (arrow) and cytoplasmic immunoreactivity for *Beta-catenin*.

confluent nodules with variable peripheral infiltration, a "fascial tail," and heterogenous T2 signal intensity (42,43). Core-needle biopsy frequently yields sufficient material for pathologic diagnosis.

Pathologic Features

Grossly, DF is occasionally circumscribed but more frequently appears as an ill-defined, infiltrative mass with a firm, tan–white cut surface (Figure 16.4b).

Microscopically, DF is characterized by long fascicles of uniform, parallel, bland spindle cells within a collagenous stroma (Figure 16.4c,d). Nuclei are oval and often vesicular with small pinpoint nucleoli. Cytoplasm is tapering with ill-defined borders (Figure 16.4e). Mitoses can number up to five per 10 high-power fields; pleomorphism and tumor necrosis are absent. Slit-like blood vessels are scattered throughout the tumor (44).

Ancillary Testing

Immunohistochemical stain for SMA is usually positive, confirming the myofibroblastic phenotype. Desmin can be focal. Caldesmon is negative. Some cases demonstrate estrogen receptor positivity, which may be relevant for treatment considerations. In the proper histologic context, nuclear expression of Beta-catenin can be confirmatory, as it is expressed in up to 80 percent of sporadic DF cases and correlates to *Beta-catenin* gene mutation (Figure 16.4f) (45,46). In FAP patients, nuclear expression is present in fewer cases (67 percent) and inactivating germline mutations of the *APC* (adenomatous polyposis coli) gene are present. *APC* and *Beta-catenin* mutations are mutually exclusive in DF and are absent in superficial fibromatosis (42,44).

Treatment and Prognosis

Many cases of stable, unsymptomatic fibromatosis can be monitored with a "watchful waiting" approach, with which some studies report progression-free survival rates of 50 percent at 5 years and spontaneous regression rates of up to 10 percent. Second-line therapy is surgical resection with a balance between microscopically negative margins and preservation of function, although positive margins do not necessarily correlate with recurrence (42). For recurrent, progressive, or otherwise inoperable disease, radiotherapy or medical therapy can be considered. Antihormonal agents (including tamoxifen) and NSAIDs are first-line medical therapies. Chemotherapy (methotrexate, vinblastine, anthracyclines) may lead to toxicity; however, pegylated liposomal doxorubicin and tyrosine kinase inhibitors (imatinib) are proving effective with less toxicity (42).

Increased recurrence risk is present in younger age, intra-abdominal/mesenteric location, FAP/Gardner syndrome, and specific S45F *Beta-catenin* mutation. The highest recurrence rates are in head and neck tumors, the lowest in pregnancy-related abdominal wall tumors (44). Metastases do not occur.

Lipoma/Liposarcoma

Overview

Adipocytic tumors occur most frequently in the extremities and retroperitoneum. Intrathoracic and intra-abdominal lipomas and liposarcomas are extremely rare, and metastasis should be excluded in malignant cases. Variants of liposarcoma include: (1) well-differentiated (WDLPS)/dedifferentiated (DDLPS), (2) myxoid/round cell, and (3) pleomorphic (47).

Clinical Features

Lipogenic tumors are most frequent in adult males (48). Common presenting symptoms include chest pain, cough, and dyspnea in intrathoracic cases and abdominal pain or fullness in intra-abdominal cases. The most common intrathoracic variants are WDLPS and myxoid; the most common intra-abdominal variants are WDLPS and DDLPS (49–51). Both lipomas and WDLPS appear similar on imaging, with a prominent fat component and occasional fibrous septae. Dedifferentiated and pleomorphic liposarcomas are both fat-poor on imaging (52). Core-needle biopsy should yield sufficient material for diagnosis in most cases.

Pathologic Features

Benign adipocytic tumors are generally smaller (< 10 cm) with circumscribed borders and homogeneously yellow, glistening cut surfaces. Histologic examination demonstrates mature adipocytes without atypia, as in conventional lipomas of soft tissue (53). Variants (such as myxolipoma or fibrolipoma) may also occur (54).

Gross and microscopic features of malignant adipocyte tumors are similar to those in the extremities and retroperitoneum. WDLPS consists of four variants: conventional adipocytic (lipoma-like), sclerosing, inflammatory, and spindle cell. All variants demonstrate mature fat, occasionally of varying sizes, with nuclear atypia in fat and/or spindle stromal cells (Figure 16.5a,b). The sclerosing variant also has a prominent collagenous background and can be fat-poor. The inflammatory variant has an abundant lymphoplasmacytic component. The rare spindle cell variant demonstrates a bland spindle cell proliferation with a fibrous or myxoid stroma and occasional lipoblasts. Lipoblasts are not normally present in the three former variants (47). DDLPS most frequently resemble a high-grade undifferentiated sarcoma (with or without an inflammatory background), but can also resemble myxofibrosarcoma or leio- or rhabdomyosarcoma (Figure 16.5c,d). In the setting of hypercellularity and absence of fat in areas of a WDLPS, mitoses of five or more per 10 high-power fields can be used to define DDLPS (55). Myxoid liposarcoma is hypocellular proliferation

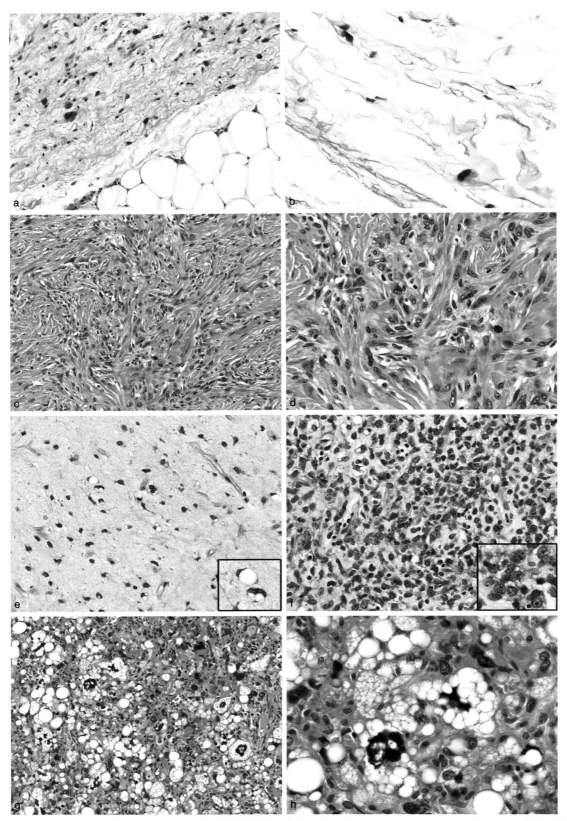

Figure 16.5 (a) Hyperchromatic stromal cells in WDLPS. (b) Atypical nuclei within mature-appearing fat are also present. (c) Storiform spindle cell growth pattern in DDLPS. (d) Numerous mitotic figures are also present. (e) Myxoid stroma, curvilinear blood vessels, and signet ring and multivacuolated lipoblasts (inset) in myxoid LPS. (f) Increasing cellularity comprising cells with scant cytoplasm and oval to round nuclei with nucleoli in round cell LPS. (g) Sheets of pleomorphic cells in pleomorphic LPS. (h) Pleomorphic lipoblasts demonstrated hyperchromatic, lobulated nuclei and multivacuolated cytoplasm.

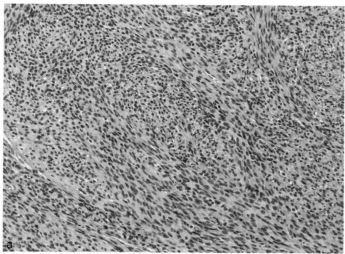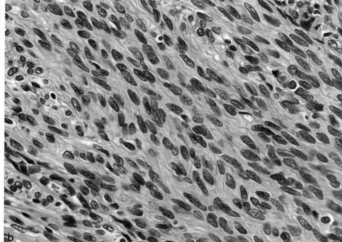

Figure 16.6 (a) Moderately cellular fascicles of spindle cells intersecting at 90 degree angles, suggestive of smooth muscle differentiation in leiomyomatosis peritonealis disseminata. (b) Spindle cells show oval, blunt nuclei and eosinophilic cytoplasm.

of bland spindle to stellate cells and lipoblasts in a myxoid stroma with abundant thin-walled branching vessels (Figure 16.5e). A round cell component in excess of 5 percent defines high-grade or round cell liposarcoma (Figure 16.5f). The histologic hallmark of pleomorphic liposarcoma is markedly irregular lipoblasts, usually in a high-grade spindle cell or epithelioid background (Figure 16.5g,h) (47).

Ancillary Testing

Both WDLPS and DDLPS are characterized by ring and/or giant marker chromosomes with amplified 12q13–15 region, which includes proto-oncogenes *MDM2*, *CDK4*, and *HMGA2*. Overexpression of *MDM2*, *CDK4*, and *HMGA2* can be detected by immunostaining and amplification detected by FISH (47). Some authors advocate a combination of MDM2, CDK4, and p16 immunostains, as 100 percent of WDLPS and 93 percent of DDLPS expressed two of these three markers (56).

Myxoid and round cell liposarcoma share balanced translocations of chromosome 12, most frequently t(12;16)(q13;p11) or t(12;22)(q13;q22), representing *DDIT3(CHOP)/FUS* or *DDIT3(CHOP)/EWSR1* fusions, respectively. Pleomorphic liposarcoma demonstrates complex karyotypic aberrations without specific cytogenetic findings (47).

Treatment and Prognosis

Well-differentiated morphology and/or radical surgery generally results in increased survival in intrathoracic tumors (52). Chemo- and/or radiotherapy are also options, but variable response rates have been observed. Dedifferentiated and pleomorphic morphology generally portend a worse prognosis (51,52).

Leiomyomatosis Peritonealis Disseminata (Diffuse Peritoneal Leiomyomatosis)

Overview

Leiomyomatosis peritonealis disseminata (LPD) is a rare benign smooth muscle tumor characterized by multiple small peritoneal nodules, often occurring in the setting of uterine leiomyomas. Malignant transformation is rare.

Clinical Features

LPD generally occurs as tens to hundreds of small (2 mm to 3 cm) peritoneal nodules in women of reproductive age, either in the pregnant or postpartum state or in the setting of uterine leiomyomas, often in women on hormonal contraceptives. In pregnancy, they are often found incidentally at cesarean section or tubal ligation. Non-pregnant women may experience pelvic discomfort or pain (57). This condition is different from parasitic leioyoma (a solitary, detached leiomyoma that attaches to the peritoneal surface and undergoes neovascularization), benign metastasizing leiomyoma (ectopic leiomyoma but usually at a distant site such as lung), and intravenous leiomyomatosis (within pelvic or other blood vessels) (58).

Pathologic Features

Grossly, they are well-circumscribed, firm nodules with a whorled, white–tan cut surface resembling leiomyomas. Microscopically, they demonstrate eosinophilic spindle cells in whorls or fascicles with elongated, blunt nuclei with small nucleoli (Figure 16.6a,b). Cytologic atypia is absent and mitoses are no more than 3 per 10 high-power fields (57). Decidual cells may be present in pregnant/postpartum women (59). A mesothelial lining is often appreciated.

Ancillary Testing

Immunohistochemical evidence of smooth muscle phenotype is present (desmin, SMA). Nuclear estrogen and progesterone receptor expression can be seen in spindle cells (60).

Treatment and Prognosis

Complete excision of all nodules is not always possible nor necessary, as they generally do not progress and may regress with withdrawal of estrogenic stimulus. Rare examples of malignant progression have been reported (61).

Angiosarcoma and Epithelioid Hemangioendothelioma

Overview

Angiosarcoma and epithelioid hemangioendothelioma (EHE) can, on occasion, arise in the pleura and have been recognized as potential mimics of mesothelioma. They are typically seen as a spectrum from epithelioid low-grade EHE, to intermediate-grade EHE, to high-grade epithelioid angiosarcoma (EAS).

Clinical Features

Patients typically present with pleural effusion, chest pain, shortness of breath, or hemoptysis. They are often found to have extensive pleural thickening on imaging studies (62,63). Rare peritoneal cases are described (62,64). Angiosarcomas can be radiation-induced (64). EHE and EAS are adult-age diseases without clear gender predilection.

Pathologic Features

Tumors often result in diffuse plaque-like thickening of the pleura or a multinodular appearance (Figure 16.7). Histologically, clusters and nests of epithelioid cells are seen. Some cases exhibit a tubulopapillary growth pattern mimicking mesothelioma. The pleural thickening is often associated with invasion into adjacent adipose tissue (62,63).

A distinction between low- and intermediate-grade EHEs has been suggested based on mitotic activity, necrosis, and nuclear pleomorphism. The distinction between high-grade EHE and EAS can be difficult. Criteria favoring EHE are intracytoplasmic lumina, nuclear cytoplasmic inclusions, and distinctive extracellular matrix with myxoid or chondroid features. Criteria favoring EAS are prominent nucleoli, high mitotic

activity, papillary growth, blood lakes, and capillary-like vasoformative spaces (63).

Ancillary Techniques

The lesional cells usually express FLI-1, CD31, CD34, ERG, and vimentin (Figure 16.7c,d). Cytokeratins and D2–40 (podoplanin) can be positive. WT-1 and calretinin are negative. The presence of a *CAMTA1–WWTR1* fusion gene is associated with EHE and may argue against a diagnosis of EAS in challenging cases (63).

EHE and EAS can mimic mesothelioma with its diffuse plaque-like growth as well as its histomorphology with epithelioid cells exhibiting areas of tubulopapillary growth. The growth of epithelioid cells expressing cytokeratins can also be mistaken for carcinoma.

Treatment and Prognosis

Suster et al. report data suggesting a relatively favorable outcome for patients with anterior mediastinal EHE (65). The outcome data in other studies is less good. Histologic grade on the outlined spectrum of epithelioid vascular lesions correlates with prognosis. Intermediate-grade EHE and EAS are aggressive diseases leading to the demise of the patients within months (62,63). Pleural involvement is a poor prognostic feature for these vascular tumors.

Ewing Family of Tumors (PNET/Ewing Sarcoma/Askin Tumor)

Overview

These neoplasms are small round cell tumors with typical molecular features that include a spectrum of manifestations historically described separately.

Clinical Features

Ewing family tumors (EFT) include Ewing sarcoma of bone, Askin tumor in the thoracopulmonary region, and peripheral neuroectodermal tumor (PNET) in the soft tissue. The definition of the underlying t(11;22) translocation has helped to confirm that these lesions are all part of the same spectrum. In addition to EFTs in the chest that were traditionally described as Askin tumor, there are rare reports of these tumors arising in the omentum or mesentery (66,67). These tumors are most common in adolescents and young adults. There is a slight male predominance. Caucasians are more commonly affected than other ethnic groups (68–71).

Pathologic Features

Grossly, the tumor is friable tan–gray or yellow–gray. Necrosis is often grossly apparent. Histologically uniform cells with

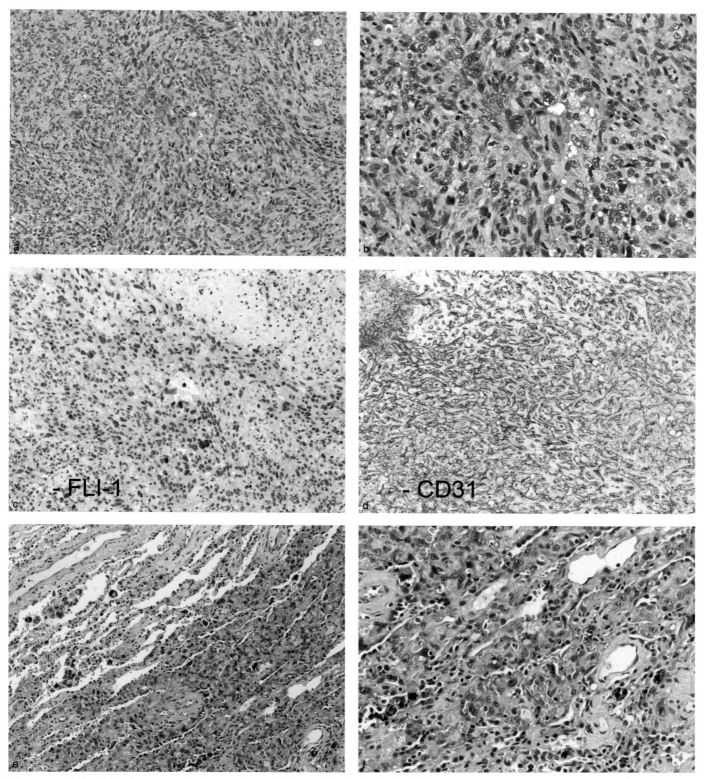

Figure 16.7 Pericardial angiosarcoma with pleomorphic spindled to epithelioid cells that focally form or line spaces containing red blood cells (a,b). These label for FLI-1 and CD31 as markers consistent with endothelial lineage (c,d). Case of pleuropulmonary angiosarcoma growing into lung parenchyma (e) that comprises epithelioid highly atypical tumor cells lining blood-filled spaces (f).

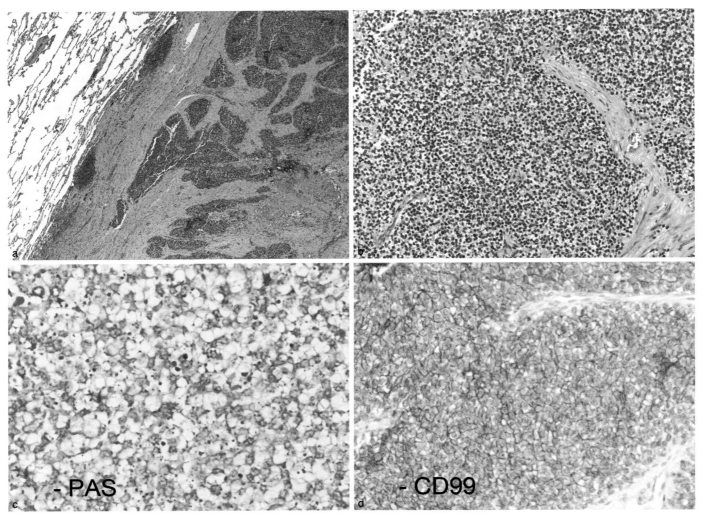

Figure 16.8 This upper chest wall Ewing sarcoma grew to compress adjacent lung (a) and comprises sheets and nests of cells. The monomorphic small round blue cells show some cytoplasmic vacuolation (b). PAS-positive cytoplasmic glycogen can be seen in the lesional cells (c). The tumor cells exhibit uniform membranous labeling for CD99 (d).

round or ovoid nuclei are arranged in sheets or lobules (Figure 16.8). Scant cytoplasm with vacuolation attributable to cytoplasmic glycogen is seen in most cases (Figure 16.8c). Some cases show "PNET-type" features with Homer Wright rosettes. Mitotic activity can be variable. Unusual variants include those with spindle cell features, adamantinoma-like features, or keratin expression (27,72,73).

Ancillary Testing

EFT exhibit staining for CD99/MIC2 with membranous accentuation and nuclear expression of FLI-1 (Figure 16.8d) (27,72,73). Many show some staining with neural markers like synaptophysin, NSE, CD57, S100, and PGP9.5. Cytokeratin expression can be found in about a quarter of cases and often goes along with focal or dot-like pattern of staining. Rare cases are desmin-positive. The diagnosis is confirmed by identify-

ing one of the described recurrent translocations that typically involved the *EWSR1* locus and a member of the ETS family. The t(11;22) translocation resulting in a *EWSR1–FLI1* fusion transcript is found in approximately 85 percent of cases. A long list of other fusion partners is also described (27,72,73).

Other small round blue cell tumors may be considered together with EFT. In younger patients these include rhabdomyosarcoma, desmoplastic small round cell tumor (DSRCT), neuroblastoma or hematopoietic tumors. In older patients the differential may also include carcinoma.

Treatment and Prognosis

Patients are treated with a combination of surgery, chemotherapy and radiation therapy. In general, the 5-year survival for EFT is close to 70 percent. Survival for metastatic or recurrent cases is still poor (73,74).

Desmoplastic Small Round Cell Tumor

Overview

Desmoplastic small round cell tumor (DSRCT) is a high-grade malignant mesenchymal neoplasm that is typically seen in children and young adults and is associated with a defining *EWSR1–WT1* fusion transcript. The WHO classifies it among the tumors of uncertain differentiation.

Clinical Features

The peak incidence is in the third decade of life. Males are more commonly affected than females. The typical location for this tumor are the abdominal cavity, retroperitoneum, or pelvis, but rare cases restricted to the thoracic cavity are described. Abdominal cases usually present with advanced disseminated disease causing vague non-specific complaints such as abdominal pain, abdominal distention, nausea, or emesis. Patients with pleural disease may present with symptoms including chest pain, scoliosis attributable to pain, and respiratory manifestations (75–77).

Pathologic Features

Grossly, the tumor usually appears as a multinodular lesion with a white–gray cut surface. Histologically, sharply defined nests and cords of small cells are found in a background of desmoplastic stroma (Figure 16.9a–d) (73,77). The lesional cells show hyperchromatic nuclei, abundant mitotic activity, and frequent apoptotic bodies. Necrosis and cystic degeneration may be found (73,77).

Ancillary Testing

DSRCT is characterized by a complex immunophenotype with expression of markers that are usually associated with different lineages of differentiation, including markers of epithelial, muscle, and neural differentiation (73,77). The tumor often shows some staining for keratins, EMA, vimentin, desmin, and NSE (Figure 16.9e,f). Myogenin and MyoD1 are negative. A few cases may express CD99 and rare ones FLI-1. DSRCT is characterized by a t(11;22) translocation that results in a *EWSR1–WT1* fusion transcript. By immunohistochemistry, staining is seen with antibodies targeting the carboxy terminus but not the amino terminus of WT-1 (73,77).

Other small round blue cell tumors may be considered together with DSRCT. In younger patients this may include rhabdomyosarcoma, EFT, neuroblastoma, or hematopoietic tumors. In older patients the differential may also include carcinoma. The complex immunophenotype can be misleading.

Treatment and Prognosis

Patients typically receive multimodal treatment with chemotherapy, radiation therapy, and surgery. Three-year survival may reach 50 percent. The long-term survival is still poor despite aggressive treatment (73,76).

Pleuropulmonary Blastoma

Overview

Pleuropulmonary blastoma is a manifestation of germline *DICER1* mutations and a sentinel lesion of the associated hereditary syndrome. The *DICER1* syndrome also includes pituitary blastoma, pineoblastoma, nasal chondromesenchymal hamartoma, cystic nephroma, botryoid-type embryonal rhabdomyosarcoma, ovarian Sertoli–Leydig cell tumor, ciliary body medulloepithelioma, and different carcinomas of the thyroid.

Clinical Features

Pleuropulmonary blastoma is commonly seen in young children. Common presenting symptoms include dry cough, dyspnea, fever, and chest pain. The tumor is typically located in the peripheral lung parenchyma adjacent to the pleura. Rare cases may arise in the parietal pleura or the diaphragm. Imaging studies help to define the location of the lesion and can aid in its classification as cystic (type I), cystic and solid (type II), or purely solid (type III). Type I lesions are seen almost exclusively in the first three years of life with a peak at one year of age, while the median age for type II and type III lesions is around 3 years of age. Rare cases are found in adolescents (78). A recent large study found germline *DICER1* mutations in 2/3 of patients with pleuropulmonary blastoma (78). No clinical differences were found between cases with and without germline mutation (79).

Pathologic Features

In principal, the tumor comprises primitive mesenchymal cells and admixed entrapped benign epithelial elements (Figure 16.10) (78,80,81). Focal rhabdomyoblastic or cartilaginous differentiation can be encountered. The cystic presumed early form (type I) of the disease can be uniloculated or multiloculated, with variable amounts of mesenchymal cells under the benign epithelial lining. With that the lesions can appear deceptively bland. In this context, cystic lesions lacking the primitive component have been classified as type Ir with an "r" indicating regression. Type II and III lesions contain solid areas with primitive or blastematous mesenchyme, rhabdomyosarcoma-like areas, fibrosarcoma-like areas, primitive sarcomatous areas, cartilaginous areas, anaplastic cells, and atypical mitoses. Type II contains residual cystic areas while type III is entirely solid. Therefore, a biopsy may not always allow distinction between these two types (82).

Ancillary Studies

The mesenchymal cells of these tumors stain for vimentin and express desmin, myogenin, and muscle-specific actin. EMA and keratin are negative in these cells but label the lining epithelium. The cases associated with germline *DICER1* mutation are

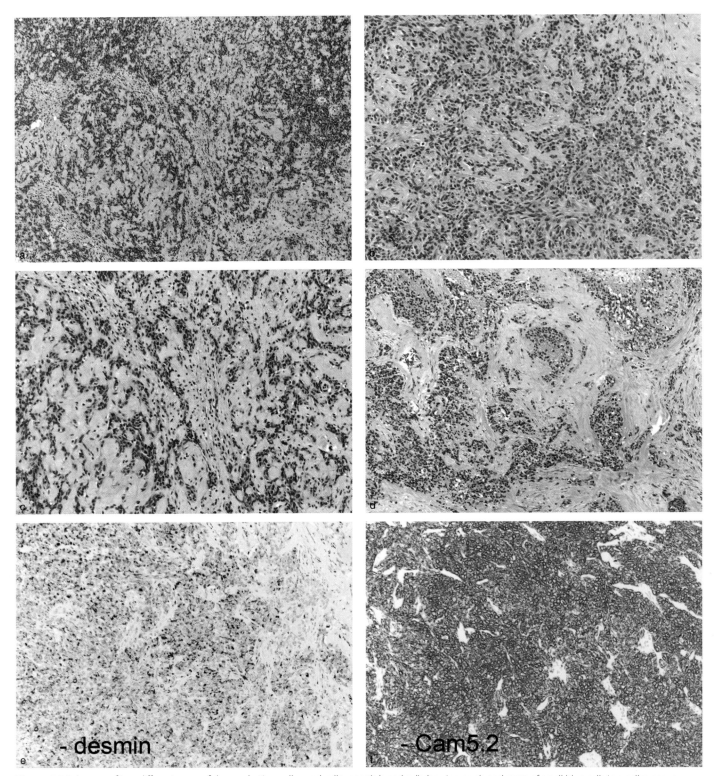

Figure 16.9 Images of two different cases of desmoplastic small round cell tumor (a,b and c,d) showing cords and nests of small blue cells in a collagenous background. The lesional cells express an unusual combination of immunohistochemical markers as illustrated by the positive labeling for desmin and cytokeratin Cam5.2 shown here (e,f).

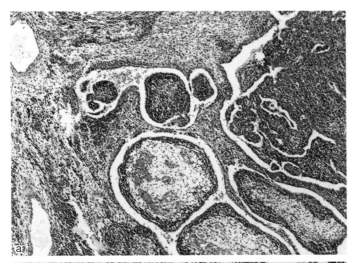

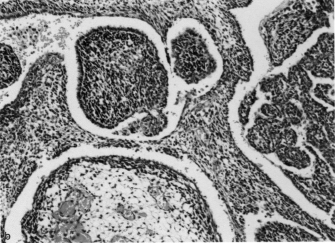

Figure 16.10 The H&E-stained sections of pulmonary blastoma show two components, immature mesenchymal cells admixed with benign entrapped epithelial cells (a,b).

assumed to carry a second-hit somatic mutation. At least some of the sporadic cases have been shown to carry two somatic *DICER1* mutations. *DICER1* mutations are thought disrupt 5p micro-RNA processing, shifting the balance between 3p and 5p miRNAs. That shift is thought to de-repress oncofetal genes. *TP53* mutations are frequent and some cases show *NRAS* or *BRAF* mutations. Cytogenetic studies have shown gains and losses of multiple chromosomes or chromosome arms including 2+, 8+, 10q–, 11q–, 17q–, and 20q+ (78,82,83).

The differential diagnosis for type I lesions may include congenital pulmonary airway malformations, while that of type II and type III lesions includes fetal lung interstitial tumor.

Treatment and Prognosis

The type I lesions do not have metastatic potential and are associated with a good survival of about 90 percent. Approximately

10 percent of patients may progress to a type II or III lesion. The role of chemotherapy in the treatment of type I lesions is still unclear and under investigation. Type II and III lesions may metastasize. Brain and bone are typical sites for metastatic disease. Type II and III lesions are regarded as aggressive tumors that require chemotherapy in addition to surgical resection. Five-year survival is in the range of 55–70 percent for these tumors (78).

Synovial Sarcoma (SS)

Overview

Historically thought to arise from the synovium, synovial sarcoma is now considered a misnomer. It is a tumor of uncertain differentiation that most frequently occurs in periarticular soft tissue but can also occur on serous membranes.

Clinical Features

Primary pleuropulmonary SS occurs with greater frequency than pericardial or mesenteric SS. Like its soft-tissue counterpart, it tends to occur in young to middle-aged adults without a gender predilection. Symptoms include chest pain and cough, pericardial effusion and shortness of breath, or abdominal pain, depending on site (84–86). Median size is approximately 10 cm. CT shows a usually solitary tumor with circumscribed borders and heterogeneous enhancement. Echocardiography can be used in pericardial cases (85). In intrathoracic cases, metastasis should be considered, as lung is the most frequent site of metastasis in soft-tissue tumors (40–50 percent of cases) (84). Fine-needle aspiration could be suggestive of spindle cell neoplasm; however, core biopsy or excision are generally required for definitive diagnosis.

Pathologic Features

Grossly, SS is usually well-circumscribed and uni- or multinodular with a variably soft to firm tan–pink cut surface. Hemorrhage or necrosis may be present.

Microscopically, most pleuroplumonary cases are monophasic; however, biphasic tumors can occur (84). Monophasic forms are composed of moderately cellular to hypercellular sheets or vague fascicles of uniform spindle cells with bland oval to elongated nuclei, scant basophilic cytoplasm, and indistinct cell borders (Figure 16.11a,b) (87). The stroma can exhibit some myxoid to collagenous change. Biphasic forms show epithelial and spindle cells in varying proportions. The epithelial component may demonstrate solid, tubulo-glandular, or papillary architecture. Thin-walled, dilated (hemangiopericytoma-like) blood vessels may be present in monophasic or biphasic forms.

Poorly differentiated SS has been described, and can manifest as three morphologic patterns: a large epithelioid cell

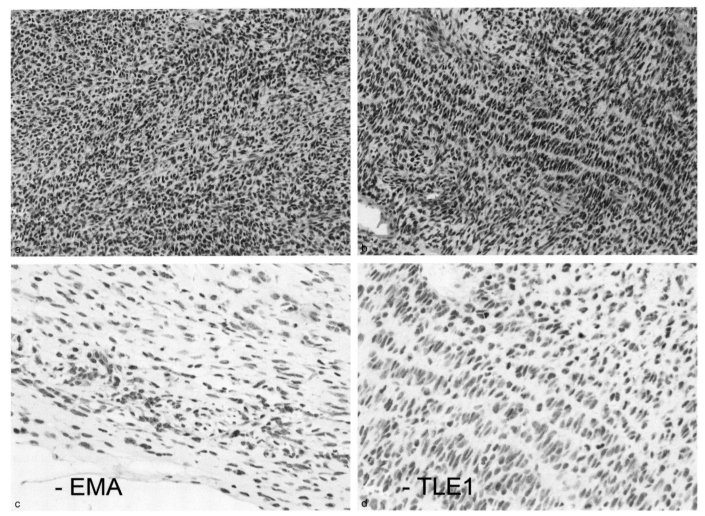

Figure 16.11 (a) A large synovial sarcoma involving the neck and mediastinum with extensive carciac extension. The lesion comprises sheets of vaguely fasciculated, monomorphic spindle cells within a somewhat myxoid stroma. (b) An unusual feature is a distinct palisaded arrangement. (c) EMA stains at least some cells. (d) Nuclear immunoreactivity for TLE-1.

variant with hypercellularity and pleomorphism; a small cell variant with occasional rosette-like structures; and a spindle cell variant with herringbone growth and increased mitotic rate (88).

Ancillary Testing

EMA is positive in the majority of SS (monophasic, biphasic, and poorly differentiated) (Figure 16.11c). Keratins are expressed frequently in biphasic and monophasic SS, with less expression in poorly differentiated SS. Nuclear TLE-1 staining is present in 80–90 percent of SS cases (Figure 16.11d), but can stain weakly with low frequency in solitary fibrous tumors and benign or malignant peripheral nerve sheath tumors (89,90).

Translocation t(X;18) between the *SYT* gene on chromosome 18 and either the *SSX1* or *SSX2* gene on chromosome X has been described in up to 90 percent of SS, and can be detected by FISH or PCR for the fusion transcript (87,88).

Treatment and Prognosis

Primary treatment includes surgical resection often followed by adjuvant radiation or chemotherapy. Local recurrence can occur in a significant number of patients (25–75 percent), with occasional metastasis. Five-year survival can range from 25 to 65 percent. Poorer prognosis has been attributed to increased tumor size ($\geq$ 9 cm), male gender, older age ($>$ 20 years), extensive tumor necrosis, and poorly differentiated morphology (87,88). Additionally, prognosis of pericardial cases is generally poor (85).

References

1. Chung EM, Biko DM, Arzamendi AM, Meldrum JT, Stocker JT. Solid tumors of the peritoneum, omentum, and mesentery in children: radiologic–pathologic correlation: from the radiologic pathology archives. *RadioGraphics*. 2015;35(2):521–46.

2. Gladish GW, Sabloff BM, Munden RF, Truong MT, Erasmus JJ, Chasen MH. Primary thoracic sarcomas. *RadioGraphics*. 2002;22(3):621–37.

3. Levy AD, Arnaiz J, Shaw JC, Sobin LH. From the archives of the AFIP: primary peritoneal tumors: imaging features with pathologic correlation. *RadioGraphics*. 2008;28(2):583–607, quiz 621–22.

4. Vicens RA, Patnana M, Le O, Bhosale PR, Sagebiel TL, Menias CO, et al. Multimodality imaging of common and uncommon peritoneal diseases: a review for radiologists. *Abdom Imaging*. 2015;40(2):436–56.

5. Joshi A, McAndrew N, Birdsall S, Attanoos RL. Clear cell sarcoma mimicking malignant pleural mesothelioma. *Histopathology*. 2008;53(3):359–61.

6. Ju HU, Seo KW, Jegal Y, Ahn JJ, Lee YJ, Kim YM, et al. A case of alveolar soft part sarcoma of the pleura. *J Korean Med Sci*. 2013;28(2):331–35.

7. Liang W, Xu S. Imaging findings from a case of pleural low-grade fibromyxoid sarcoma similar to mesothelioma with pleural effusion. *Clin Respir J*. 2016;10(1):120–24.

8. Lee CH, Park CR, Kim JW, Suh JH, Lee YJ, Jung JP. Extraskeletal osteosarcoma arising from the pleura. *Korean J Thorac Cardiovasc Surg*. 2014;47(3):320–24.

9. Cagle PT, Allen TC. Pathology of the pleura: what the pulmonologists need to know. *Respirology*. 2011;16(3):430–38.

10. Marak CP, Dorokhova O, Guddati AK. Solitary fibrous tumor of the pleura. *Med Oncol*. 2013;30(2):573.

11. Cardillo G, Lococo F, Carleo F, Martelli M. Solitary fibrous tumors of the pleura. *Curr Opin Pulm Med*. 2012;18(4):339–46.

12. Lee KH, Song KS, Kwon Y, Lee I, Lee JS, Lim TH. Mesenchymal tumours of the thorax: CT findings and pathological features. *Clin Radiol*. 2003;58(12):934–44.

13. Vogels RJ, Vlenterie M, Versleijen-Jonkers YM, Ruijter E, Bekers EM, Verdijk MA, et al. Solitary fibrous tumor – clinicopathologic, immunohistochemical and molecular analysis of 28 cases. *Diagn Pathol*. 2014;9(1):224.

14. Rao N, Colby TV, Falconieri G, Cohen H, Moran CA, Suster S. Intrapulmonary solitary fibrous tumors: clinicopathologic and immunohistochemical study of 24 cases. *Am J Surg Pathol*. 2013;37(2):155–66.

15. Vallat-Decouvelaere AV, Dry SM, Fletcher CD. Atypical and malignant solitary fibrous tumors in extrathoracic locations: evidence of their comparability to intra-thoracic tumors. *Am J Surg Pathol*. 1998;22(12):1501–11.

16. England DM, Hochholzer L, McCarthy MJ. Localized benign and malignant fibrous tumors of the pleura. A clinicopathologic review of 223 cases. *Am J Surg Pathol*. 1989;13(8):640–58.

17. de Perrot M, Fischer S, Bründler M-A, Sekine Y, Keshavjee S. Solitary fibrous tumors of the pleura. *Ann Thorac Surg*. 2002;74(1):285–93.

18. Tapias LF, Mercier O, Ghigna MR, Lahon B, Lee H, Mathisen DJ, et al. Validation of a scoring system to predict recurrence of resected solitary fibrous tumors of the pleura. *Chest*. 2015;147(1):216–23.

19. Schmid S, Csanadi A, Kaifi JT, Kübler M, Haager B, Kayser G, et al. Prognostic factors in solitary fibrous tumors of the pleura. *J Surg Res*. 2015;195(2):580–87.

20. Mosquera J-M, Fletcher CDM. Expanding the spectrum of malignant progression in solitary fibrous tumors: a study of 8 cases with a discrete anaplastic component–is this dedifferentiated SFT? *Am J Surg Pathol*. 2009;33(9):1314–21.

21. Doyle LA, Vivero M, Fletcher CD, Mertens F, Hornick JL. Nuclear expression of STAT6 distinguishes solitary fibrous tumor from histologic mimics. *Mod Pathol*. 2014;27(3):390–95.

22. Ng TL, Gown AM, Barry TS, Cheang MCU, Chan AKW, Turbin DA, et al. Nuclear beta-catenin in mesenchymal tumors. *Mod Pathol*. 2005;18(1):68–74.

23. Langman G, Rathinam S, Papadaki L. Primary localised pleural neurofibroma: expanding the spectrum of spindle cell tumours of the pleura. *J Clin Pathol*. 2010;63(2):116–18.

24. Miguchi M, Takakura Y, Egi H, Hinoi T, Adachi T, Kawaguchi Y, et al. Malignant peripheral nerve sheath tumor arising from the greater omentum: case report. *World J Surg Oncol*. 2011;9:33.

25. Boland JM, Colby TV, Folpe AL. Intrathoracic peripheral nerve sheath tumors – a clinicopathological study of 75 cases. *Hum Pathol*. 2015;46(3):419–25.

26. Antonescu CR, Perry A, Woodruff JM. Schwannoma (including variants). In: Fletcher CDM, Bridge JA, Hogdendoorn PCW, Mertens F, Bosman FT, Jaffe ES, et al., editors. *WHO classification of tumours of soft tissue and bone*. Lyon: International Agency for Research on Cancer; 2013: 170–72.

27. Goldblum JR, Folpe AL, Weiss SW. *Enzinger and Weiss's soft tissue tumors*. 6th edition. Philadelphia, PA: Elsevier; 2014.

28. Nascimento AF, Fletcher CD. The controversial nosology of benign nerve sheath tumors: neurofilament protein staining demonstrates intratumoral axons in many sporadic schwannomas. *Am J Surg Pathol*. 2007;31(9):1363–70.

29. Wu J, Zhu H, Li K, Yuan CY, Wang YF, Lu GM. Imaging observations of pulmonary inflammatory myofibroblastic tumors in patients over 40 years old. *Oncol Lett*. 2015;9(4):1877–84.

30. Coffin CM, Hornick JL, Fletcher CDM. Inflammatory myofibroblastic tumor: comparison of clinicopathologic, histologic, and immunohistochemical features including *ALK* expression in atypical and aggressive cases. *Am J Surg Pathol*. 2007;31(4):509–20.

31. Panagiotopoulos N, Patrini D, Gvinianidze L, Woo WL, Borg E, Lawrence D. Inflammatory myofibroblastic tumour of the lung: a reactive lesion or a true neoplasm? *J Thorac Dis*. 2015;7(5):908–11.

32. Siminovich M, Galluzzo L, López J, Lubieniecki F, de Dávila MTG. Inflammatory myofibroblastic tumor of the lung in children: anaplastic

lymphoma kinase (*ALK*) expression and clinico-pathological correlation. *Pediatr Dev Pathol.* 2012;15(3):179–86.

33. Oguz B, Ozcan HN, Omay B, Ozgen B, Haliloglu M. Imaging of childhood inflammatory myofibroblastic tumor. *Pediatr Radiol.* 2015;45(11):1672–81.

34. Coffin CM, Humphrey PA, Dehner LP. Extrapulmonary inflammatory myofibroblastic tumor: a clinical and pathological survey. *Semin Diagn Pathol.* 1998;15(2):85–101.

35. Coffin CM, Watterson J, Priest JR, Dehner LP. Extrapulmonary inflammatory myofibroblastic tumor (inflammatory pseudotumor). A clinicopathologic and immunohistochemical study of 84 cases. *Am J Surg Pathol.* 1995;19(8):859–72.

36. Antonescu CR, Suurmeijer AJH, Zhang L, Sung YS, Jungbluth AA, Travis WD, et al. Molecular characterization of inflammatory myofibroblastic tumors with frequent *ALK* and *ROS1* gene fusions and rare novel *RET* rearrangement. *Am J Surg Pathol.* 2015;39(7):957–67.

37. Lovly CM, Gupta A, Lipson D, Otto G, Brennan T, Chung CT, et al. Inflammatory myofibroblastic tumors harbor multiple potentially actionable kinase fusions. *Cancer Discov.* 2014;4(8):889–95.

38. Cook JR, Dehner LP, Collins MH, Ma Z, Morris SW, Coffin CM, et al. Anaplastic lymphoma kinase (*ALK*) expression in the inflammatory myofibroblastic tumor: a comparative immunohistochemical study. *Am J Surg Pathol.* 2001;25(11):1364–71.

39. Hornick JL, Sholl LM, Dal Cin P, Childress MA, Lovly CM. Expression of ROS1 predicts *ROS1* gene rearrangement in inflammatory myofibroblastic tumors. *Mod Pathol.* 2015;28(5):732–39.

40. Kovach SJ, Fischer AC, Katzman PJ, Salloum RM, Ettinghausen SE, Madeb R, et al. Inflammatory myofibroblastic tumors. *J Surg Oncol.* 2006;94(5):385–91.

41. Tothova Z, Wagner AJ. Anaplastic lymphoma kinase-directed therapy in inflammatory myofibroblastic tumors. *Curr Opin Oncol.* 2012;24(4):409–13.

42. Kasper B, Baumgarten C, Bonvalot S, Haas R, Haller F, Hohenberger P, et al. Management of sporadic desmoid-type fibromatosis: a European consensus approach based on patients "and professionals" expertise – a sarcoma patients EuroNet and European Organisation for Research and Treatment of Cancer/Soft Tissue and Bone Sarcoma Group initiative. *Eur J Cancer.* 2015;51(2):127–36.

43. Otero S, Moskovic EC, Strauss DC, Benson C, Miah AB, Thway K, et al. Desmoid-type fibromatosis. *Clin Radiol.* 2015;70(9):1038–45.

44. Fisher C, Thway K. Aggressive fibromatosis. *Pathology.* 2014;46(2):135–40.

45. Carlson JW, Fletcher CDM, Fletcher C. Immunohistochemistry for β-catenin in the differential diagnosis of spindle cell lesions: analysis of a series and review of the literature. *Histopathology.* 2007;51(4):509–14.

46. Bhattacharya B, Dilworth HP, Iacobuzio-Donahue C, Ricci F, Weber K, Furlong MA, et al. Nuclear β-catenin expression distinguishes deep fibromatosis from other benign and malignant fibroblastic and myofibroblastic lesions. *Am J Surg Pathol.* 2005;29(5):653–59.

47. Dei Tos AP. Liposarcomas: diagnostic pitfalls and new insights. *Histopathology.* 2014;64(1):38–52.

48. Okby NT, Travis WD. Liposarcoma of the pleural cavity: clinical and pathologic features of 4 cases with a review of the literature. *Arch Pathol Lab Med.* 2000;124(5):699–703.

49. Wong WW, Pluth JR, Grado GL, Schild SE, Sanderson DR. Liposarcoma of the pleura. *Mayo Clin Proc.* 1994;69(9):882–85.

50. Grifasi C, Calogero A, Carlomagno N, Campione S, D'Armiento FP, Renda A. Intraperitoneal dedifferentiated liposarcoma showing MDM2 amplification: case report. *World J Surg Oncol.* 2013;11:305.

51. Hasegawa T, Seki K, Hasegawa F, Matsuno Y, Shimodo T, Hirose T, et al. Dedifferentiated liposarcoma of retroperitoneum and mesentery: varied growth patterns and histological grades – a clinicopathologic study of 32 cases. *Hum Pathol.* 2000;31(6):717–27.

52. Chen M, Yang J, Zhu L, Zhou C, Zhao H. Primary intrathoracic liposarcoma: a clinicopathologic study and prognostic analysis of 23 cases. *J Cardiothorac Surg.* 2014;9:119.

53. Zidane A, Atoini F, Arsalane A, Traibi A, Hammoumi M, Ouariachi F, et al. Parietal pleura lipoma: a rare intrathoracic tumor. *Gen Thorac Cardiovasc Surg.* 2011;59(5):363–66.

54. Sakurai H, Kaji M, Yamazaki K, Suemasu K. Intrathoracic lipomas: their clinicopathological behaviors are not as straightforward as expected. *Ann Thorac Surg.* 2008;86(1):261–65.

55. Evans HL. Atypical lipomatous tumor, its variants, and its combined forms: a study of 61 cases, with a minimum follow-up of 10 years. *Am J Surg Pathol.* 2007;31(1):1–14.

56. Thway K, Flora R, Shah C, Olmos D, Fisher C. Diagnostic utility of p16, CDK4, and MDM2 as an immunohistochemical panel in distinguishing well-differentiated and dedifferentiated liposarcomas from other adipocytic tumors. *Am J Surg Pathol.* 2012;36(3):462–69.

57. Tavassoli FA, Norris HJ. Peritoneal leiomyomatosis (leiomyomatosis peritonealis disseminata): a clinicopathologic study of 20 cases with ultrastructural observations. *Int J Gynecol Pathol.* 1982;1(1):59–74.

58. Al-Talib A, Tulandi T. Pathophysiology and possible iatrogenic cause of leiomyomatosis peritonealis disseminata. *Gynecol Obstet Invest.* 2010;69(4):239–44.

59. Parmley TH, Woodruff JD, Winn K, Johnson JW, Douglas PH. Histogenesis of leiomyomatosis peritonealis disseminata (disseminated fibrosing deciduosis). *Obstet Gynecol.* 1975;46(5):511–16.

60. Düe W, Pickartz H. Immunohistologic detection of estrogen and progesterone receptors in disseminated peritoneal leiomyomatosis. *Int J Gynecol Pathol.* 1989;8(1):46–53.

61. Bekkers RL, Willemsen WN, Schijf CP, Massuger LF, Bulten J, Merkus JM. Leiomyomatosis peritonealis disseminata: does malignant transformation occur? A literature review. *Gynecologic Oncology.* 1999;75(1):158–63.

62. Lin BT, Colby T, Gown AM, Hammar SP, Mertens RB, Churg A, et al. Malignant vascular tumors of the serous membranes mimicking mesothelioma. A report of 14 cases. *Am J Surg Pathol.* 1996;20(12): 1431–39.

63. Anderson T, Zhang L, Hameed M, Rusch V, Travis WD, Antonescu CR. Thoracic epithelioid malignant vascular tumors: a clinicopathologic study of 52 cases with emphasis on pathologic grading and molecular studies of *WWTR1–CAMTA1* fusions. *Am J Surg Pathol*. 2015;39(1):132–39.

64. Suzuki F, Saito A, Ishi K, Koyatsu J, Maruyama T, Suda K. Intra-abdominal angiosarcomatosis after radiotherapy. *J Gastroenterol Hepatol*. 1999;14(3):289–92.

65. Suster S, Moran CA, Koss MN. Epithelioid hemangioendothelioma of the anterior mediastinum. Clinicopathologic, immunohistochemical, and ultrastructural analysis of 12 cases. *Am J Surg Pathol*. 1994;18(9):871–81.

66. Khong PL, Chan GC, Shek TW, Tam PK, Chan FL. Imaging of peripheral PNET: common and uncommon locations. *Clin Radiol*. 2002;57(4):272–77.

67. Tanida S, Tanioka F, Inukai M, Yoshioka N, Saida Y, Imai K, et al. Ewing's sarcoma/peripheral primitive neuroectodermal tumor (pPNET) arising in the omentum as a multilocular cyst with intracystic hemorrhage. *J Gastroenterol*. 2000;35(12):933–40.

68. Askin FB, Rosai J, Sibley RK, Dehner LP, McAlister WH. Malignant small cell tumor of the thoracopulmonary region in childhood: a distinctive clinicopathologic entity of uncertain histogenesis. *Cancer*. 1979;43(6):2438–51.

69. Angervall L, Enzinger FM. Extraskeletal neoplasm resembling Ewing's sarcoma. *Cancer*. 1975;36(1):240–51.

70. Aurias A, Rimbaut C, Buffe D, Zucker JM, Mazabraud A. Translocation involving chromosome 22 in Ewing's sarcoma. A cytogenetic study of four fresh tumors. *Cancer Genet Cytogenet*. 1984;12(1):21–25.

71. Whang-Peng J, Triche TJ, Knutsen T, Miser J, Douglass EC, Israel MA. Chromosome translocation in peripheral neuroepithelioma. *N Engl J Med*. 1984;311(9):584–85.

72. Folpe AL, Goldblum JR, Rubin BP, Shehata BM, Liu W, Dei Tos AP, et al. Morphologic and immunophenotypic diversity in Ewing family tumors: a study of 66 genetically confirmed cases. *Am J Surg Pathol*. 2005;29(8):1025–33.

73. Tsokos M, Alaggio RD, Dehner LP, Dickman PS. Ewing sarcoma/peripheral primitive neuroectodermal tumor and related tumors. *Pediatr Dev Pathol*. 2012;15(1 Suppl):108–26.

74. Subbiah V, Anderson P, Lazar AJ, Burdett E, Raymond K, Ludwig JA. Ewing's sarcoma: standard and experimental treatment options. *Curr Treat Options Oncol*. 2009;10(1–2): 126–40.

75. Prat J, Matias-Guiu X, Algaba F. Desmoplastic small round-cell tumor. *Am J Surg Pathol*. 1992;16(3):306–07.

76. Karavitakis EM, Moschovi M, Stefanaki K, Karamolegou K, Dimitriadis E, Pandis N, et al. Desmoplastic small round cell tumor of the pleura. *Pediatr Blood Cancer*. 2007;49(3):335–38.

77. Antonescu CR, Ladanyi M. Desmoplastic small round cell tumour. In: Fletcher CDM, Bridge JA, Hogdendoorn PCW, Mertens F, Bosman FT, Jaffe ES, et al., editors. *WHO classification of tumours of soft tissue and bone*. Lyon: International Agency for Research on Cancer; 2013: 225–27.

78. Messinger YH, Stewart DR, Priest JR, Williams GM, Harris AK, Schultz KA, et al. Pleuropulmonary blastoma: a report on 350 central pathology-confirmed pleuropulmonary blastoma cases by the International Pleuropulmonary Blastoma Registry. *Cancer*. 2015;121(2):276–85.

79. Doros L, Schultz KA, Stewart DR, Bauer AJ, Williams G, Rossi CT, et al. *DICER1*-related disorders. In: Pagon RA, Adam MP, Ardinger HH, Wallace SE, Amemiya A, Bean LJH, et al., editors. *GeneReviews(R)*. Seattle, WA; 1993.

80. Hachitanda Y, Aoyama C, Sato JK, Shimada H. Pleuropulmonary blastoma in childhood. A tumor of divergent differentiation. *Am J Surg Pathol*. 1993;17(4):382–91.

81. Manivel JC, Priest JR, Watterson J, Steiner M, Woods WG, Wick MR, et al. Pleuropulmonary blastoma. The so-called pulmonary blastoma of childhood. *Cancer*. 1988;62(8):1516–26.

82. de Krijger RR, Claessen SM, van der Ham F, van Unnik AJ, Hulsbergen-van de Kaa CA, van Leuven L, et al. Gain of chromosome 8q is a frequent finding in pleuropulmonary blastoma. *Mod Pathol*. 2007;20(11):1191–99.

83. Pugh TJ, Yu W, Yang J, Field AL, Ambrogio L, Carter SL, et al. Exome sequencing of pleuropulmonary blastoma reveals frequent biallelic loss of *TP53* and two hits in *DICER1* resulting in retention of 5p-derived miRNA hairpin loop sequences. *Oncogene*. 2014;33(45):5295–302.

84. Kim GH, Kim MY, Koo HJ, Song JS, Choi C-M. Primary pulmonary synovial sarcoma in a tertiary referral center: clinical characteristics, CT, and 18F-FDG PET findings, with pathologic correlations. *Medicine (Baltimore)*. 2015;94(34):e1392.

85. Goldblatt J, Saxena P, McGiffin DC, Zimmet A. Pericardial synovial sarcoma: a rare clinical entity. *J Card Surg*. 2015;30(11):801–04.

86. Hemmings C, Fisher C. Primary omental synovial sarcoma: a case with cytogenetic confirmation. *Pathology*. 2004;36(2):208–11.

87. Mirzoyan M, Muslimani A, Setrakian S, Swedeh M, Daw HA. Primary pleuropulmonary synovial sarcoma. *Clin Lung Cancer*. 2008;9(5):257–61.

88. van de Rijn M, Barr FG, Xiong QB, Hedges M, Shipley J, Fisher C. Poorly differentiated synovial sarcoma: an analysis of clinical, pathologic, and molecular genetic features. *Am J Surg Pathol*. 1999;23(1):106–12.

89. Foo WC, Cruise MW, Wick MR, Hornick JL. Immunohistochemical staining for *TLE1* distinguishes synovial sarcoma from histologic mimics. *Am J Clin Pathol*. 2011;135(6):839–44.

90. Kosemehmetoglu K, Vrana JA, Folpe AL. *TLE1* expression is not specific for synovial sarcoma: a whole section study of 163 soft tissue and bone neoplasms. *Mod Pathol*. 2009;22(7):872–78.

Index